Deep Learning Applications in Medical Image Segmentation

IEEE Press
445 Hoes Lane
Piscataway, NJ 08854

Deep Learning Applications in Medical Image Segmentation

Overview, Approaches, and Challenges

Edited by

Sajid Yousuf Bhat
Department of Computer Science
University of Kashmir
Srinagar
India

Aasia Rehman
Department of Computer Science
University of Kashmir
Srinagar
India

Muhammad Abulaish
Department of Computer Science
South Asian University
New Delhi
India

IEEE*Press*
WILEY

Published by John Wiley & Sons, Inc., Hoboken, New Jersey.
Published simultaneously in Canada.

Library of Congress Cataloging-in-Publication Data applied for

Hardback ISBN: 9781394245338

Cover Design: Wiley
Cover Images: © MR.Cole_Photographer/Getty Images, © Krongkaew/Getty Images

Set in 9.5/12.5pt STIXTwoText by Straive, Chennai, India

Contents

Acknowledgments

The journey to completing *Deep Learning Applications in Medical Image Segmentation* has been deeply collaborative, and we are immensely grateful to all those who have made significant contributions to this work.

First and foremost, we express our sincere appreciation to the contributing authors. Their dedication, expertise, and hard work have been the foundation of this book. Their insightful chapters have enriched this volume and made it a comprehensive resource for the field of medical image segmentation.

We are also thankful to the reviewers whose valuable feedback and constructive suggestions were instrumental in refining the content. Their critical insights ensured the highest standard of quality, and their contributions are greatly appreciated.

Lastly, we acknowledge our families and friends for their unwavering support and encouragement during the preparation of this book. Their understanding and patience have been a source of strength and motivation.

List of Contributors

Zachariah C. Alex
School of Electronics Engineering
VIT University
Vellore
India

Tairah Andrabi
Department of Computer Science
University of Kashmir
Srinagar
Jammu and Kashmir
India

Mudasir Ashraf
School of Computer Science & IT
Univeristy of the People
CA
USA

Rita Banik
Department of Electrical Engineering
ICFAI University Tripura
Kamalghat
West Tripura
India

Rejaul Karim Barbhuiya
Central Institute of Educational
Technology (CIET)
National Council of Educational
Research and Training (NCERT)
New Delhi
India

Sajid Yousuf Bhat
Department of Computer Science
University of Kashmir
Srinagar
Jammu and Kashmir
India

Roshan Birjais
Department of Electrical, Computer
and Software Engineering
Faculty of Engineering
The University of Auckland
Auckland
New Zealand

Ankur Biswas
Department of Computer Science and Engineering
Tripura Institute of Technology
Narsingarh
West Tripura
India

Manzoor Chachoo
Department of computer science
University of Kashmir
Srinagar
Jammu and Kashmir
India

Anupama Chandrasekharan
Department of Radiology
Sri Ramachandra University
Chennai
India

Chelli N. Devi
Department of Biomedical Engineering
Kalasalingam Academy of Research and Education
Srivilliputhur

Vani Malagar
Model Institute of Engineering and Technology
Department of Computer Science and Engineering
Jammu
India

Aijaz Mir
Department of Computer Science
University of Kashmir
Srinagar
Jammu and Kashmir
India

Suhail Qadir Mir
Department of Informatics and Computer Systems
King Khalid University
Abha
Saudi Arabia

Chayan Paul
Department of Computer Science and Engineering
Swami Vivekananda University
Barakpore
West Bengal
India

Aasia Rehman
Department of Computer Science
University of Kashmir
Srinagar
Jammu and Kashmir
India

Lubna Riyaz
Department of Computer Science
University of Kashmir
Srinagar
Jammu and Kashmir
India

Mekhla Sharma
Model Institute of Engineering and Technology
Department of Computer Science and Engineering
Jammu
India

Ishfaq Sheikh
Department of Computer Science
University of Kashmir
Srinagar
Jammu and Kashmir
India

Bisma Sultan
Department of Computer Science
University of Kashmir
Srinagar
Jammu and Kashmir
India

V. K. Sundararaman
Independent Consultant
MR Imaging and Former Adjunct Professor
VIT University
Vellore
India

Navin Mani Upadhyay
Model Institute of Engineering and Technology
Department of Computer Science and Engineering
Jammu
India

Majid Zaman
Scientist D
University of Kashmir
Jammu and Kashmir
India

Preface

The field of medical image segmentation has seen tremendous advancements over the past decade, driven largely by the rapid development of deep learning technologies. These advancements have enabled the medical community to achieve levels of precision and efficiency in image analysis that were once thought impossible. Recognizing the profound impact of these technologies, we set out to create a comprehensive resource that would serve as both an introduction to the field and a guide to the latest research and techniques.

Deep Learning Applications in Medical Image Segmentation was conceived with the vision of providing readers with a thorough understanding of how deep learning is revolutionizing the way we approach medical image segmentation. This book brings together contributions from experts in the field, each offering their unique insights into various aspects of deep learning and its application to medical imaging.

The book is organized to guide readers from foundational concepts to advanced techniques. It begins with an introduction to the basics of medical image segmentation, including key datasets, data augmentation methods, and evaluation metrics. As readers progress, they will encounter discussions on traditional segmentation approaches, providing a historical context that highlights the evolution of methodologies leading to the current state-of-the-art deep learning models.

In subsequent chapters, the book delves into specific applications of deep learning in medical imaging, covering critical areas such as brain tumor segmentation, retinal vessel segmentation, and early detection of diabetic retinopathy. These chapters not only explore the techniques employed but also address the challenges and limitations that researchers face in these specialized domains.

The book also covers cutting-edge topics such as the use of generative adversarial networks (GANs) for image segmentation and collaborative models for cell image segmentation. By including these advanced topics, we aim to provide readers with a forward-looking perspective on the future of medical image segmentation.

We believe this book will serve as a valuable resource for a wide audience, including researchers, practitioners, and students. It is designed to equip readers with both the theoretical knowledge and practical insights needed to navigate the rapidly evolving landscape of medical image segmentation. Our hope is that this book will inspire further research and innovation in this vital field, ultimately contributing to improved healthcare outcomes.

As editors, we are deeply grateful to the contributing authors, reviewers, and all those who have supported this project. Their expertise, dedication, and collaborative spirit have been instrumental in bringing this book to fruition. We trust that readers will find this book to be an informative and enriching resource that will aid them in their professional development and research endeavors.

Introduction

Medical image segmentation is a critical component in the field of medical imaging, enabling precise identification and analysis of anatomical structures and abnormalities. With the exponential growth in imaging technologies and the availability of vast medical datasets, the need for accurate, efficient, and automated segmentation methods has never been more pressing. Deep learning, a subset of artificial intelligence, has emerged as a transformative approach, offering unprecedented capabilities in processing and interpreting complex medical images.

This book, titled *Deep Learning Applications in Medical Image Segmentation*, aims to provide a comprehensive and in-depth exploration of how deep learning models are revolutionizing this field. By consolidating the latest research, methodologies, and practical applications, it serves as a one-stop resource for readers seeking to understand the challenges and advancements in medical image segmentation using deep learning architectures.

The book begins with a foundational overview of medical image segmentation, discussing various imaging modalities, benchmark datasets, data augmentation techniques, and evaluation metrics essential for developing robust segmentation models. It then delves into the historical context and traditional approaches that laid the groundwork for modern techniques, offering valuable insights into the evolution of this field.

Subsequent chapters focus on the application of deep learning models to specific areas of medical imaging, including brain tumor segmentation, retinal vessel segmentation, inner ear segmentation, and early detection of diabetic retinopathy. Each chapter provides a thorough examination of the methodologies, challenges, and future directions in these specialized areas, highlighting the practical impact of deep learning in improving patient outcomes.

The book also explores advanced topics such as the use of generative adversarial networks (GANs) in medical image segmentation, collaborative models for cell image segmentation, and the ongoing challenges faced by researchers in this rapidly evolving domain. The final chapters provide a forward-looking perspective, discussing the future prospects of deep learning in medical imaging and the potential hurdles that must be overcome to fully realize its potential.

Through this comprehensive approach, *Deep Learning Applications in Medical Image Segmentation* equips readers with the knowledge and tools necessary to navigate and contribute to this dynamic field. Whether you are a researcher, practitioner, or student, this book offers valuable insights into the application of deep learning to one of the most challenging and impactful areas of medical science.

1

Introduction to Medical Image Segmentation: Overview of Modalities, Benchmark Datasets, Data Augmentation Techniques, and Evaluation Metrics

Aasia Rehman[1] *and Suhail Qadir Mir*[2]

[1] *Department of Computer Science, University of Kashmir, Srinagar, Jammu and Kashmir, India*
[2] *Department of Informatics and Computer Systems, King Khalid University, Abha, Saudi Arabia*

1.1 Introduction

Medical image analysis is an essential part of monitoring the clinical progression of the disease and how the patient is responding to a certain kind of treatment and thus helps in further planning of treatment for patients. Medical imaging has sped up the diagnosis and treatment of a number of illnesses. There are generally many different kinds of medical imaging modalities that make use of different techniques to produce images for various purposes. Figure 1.1 shows the examples of different medical images. In today's clinical practice, imaging modalities such as X-ray, computed tomography (CT), magnetic resonance imaging (MRI), and US are commonly used. These medical images either examine multiple organs (e.g. MRI and CT) or are specific to particular organs (e.g. retinal images, mammograms, dermoscopy, and colonoscopy). The volume of data produced from each modality also varies (Shen et al. 2017). Each imaging modality offers distinct advantages for various applications and diagnostic objectives, as well as limits in revealing the internal structure and functions of the many organs of the body. X-ray, CT, MRI, US, dermoscopy, colonoscopy, microscopic images, and optical coherence tomography (OCT) are just a few examples of the most widely used medical imaging modalities that will be discussed in this chapter. In addition to this, we discuss their basic principle of working along with their usage.

1.1.1 X-Rays

In the medical field, X-ray imaging is employed to generate detailed images of internal anatomical structures, such as bones, aiding in the diagnostic process.

Deep Learning Applications in Medical Image Segmentation: Overview, Approaches, and Challenges,
First Edition. Edited by Sajid Yousuf Bhat, Aasia Rehman, and Muhammad Abulaish.

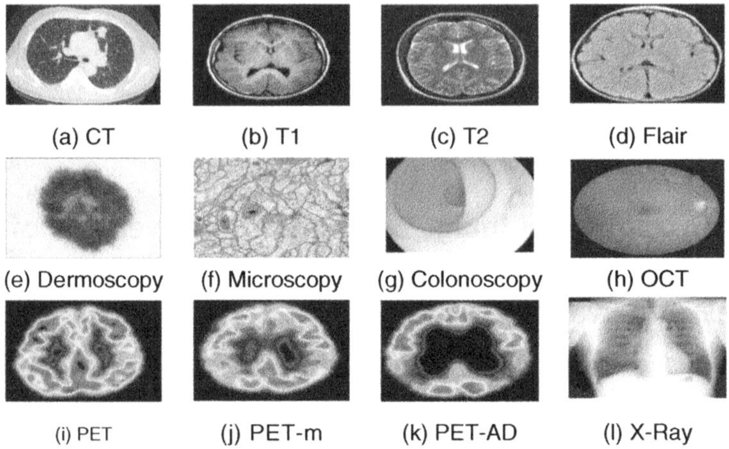

Figure 1.1 Different kinds of medical imaging modalities.

X-rays, classified as electromagnetic waves, possess the capability to penetrate various solid objects, including the human body. Among the common imaging modalities, X-rays are frequently utilized to visualize internal bodily structures. The procedure involves directing a focused beam of X-rays toward the specific region of interest within the body. Upon traversing through the body, the X-rays are captured by a sensitive detector, such as film or a digital sensor. Different tissues within the body interact with X-rays differently; softer tissues, like muscles and organs, absorb fewer X-rays, resulting in darker shades on the resultant image, while denser tissues, like bones, absorb more X-rays, manifesting as white areas on the image. A proper amount of radiation must be used, and the body component must be at the ideal location relative to the X-ray beam, for a clear image to be produced. To get a more accurate depiction of the body's three-dimensional (3D) structure, many pictures of the same location are acquired from different angles and superimposed to create a two-dimensional (2D) image. A radiologist, a specialized medical practitioner, focuses on analyzing medical images to diagnose various conditions such as fractures, cancers, and other ailments by interpreting the visual information depicted in the images. An X-ray is electromagnetic radiation that is produced in a glass tube that has been evacuated. A cathode and an anode create a voltage gap, which propels electrons across the vacuum of the tube and toward the revolving tungsten anode. When electrons impact the anode, they generate both X-rays and heat. X-rays are exclusively produced when there is a voltage differential applied across the cathode and anode, rendering the X-ray tube inert until activated by the medical radiation technologist. X-ray, CT, fluoroscopy, and angiography are all types of imaging that employ this physical on/off setup. X-rays are commonly employed to capture images of bones, primarily to assess for fractures or other abnormalities. Additionally, dentists and orthodontists utilize X-rays to obtain detailed views of teeth. Moreover, X-rays are instrumental in detecting tumors or abnormalities in bones. They are also used to guide surgeons during surgery. X-ray images of the breast are obtained during mammography to find and assess anomalies like tumors or microcalcifications. As it can spot probable cancer signals before they can be felt during a physical examination, it is a crucial tool in the early identification and prevention of breast cancer. X-rays are not only utilized for imaging the bones but also the chest and lungs to diagnose diseases, including pneumonia, lung cancer, and emphysema. In addition to detecting gallstones, kidney stones, and intestinal obstruction, X-ray imaging can be used to evaluate abdominal organs such as the liver, spleen, and kidneys. Figure 1.11 represents an example of chest X-ray. Due to its broad accessibility, speed, and affordability, X-ray imaging stands as a widely favored diagnostic method. It is a noninvasive procedure, eliminating the need for incisions or injections, thus ensuring a reasonably safe and comfortable experience for the patient. Low tissue contrast is one of the drawbacks of X-ray imaging. Distinguishing between malignancies and healthy tissue is more difficult than with other modalities. X-ray imaging also has the drawback of only providing a 2D picture of the body's 3D structure, which might make it impossible to see certain internal structures, especially in inaccessible locations. Some aspects of interior structures can be obscured by the lack of depth in the 2D image, making it harder to make accurate diagnoses.

1.1.2 Computed Tomography (CT)

A CT scan, or computerized tomography scan, generates intricate images of the body's internal structures by combining X-rays and computer technology. Unlike traditional X-rays, CT scans produce cross-sectional images, offering a different perspective of the body. These scans are noninvasive, ensuring a painless experience for the patient. By aiming X-rays at the body from various angles and measuring the intensity of the X-rays as they move through the body with detectors, CT scans can provide high-resolution images of internal anatomy. CT scans use a multi-slice detector, a specialized sort of X-ray detector that can gather many images simultaneously from different angles to provide detailed cross-sectional views of the body. Spatial filtering, which reduces noise and boosts contrast, and multi-energy imaging, which employs X-rays of varying energies to record distinct data and enhance contrast, are two more methods used in CT scans to improve image quality. CT scans produce images that can be viewed in a variety of formats, including cross-sectional slices, 3D images, and even virtual reality images, thanks to computer processing. Radiologic technologists do CT scans, while radiologists, medical specialists with training in image interpretation, decipher the results. When using a CT scanner, the patient will lie on a table that will be moved into the center of a machine in the shape of a doughnut. The scanner's internal X-ray tube spins to produce a sequence of X-ray beams at varying angles as it rounds the patient. The X-ray light creates a pattern of attenuation as it goes through the body because it is absorbed at different rates by various tissues. An array of detectors positioned opposite the X-ray tube picks up the pattern of attenuated X-rays and turns them into electrical impulses. The data from these electrical signals is then transferred to a computer, where complex algorithms are used to reassemble the information as a 3D image. CT scans are employed to enhance the examination of soft tissues and intricate areas of the image that may not be clearly defined by traditional X-rays. They are commonly employed to visualize and assess blood vessels, internal organs, bones, the brain, neck, spine, and chest. CT scans aid medical professionals in various diagnostic tasks, including tumor detection, fracture evaluation, and monitoring the impact of cancer treatment on patients.

Figure 1.1a shows an example of a CT scan of the lungs. CT imaging's high resolution is a big benefit since it allows doctors to see anatomical details such as bone structure, organ function, and blood vessel structure. This makes it beneficial for diagnosing a large variety of illnesses. In addition to its usefulness as a diagnostic tool, CT imaging technology is commonly available in settings such as hospitals, clinics, and doctors' offices. In addition, CT imaging is quick and efficient, with data typically being made available in a short amount of time. Ionizing radiation exposure is a key concern with CT imaging since it can increase the risk of cancer and other health issues, especially with repeated scans or in pregnant women. CT scanners also represent a large financial commitment, which can be out of reach for some hospitals. Because of this, some patients may not be able to get their hands on this form of imaging. The advantages and disadvantages of CT scans must be weighed carefully, and when possible, other imaging methods should be considered.

1.1.3 Medical Resonance Imaging (MRI)

MRI, or magnetic resonance imaging, shares similarities with CT scans but offers superior quality, producing detailed cross-sectional images of body structures. Similar to CT scans, MRIs are painless and safe, as magnetic fields and radio waves do not pose any adverse effects on patients. MRI utilizes a robust magnetic field to align the nuclei of hydrogen atoms within the body, enabling the generation of precise images of internal structures. This generates a minute magnetic moment that can be exploited to provide accurate representations of the body's internal anatomy. First, a weak radio signal is emitted from the rearranged hydrogen nuclei thanks to the use of radiofrequency (RF) pulses. A detector picks up on these signals, and after being analyzed by a computer, we get clear pictures of the body's inner workings. The hydrogen atoms in a patient's body are rearranged when patients enter an MRI machine and are subjected to a powerful magnetic field. Then, a weak radio signal is produced by the aligned hydrogen atoms after radio waves are delivered through the body. An antenna picks up the radio wave, and the information is transmitted to a computer for processing. The data is processed by sophisticated algorithms to create a 3D model of the body's internal anatomy. Hydrogen atoms, which are present in every cell in the body, are found in variable concentrations depending on the kind of tissue. Axial, sagittal, and coronal pictures can be generated in an MRI, giving a full 3D picture of the patient's anatomy.

MRIs are employed for observing the inner composition of the brain, spinal cord, bones, heart, blood vessels, and various other internal bodily structures. In Figure 1.1b–d represent an example of MR T1-weighted, T2-weighted, and Flair, respectively. MRI is favored over alternative imaging methods such as X-rays and CT scans due to its avoidance of harmful ionizing radiation exposure to patients. Soft tissues, including muscles, tendons, and ligaments, can also be seen in exquisite detail by these instruments. They can provide images on different planes, providing a more comprehensive view of internal structures. In addition to its other benefits, MRI's ability to deliver microscopic resolution without causing any damage or discomfort is a major selling point. Nonetheless, MRI scanners are responsive to metal; thus, individuals with specific implants, such as pacemakers, are ineligible for MRI scans.

Scanners can be a considerable investment due to their high cost, making them out of reach for some establishments. Examination times may also be greater compared to those of X-rays or CT scans.

1.1.4 Positron Emission Tomography (PET)

A PET scan produces a 3D image of the inner body parts. To see and quantify metabolic and functional activities taking place inside the body, doctors use PET scans. In the medical field, it is frequently employed for the detection, classification, and follow-up of a wide range of conditions, including cancer and neurological diseases. A PET scan works by looking for radiotracers that release positrons. These radiotracers are substances that are injected into the body and emit positrons, which are positively charged particles. When a positron meets an electron within the body, they mutually annihilate, generating two gamma rays that propagate in opposing directions. These gamma rays are identified by the PET scanner and employed to construct 3D images depicting the distribution of the radiotracer within the body. PET scans are widely used in oncology to assess tumor growth, evaluate treatment response, and detect metastases. PET scans serve various purposes, notably in generating high-resolution brain images and forecasting cancer progression. They are commonly employed for patients already diagnosed with cancer, as PET scans can accurately illustrate the extent of cancer spread and evaluate the efficacy of chemotherapy. Additionally, PET scans aid in pre-surgical planning for procedures involving the brain or heart. Moreover, conditions such as Alzheimer's disease, epilepsy, and Parkinson's disease can be diagnosed using PET scans, as they provide clear insights into changes in brain functionality. In Figure 1.1i–k represent an example of PET scans for normal, mild cognitive impairment, and Alzheimer's disease, respectively. PET scans can detect functional and metabolic changes in tissues before structural abnormalities become apparent through other imaging techniques. PET scans can offer a thorough assessment of the entire body, allowing for the detection of metastatic disease or the evaluation of multiple organ systems simultaneously. Unlike other imaging techniques, PET scans provide information about the physiological and biochemical processes occurring within the body, enabling a better understanding of disease mechanisms. PET scans involve the use of radioactive substances, which expose the patient to a small amount of ionizing radiation. While the radiation dose is generally considered safe, it is still a factor to consider, especially for pregnant women and children. It may be difficult to correctly localize tiny lesions on PET scans because of their potentially inferior spatial resolution compared to other forms of imaging like CT or MRI. PET scans can be more expensive than other imaging techniques, mainly due to the production and administration of radiotracers, as well as the specialized equipment required for scanning and image analysis. PET scanners are not as widely available as other imaging modalities, which can limit access to this technology in certain areas. It is important to note that PET scans are typically used in conjunction with other imaging modalities to provide a more comprehensive evaluation of a patient's condition. The decision to use a PET scan is made by a physician based on the specific clinical scenario and the potential benefits outweighing the risks and costs associated with the procedure.

1.1.5 Ultrasound (US) Images

US, also known as a sonogram, utilizes high-frequency waves to visualize internal body structures. In this medical imaging technique, a transducer emits high-frequency sound waves and captures the returning echoes from internal structures to create images. Some of the sound waves that are transmitted into the body are reflected back to the transducer as they cross a line separating various types of tissue. The transducer receives these echoes, converts them into electrical signals, and transmits them to a computer for analysis, resulting in high-resolution images of the body's internal structures. Depth information is obtained by measuring the time delay between the emitted US wave and the reflected wave from each layer of the sample, enabling the creation of 2D- or 3D images. US is frequently used to monitor the growth of unborn babies, providing real-time imaging. It is typically unsuitable for imaging bones or air-containing tissues such as lungs but finds extensive application in abdominal, vascular, and thyroid examinations. In abdominal imaging, US is commonly used to examine the organs of the digestive system, including the gallbladder, pancreas, spleen, and kidneys. As a medical imaging technique, US has a number of benefits. The portability of the tools makes it possible to do imaging procedures anywhere, not just at a hospital. Furthermore, employing US offers the benefits of speed and radiation-free imaging. As it does not utilize potentially harmful ionizing radiation, it is also favored over other imaging methods like X-ray and CT scans. The capability to produce real-time images also enables the dynamic evaluation of internal structures and functions. US imaging, however, has a number of drawbacks. The inability to picture structures under the surface or behind opaque media (such as bone or gas) is a major drawback. Aberrations like bone or air echoes can further distort images, making it difficult to make out inner structures. US images and the precision of the diagnosis may also be affected by the US technician's level of expertise.

1.1.6 Colonoscopy

Virtual colonoscopy, also referred to as CT colonoscopy, allows medical professionals to examine the large intestine for colon or rectal cancer, as well as growths called polyps, as demonstrated in a study (Nguyen and Lee 2019). The principle behind colonoscopy is the insertion of a colonoscope into the rectum and through the colon. The colonoscope is a long, flexible tube equipped with a light source and a camera at the tip. It allows the physician to visualize the colon lining in real time and detect any abnormalities such as polyps, ulcers, inflammation, or tumors. During the procedure, the physician can also perform therapeutic interventions, such as polyp removal or tissue biopsies, if necessary. Figure 1.1g represents an example of colonoscopy. Colonoscopy is an effective diagnostic tool for identifying colorectal cancer, inflammatory bowel disease (e.g. ulcerative colitis and Crohn's disease), and other conditions affecting the colon and rectum. Colonoscopy allows for the detection and removal of polyps, which are abnormal growths that may develop into cancer over time. Colonoscopy has a high diagnostic accuracy for colorectal cancer and other gastrointestinal (GI) conditions, helping to guide appropriate treatment plans. A colonoscopy is an invasive procedure that requires the insertion of a flexible tube into the rectum and colon, which can cause discomfort or pain for the patient. It is important to discuss the risks, benefits, and alternatives of colonoscopy with a healthcare professional to make an informed decision about the procedure based on individual circumstances and medical history.

1.1.7 Dermoscopy

Dermoscopy is a noninvasive imaging technique used to evaluate skin lesions. It is also known as dermatoscopy or epiluminescence microscopy. This process entails inspecting the skin with a dermatoscope, a portable instrument fitted with magnifying lenses and illumination. Dermoscopy allows dermatologists to observe skin structures and patterns that are not visible to the naked eye, assisting in the identification and treatment of various skin conditions, notably melanoma and other forms of skin cancer. The principle behind dermoscopy is the use of polarized or non-polarized light to illuminate the skin and magnify the surface and subsurface features. The dermatoscope eliminates the surface reflection of the skin, allowing for a clearer view of the deeper layers. Dermoscopy also utilizes liquid immersion or contact dermoscopy, in which a gel or oil is applied to the skin to eliminate the air gap between the dermatoscope and the skin, further improving image quality. Dermoscopy plays a crucial role in the early detection of melanoma, the deadliest form of skin cancer. It helps dermatologists assess the morphological characteristics of pigmented skin lesions and differentiate between benign and malignant lesions. It aids in distinguishing between different types of skin lesions and guiding appropriate treatment plans. In Figure 1.1e represents an example of a skin lesion. Dermoscopy can be used to monitor changes in skin lesions over time, particularly in individuals with a history of skin cancer or atypical moles. It helps identify any signs of progression or regression, aiding in the decision-making process for further management. Dermoscopy improves the diagnostic accuracy of skin lesions, particularly in differentiating between benign and malignant lesions. Dermoscopy is a noninvasive procedure that does not require any incisions or tissue sampling. It can be performed quickly and easily in an outpatient setting. Dermoscopy can reduce the need for unnecessary biopsy of benign lesions, leading to cost savings in healthcare resources. The quality and capabilities of the dermatoscope used can influence the accuracy and reliability of dermoscopic images. High-quality equipment with appropriate magnification and lighting is essential for optimal results.

1.1.8 Microscopic Images

Microscopic imaging refers to the use of microscopes to visualize and examine objects at a microscopic level. It involves the magnification of objects that are too small to be seen with the naked eye, allowing for a detailed examination of their structure and features. Science and medicine rely heavily on microscopic imaging for a wide range of purposes, including the study, diagnosis, and analysis of tiny materials, organisms, and other specimens. The principle behind microscopic imaging is based on the interaction of light or electrons with the sample being observed. There are different types of microscopes used for imaging, including optical microscopes and electron microscopes. Tissue samples are commonly obtained through a biopsy for examination, with small sections of the tissue subsequently stained and colored to reveal cellular features. Counterstains are employed to enhance the color, visibility, and contrast of the images. Such images are commonly utilized in cancer identification, with characteristics such as cell size, shape, and distribution typically scrutinized. Figure 1.1f represents an example of a microscopic image. Microscopic imaging is crucial in medical diagnostics and pathology. It allows for the examination of biopsy samples, the identification of cellular abnormalities, and the diagnosis of various diseases and conditions. Microscopic imaging techniques, such as optical microscopy, allow for nondestructive examination of samples. This means that samples can be observed without altering their structure or composition, enabling further analysis or experimentation. Advanced microscopic imaging equipment, such as electron microscopes, can be expensive to acquire and maintain. Each microscopic imaging technique has its specific limitations in terms of resolution, depth of field, and contrast. Choosing the appropriate imaging technique for a specific application is important to obtain accurate and reliable results.

1.1.9 Optical Coherence Tomography (OCT)

OCT is a noninvasive imaging method that utilizes light waves to produce detailed cross-sectional images of biological tissues. The principle behind OCT is based on the interference of light waves. The technique employs low-coherence interferometry, where a near-infrared light beam emitted by a light source is divided into two paths: a reference arm and a sample arm. The reference arm includes a mirror, while the sample arm directs the light toward the tissue under examination. The light reflected back from both arms is recombined, and interference occurs between the reference and sample beams. The interference pattern is detected and analyzed to reconstruct a depth-resolved image of the tissue. Through measuring the time delay of reflected light, OCT can ascertain the depth of various tissue layers or structures within the sample, which is then utilized to produce a detailed cross-sectional image of the tissue. OCT finds widespread application in diagnosing and treating various eye conditions such as macular degeneration, diabetic retinopathy, glaucoma, and retinal detachment. It provides detailed images of the layers within the retina, allowing for early detection and monitoring of eye diseases. Figure 2.1h represents an example of OCT of an eye. In cardiology, OCT is used to visualize and assess coronary arteries. It helps in diagnosing and characterizing coronary artery disease, detecting plaque buildup, and guiding interventions such as stent placement. OCT provides detailed, high-resolution images of tissue structures, enabling the visualization of fine details and abnormalities. It provides real-time imaging, allowing for immediate evaluation and assessment. The penetration depth of OCT is limited to a few millimeters, depending on the tissue being imaged. This restricts its application in imaging deeper tissues or structures. Advanced OCT systems can be expensive, limiting their accessibility in certain healthcare settings. However, the technology has become more widely available over time.

1.2 Datasets for Segmentation of Medical Images

Segmentation using deep learning methods requires high-quality and diverse datasets for training and evaluation. In this section, we discuss the datasets commonly used in the field of segmentation and their characteristics. Researchers can build and test their deep learning models with the help of these datasets. The performance and generalizability of the created models can be better understood by learning more about the qualities and challenges of these datasets. Domain specialists oversee the creation and annotation of these datasets. The details of each of these datasets are described in the subsections below, and metadata is provided in Table 1.1.

Table 1.1 Datasets for segmentation of medical images.

Dataset	Modality	Organ	Url
LiTS (Bilic, P., 2023)	CT	Liver	https://competitions.codalab.org/
KiTS (Heller et al. 2019)	CT	Kidney	https://wiki.cancerimagingarchive.net/
Brats (Menze et al. 2015)	MR	Brain	https://www.kaggle.com/brats2020- training-data
LIDCIDRI (Armato et al. 2011)	CT	Lung	https://wiki.cancerimagingarchive.net/LIDCIDRI
ISIC (Codella et al. 2018; Tschandl et al. 2018)	Dermoscopy	Skin	https://challenge.isic-archive.com/
BUSI (Al-Dhabyani et al. 2020)	Ultrasound	Breast	https://scholar.cu.edu.eg/?q=afahm
KvasirSEG (Jha et al. 2020)	Colonoscopy	Polyps	https://datasets.simula.no/kvasir-seg/
CVCClinicDB (Bernal et al. 2015)	Colonoscopy	Polyps	https://www.kaggle.com/cvcclinicdb

1.2.1 Multimodal Brain Tumor Segmentation Challenge (BraTS) Dataset

The BraTS dataset is a widely used dataset for brain lesion segmentation that has been merged with the Medical Image Computing and Computer-Assisted Intervention (MICCAI) conference. The BraTS dataset is a vast compilation of different patients' MRI scans of the brain. Different versions of the dataset may include a different number of images. However, hundreds of scenarios are frequently included for both training and testing. Multiple imaging modalities, including T1-weighted, T2-weighted, and contrast-enhanced T1-weighted images, are routinely included in each MRI scan in the BraTS collection. These images can be of any size, although they are often 3D volumes with spatial dimensions of $240 \times 240 \times 155$ voxels or larger. The enhancing tumor core, peritumoral edema, and necrotic regions are all annotated in this dataset with their true labels. This enables the evaluation and comparison of segmentation algorithms on specific tumor components. Different types of cancers are present in this dataset, as are a wide range of tumor sizes and forms, as well as the need to precisely segment tumors in the presence of other brain structures. Several challenges on the Kaggle platform have centered on the BraTS dataset. The BraTS 2020 Kaggle Challenge is one noteworthy competition that attempted to progress the domain of brain lesion segmentation through deep learning techniques. A subset of the BraTS dataset was made available to challenge participants for practice and assessment.

1.2.2 LIDC-IDRI (Lung Image Database Consortium Image Collection) Dataset

The LIDC/IDRI database is a well-known dataset for lung lesion segmentation and diagnosis. It is a globally accessible online platform designed for developing, training, and assessing computer-assisted diagnostic (CAD) techniques aimed at the early detection and diagnosis of lung cancer. The 1018 cases in this data set represent the combined efforts of eight medical imaging companies and seven educational institutions. Images from a clinical thoracic CT scan and the results of a two-stage image annotation technique performed by four experienced thoracic radiologists are included for each individual in an Extensible Markup Language (XML) file. During the initial round of blinded reading, radiologists evaluated all CT scans separately and categorized lesions as "nodule > or = 3 mm," "nodule < 3 mm," or "non-nodule > or = 3 mm." After the blinded-read phase, each radiologist evaluated his or her own mask and the masks of the other three radiologists to reach a conclusion. The LIDC/IDRI database contains a total of 2, 44, and 527 CT scan images. Each CT scan typically consists of a series of axial slices, resulting in a 3D volume representation of the lungs. The size of the CT images may vary, but they are usually high-resolution axial slices with dimensions of around 512×512 pixels.

1.2.3 LiTS (Liver Tumor Segmentation) Dataset

The LiTS dataset is a widely used dataset for liver lesion segmentation, focusing on the segmentation of liver tumors. The LiTS dataset focuses specifically on LiTS, providing CT scans that include both malignant and benign liver lesions. The dataset offers voxel-level annotations, enabling precise segmentation and analysis of liver tumors. It provides a diverse collection of cases, capturing variations in tumor size, shape, location, and appearance within the liver. Automatic segmentation of tumor lesions is difficult due to their heterogeneous and diffusive structure. There are 200 liver CT scans included in the LiTS dataset. There are 130 CT scans in the training set and 70 in the test set. Each CT scan contains multiple axial slices, resulting in a large number of images for analysis. The size of the CT images in the LiTS dataset can vary but are usually high-resolution axial slices with dimensions around 512×512 pixels. To encourage the study and development of techniques for segmenting liver lesions, the LiTS Challenge was created as a competition. The competition utilizes data and CT scan slices contributed by various clinical sites worldwide.

1.2.4 KiTS (Kidney Tumor Segmentation) Dataset

The KiTS dataset is a collection of medical imaging data specifically focused on KiTS. More than 400 thousand people are diagnosed with kidney cancer every year, and the most common method of therapy is surgery. There is presently a growing fascination with the correlation between tumor morphology and surgical results, leading to the development of advanced surgical planning methods. This interest stems from the considerable diversity observed in the morphology of kidney and renal tumors. The KiTS19 challenge, or the KiTS challenge 2019, was a contest centered on segmenting kidney tumors depicted in contrast-enhanced CT images.

The challenge aimed to encourage the development of accurate and robust algorithms for KiTS. Expertly labeled CT scans of the abdomen taken during the arterial phase were included in the data set, which included 300 individuals. 70%, or 210, were made available for use as a training set, while the remaining 30%, or 90, were saved for use as a test set. Automatic semantic segmentation of kidneys, renal tumors, and renal cysts is a hot topic in the medical imaging research community, and the KiTS23 challenge in 2023 will place teams against one another to see who can develop the most successful system in this area. KiTS23 is the third edition of the KiTS challenge, following previous competitions held in 2019 and 2021.

1.2.5 ISIC (International Skin Imaging Collaboration) Dataset

The ISIC dataset is commonly used for segmenting and classifying skin lesions. Segmentation and categorization of skin lesions, including malignant melanoma, benign lesions, and others, are the main topics of the ISIC dataset. It offers a diverse collection of images captured through dermoscopy, allowing for the exploration of different skin lesion characteristics, such as color, shape, texture, and size. The dataset provides ground truth annotations for lesion boundaries, enabling precise segmentation and analysis of skin lesions. The ISIC2018 dataset includes a subset specifically designed for lesion segmentation tasks. The ISIC2018 dataset for lesion segmentation consists of 2594 dermoscopic images. These images cover a variety of skin lesions, including melanoma, nevi, basal cell carcinoma, and other lesion types. The dataset enables researchers to develop and evaluate algorithms and models for automated lesion boundary delineation. The ISIC challenge is an integral part of the ISIC2018 dataset, providing a platform for researchers and data scientists to showcase their expertise in skin lesion analysis. The challenge invites participants to develop innovative solutions for various tasks, including lesion segmentation, classification, and detection. It provides an opportunity for researchers and data scientists to evaluate and compare their algorithms against a standardized benchmark, fostering collaboration and knowledge sharing in the field. By tackling the difficult problems of precise segmentation, classification, and detection of skin lesions, the ISIC Challenge hopes to improve the field of automated skin lesion analysis. Participants are encouraged to develop algorithms that can assist clinicians in diagnosing and managing skin conditions, ultimately improving patient care and outcomes.

1.2.6 BUSI (Breast Ultrasound) Dataset

The BUSI dataset is commonly employed for segmenting breast lesions in US images. Breast cancer stands as one of the primary causes of female mortality worldwide. However, death rates can be lowered with early detection. The BUSI dataset is categorized into three groups: images depicting normal, benign, and malignant conditions. Utilizing machine learning or deep learning in conjunction with BUSI images can yield promising outcomes in the classification, detection, and segmentation of breast cancer. The baseline data collection involved obtaining BUSI images from women aged 25 to 75 years. Six hundred female patients were included in the 2018 data set. The collection contains 780 Portable Network Graphics (PNG) images with a standard size of 500×500 pixels. Grayscale is the most common color scheme for US images. They were gathered and saved in the Digital Imaging and Communications in Medicine (DICOM) format at Baheya

Hospital. The scanning procedure employed the LOGIQ E9 US system and the LOGIQ E9 Agile US system. These state-of-the-art instruments are commonly utilized for high-quality imaging in radiology, cardiac, and vascular applications. They offer an image resolution of 1280×1024 pixels. The $ML6-15-D$ Matrix linear probe utilized transducers with a frequency range of 1–5 MHz. To enhance the usefulness of the dataset, several necessary tasks were undertaken. The dataset contained duplicated images, which were subsequently eliminated. Additionally, the annotations were thoroughly reviewed and corrected by radiologists from Baheya Hospital. To facilitate compatibility, the DICOM images were converted to PNG format using a specialized DICOM converter application. The dataset provides annotations or ground truth masks for segmenting breast lesions, enabling the evaluation of segmentation algorithms. The dataset includes US images acquired from different medical centers, introducing variability in imaging conditions, equipment, and patient populations.

1.2.7 Colonoscopy Datasets

The human GI tract consists of various segments, including the large bowel, which can be affected by different anomalies and diseases, including colorectal cancer. Both women and men are at increased risk for developing colorectal cancer, making it the third most frequent form of cancer overall. Polyps, which are pre-cursors to colorectal cancer, are found in almost half of individuals aged 50 or above during screening colonoscopies, and their prevalence increases with age. Colonoscopy is considered the standard method for detecting and assessing these polyps, followed by biopsy and removal. Early detection of diseases significantly impacts the survival rate for colorectal cancer, making polyp detection crucial. The chance of developing colorectal cancer can be reduced by improving polyp detection. Therefore, early automated diagnosis of polyps can help prevent colorectal cancer and increase survival rates. There are multiple datasets available for colonoscopy-related research, such as the Computer Vision Center (CVC) CVC-ClinicDB, CVC-ColonDB, Kvasir-SEG, and ETIS-Larib datasets. We will briefly discuss some of them here:

1.2.7.1 Kvasir-SEG

The Kvasir-SEG dataset is tailored specifically for the segmentation of polyps in GI endoscopy images. It offers freely accessible GI polyp images accompanied by their respective segmentation masks. These annotations have been meticulously crafted and validated by an expert gastroenterologist. The dataset, with a size of 46.2 MB, comprises 1000 polyp images alongside their corresponding ground truth sourced from the Kvasir Dataset v2. The images within Kvasir-SEG exhibit varying resolutions, spanning from 332×487 to 1920×1072 pixels. Organized into two distinct folders, the dataset features image files and their associated masks sharing identical filenames. The image files utilize JPEG compression for efficient storage and seamless online browsing capabilities. Researchers and educators can easily access and download this open-access dataset for research and educational purposes. The Kvasir-SEG dataset serves as a valuable resource for researchers and developers aiming to advance the field of polyp segmentation, detection, localization, and classification. With the need for multiple datasets to compare computer vision algorithms, this dataset can be used effectively for both training and validation purposes. It enables the development of cutting-edge solutions specifically tailored to colonoscopy images captured by various manufacturers. Further exploration in this area holds the potential to reduce the polyp miss rate and enhance the quality of examinations. Moreover, the versatility of the Kvasir-SEG dataset extends beyond its primary focus, making it suitable for general segmentation and bounding box detection research. Its availability alongside numerous datasets from diverse fields, including medical and nonmedical domains, adds to its value and applicability.

1.2.7.2 CVC-ClinicDB and CVC-ColonDB

CVC-ClinicDB and CVC-ColonDB are datasets specifically designed for polyp segmentation in endoscopic images. The CVC-ClinicDB collection includes 29 distinct sequences totaling 612 still images at a resolution of 384×288. Every image in the dataset is accompanied by a meticulously annotated ground truth that accurately delineates the boundaries of the polyp. CVC-ClinicDB contains endoscopic images captured during routine colonoscopy examinations. On the other hand, the CVC-ColonDB dataset contains 380 images. The images in CVC-ColonDB have a resolution of 576×720 pixels. The images of both these datasets exhibit a variety of polyp types, sizes, shapes, and textures. The challenges in the CVC-ClinicDB as well as in the CVC-ColonDB dataset include polyp detection, accurate delineation of polyp boundaries, and differentiating polyps from other structures or artifacts.

1.3 Augmentation Techniques Used in Medical Image Segmentation

Developing deep learning methods using medical images has long been an appealing avenue of study, aiming to aid clinicians in swift examinations and precise diagnoses. However, these methods require extensive datasets encompassing diverse variations during training. Unfortunately, medical image availability is often limited due to various factors like insufficient patient numbers for certain conditions, reluctance from patients to share their images, and shortages of medical equipment. Consequently, this scarcity leads to dataset bias, overfitting, and inaccurate outcomes. To mitigate these challenges, data augmentation emerges as a common remedy, with various techniques applied across different image types in existing literature. Nevertheless, determining the most effective augmentation technique for specific image types remains ambiguous due to variations in diseases, network architectures, and dataset sizes used in different studies. In this section, we will discuss some of the augmentation techniques used in medical image segmentation.

Rotation

Rotation-based image augmentations entail rotating an image while preserving its initial orientation. This rotation takes place within a fresh coordinate system, ensuring the retention of the pixels' relative positions. The rotation may proceed either clockwise or counterclockwise around an axis within a range spanning from 1° to 359°. Nevertheless, with increasing rotation angles, there is a potential risk of losing image labels. Consequently, the reliability of this augmentation technique hinges on the extent of rotation. While rotation transformations might not be ideal for recognizing digits 6 and 9 in digit recognition tasks, they are typically deemed safe for medical images.

Flipping

Flipping is a method that produces a mirrored version of an image by reversing the positions of its pixels relative to one of the two axes (in the case of 2D images). Although it can be performed along either the vertical or the horizontal axis, vertical flipping is seldom preferred due to potential inconsistencies in the interchange of the top and bottom regions of an image (Nalepa et al. 2019).

Translation

Translation entails moving images along an axis by implementing a translation vector. This approach preserves the relative pixel positions, thereby reducing positional bias (Shorten and Khoshgoftaar 2019) and preventing models from excessively focusing on features in a specific spatial location (Nalepa et al. 2019).

Scaling

Images are subjected to scaling along different axes through the application of scaling factors, which might differ or remain uniform across each axis. Specifically, scaling modifications can be described as either reducing in size (when the scaling factor <1) or enlarging (when the scaling factor >1).

Shearing

This translation moves one edge of an image along either the vertical or the horizontal axis, leading to a parallelogram shape. Vertical shear displaces an edge along the vertical axis, while horizontal shear shifts an edge along the horizontal axis. The extent of shear is dictated by a shear angle.

Augmentation Using Intensities

This augmentation includes modifying contrast or brightness, blurring, standardizing intensity, histogram equalization, sharpening, and introducing noise.

Gaussian noise alters intensity values by randomly sampling from a Gaussian distribution. Salt-and-pepper noise randomly assigns pixel values to either white or black. Uniform noise is incorporated by adjusting pixel values through random sampling from a uniform distribution.

Random Cropping and Erasing

Random cropping augmentation entails choosing a small section from the original image and resizing it to match the original image's dimensions. As a result, this augmentation technique can also be termed scaling or zooming. Random erasing augmentation involves randomly eliminating sections of the image.

Color Modification

Color modification for image augmentation encompasses various techniques. For instance, an RGB-colored image is represented as an array, with three color channels denoting red, green, and blue intensity levels. This setup allows for altering the image's color while retaining its spatial characteristics. This process, known as color space shifting, can be executed across multiple color spaces, as the original color channels are combined differently in each space. One approach to augmenting an RGB-colored image through color modification involves transforming the pixel values within the image's color channels using filters applied to a histogram, thereby creating new images with altered color space attributes. Another method involves applying three shifts (integer values) from RGB filters and incorporating each shift into a channel within the original image. Additionally, image augmentation can involve adjusting hue, saturation, and value components, isolating specific color channels (e.g. blue, red, or green), and converting between different color spaces. However, converting a color image to grayscale should be done cautiously, as this conversion may reduce performance by up to 3% (Chatfield et al. 2014).

Generative Models

Basic data augmentation methods outlined earlier are inadequate when handling intricate data such as medical images. Several studies have been conducted to propose data augmentation techniques more appropriate for medical applications. The overarching objective is to replicate a data distribution that closely resembles real-world data, making it challenging, if not impossible, to differentiate between newly generated samples and authentic data. Recent advancements in deep generative models have rendered them especially appealing for facilitating data augmentation tasks. For instance, generative adversarial networks (GANs) (Goodfellow et al. 2020) have showcased their capacity to produce lifelike images, leading to their widespread adoption in medical applications (Sandfort et al. 2019; Mahapatra et al. 2019). However, GANs also come with their limitations, including issues like learning instability, challenges in convergence, and susceptibility to mode collapse (Mescheder et al. 2018), wherein the generator generates only a limited set of samples. Variational autoencoders (VAEs) (Kingma and Welling 2014) represent another category of deep generative models, albeit receiving less focus in the realm of data augmentation. VAEs excel in output diversity compared to GANs and avoid mode collapse. However, a notable drawback is their tendency to often produce blurred and unclear output images, which arises from the regularization term incorporated in the loss function. In recent times, a novel category of deep generative models known as diffusion models (DMs) (Sohl-Dickstein et al. 2015; Ho et al. 2020) has surfaced, showing considerable potential in generating varied and lifelike outputs. Despite this promise, DMs are still in the early stages of development and have not gained significant traction in medical applications. However, they are anticipated to offer a compelling alternative to existing generative models. A drawback of DMs is their substantial computational expense and lengthy sampling duration. Table 1.2 presents cutting-edge deep learning models centered on three categories of deep generative models for augmenting medical

Table 1.2 Some of the state-of-the-art deep generative models for data augmentation in medical image segmentation.

Reference	Model	Dataset	Modality	Evaluation metric
(Guibas et al. 2017)	CGAN	DRIVE	Fundus photography	KLD, $F1$
(Shin et al. 2018)	Pix2Pix	BraTS2015, ADNI	MR	Dice
(Qasim et al. 2020)	Red-GAN	BraTS2015, ISIC	MR	Dice
(Shi et al. 2020)	StyleGAN	LIDC-IDRI	CT	Dice, pres., sens
(Platscher et al. 2022)	Pix2Pix, SPADE, CycleGAN	Private	MR	Dice
(Liang and Chen 2021)	VAE-GAN	Private	Ultrasound	MMD, 1-NN, MS-SSIM
(Gan and Wang 2022)	AL-VAE	Private	OCT	MMD, MS, WD
(Huo et al. 2022)	PA-VAE	Private	MR	PSNR, SSIM, dice NMSE, jacc.
(Khader et al. 2023)	DDPM	ADNI, MRNet, LIDC-IDRI	MR, CT	Dice
(Fernandez et al. 2022)	brainSPADE	SABRE, BraTS2015	MR	Dice, accuracy
(Wolleb et al. 2022)	IITM-Diffusion	BraTS2020	MR	—

images. Guibas et al. (Guibas et al. 2017) suggest a two-step process for creating artificial fundus photographs along with corresponding blood vessel segmentation masks. The authors exclusively evaluated the generated images based on a segmentation task, attaining an $F1$ score of 0.887 as opposed to 0.898 achieved with real images. This marginal difference indicates the comparable quality of the generated images. Platscher et al. (Platscher et al. 2022) conducted a comparative evaluation of these three frameworks, demonstrating their capacity to generate high-fidelity images ideal for medical image segmentation and translation tasks, leading to a 9.1% improvement in Dice score. These frameworks hold the potential to substantially decrease the necessity for manual annotation of medical images, consequently reducing the time and cost associated with data annotation. Huo et al. (Huo et al. 2022) introduce a progressive VAE-based framework (PAVAE) intended for creating artificial brain lesions alongside their associated segmentation masks. The authors propose a two-phase strategy, where the first phase involves generating synthetic segmentation masks using a conditional adversarial VAE. In the following stage, photorealistic lesion images are generated by incorporating them with the lesion mask through "mask embedding blocks." These blocks embed the lesion mask into the feature space during generation, similar to the approach used in Spatially-Adaptive Denormalization (SPADE). A segmentation network is trained using a combination of genuine and synthetic lesions, resulting in an enhanced Dice score compared to a model trained solely on authentic images from 66.69% to 74.18%. Fernandez and colleagues (Fernandez et al. 2022) present brainSPADE, a generative model designed to create labeled brain MRI images suitable for training segmentation models. This model merges a DM with a VAE-GAN, leveraging SPADE normalization in the GAN component to integrate the segmentation mask effectively. The model comprises two main parts: a segmentation map generator and an image generator. The segmentation map generator, a VAE, initially processes a segmentation map, extracting and structuring its latent space. This space is refined via diffusion and denoising with Latent Diffusion Models (LDMs) to emphasize meaningful information while filtering out noise.

A VAE decoder subsequently generates an artificial segmentation map from this refined latent space. The image generator, a SPADE model, establishes a style latent space from any provided style and incorporates it with the artificial segmentation map to produce the ultimate output image. The effectiveness of brainSPADE is evaluated in a segmentation task using nnU-Net, showcasing similar performance when trained on synthetic data as compared to real data, with a notable performance improvement observed when both types of data are merged. When discussing the application of generative models in medical data augmentation, several factors merit attention. First, integrating domain-specific techniques and knowledge, like anatomy and physiology, enhances the authenticity and usefulness of generated data (He et al. 2022). Second, ethical considerations, including the risk of biased or unrealistic data and the necessity for thorough validation, are crucial. Furthermore, researchers are exploring synergies between generative models and methods like transfer learning (Shorten and Khoshgoftaar 2019; Talo et al. 2019) or active learning (Ren et al. 2022; Rahimi et al. 2021) to enhance augmentation effectiveness. The importance of interpretability and explainability, particularly for clinical decisions and regulatory compliance, should not be overlooked. Beyond augmentation, generative models hold promise for various medical tasks, such as synthesizing patient records or generating images from non-image data (Chambon et al. 2022).

1.4 Performance Metrics for Evaluating Segmentation Models

Performance metrics for the segmentation of medical images are used to evaluate the accuracy and quality of segmentation algorithms applied to medical imaging data. According to the system's functionality, a number of variables influence the choice of a suitable evaluation metric. In this section, we go through a few of the most popular performance indicators that may be used to assess how accurately the deep learning models segment images. Here TP, TN, FP, FN, and GT stand for true positive, true negative, false positive, false negative, and ground truth, respectively:

1.4.1 Dice Similarity Coefficient (DSC)

The DSC evaluates how much of the ground truth region overlaps with the segmented region. It is calculated as the ratio of twice the intersection of the segmented and ground truth regions to the sum of their sizes. A higher DSC value indicates better segmentation accuracy. The Dice coefficient can be mathematically stated as illustrated in Eq (1.1):

$$\mathrm{DSC} = \left| \frac{2 \times S_{\mathrm{GT}} \cap S_{\mathrm{Segmented}}}{|S_{\mathrm{GT}}| + |S_{\mathrm{Segmented}}|} \right| = \frac{2 \times \mathrm{TP}}{2\mathrm{TP} + \mathrm{FP} + \mathrm{FN}} \tag{1.1}$$

When compared to overall pixel accuracy, the DSC is preferable since it accounts for false alarms and missed values within each class. It is preferable because it not only checks whether or not pixels have been correctly labeled but also checks whether or not segmentation boundaries have been correctly drawn. In addition, DSC is often used to evaluate the reliability of a network's performance through the implementation of cross-validation strategies.

1.4.2 Intersection over Union (IoU)

The IoU, which is also called the Jaccard Index (JI), measures how much the expected segmentation and the ground truth segmentation overlap by figuring out the ratio of the area where they overlap to the area where they join. JI shares similarities with the DSC since they exhibit a monotonic or positive correlation, as demonstrated by the following Eq. (1.2).

$$\text{JI} = \frac{S_{\text{GT}} \cap S_{\text{Segmentec}}}{S_{\text{GT}} \cup S_{\text{Segmented}}} = \frac{\text{TP}}{\text{TP} + \text{FP} + \text{FN}} \tag{1.2}$$

1.4.3 Precision

Precision, also known as true predictive assessment, is calculated as the ratio of true positives to the combined total of false positives and true positives. True positive refers to the correct identification of instances from the positive class, while false positive represents instances incorrectly predicted from the positive class. Precision is a valuable metric for assessing the success of predictions. It precisely states the percentage of reliable positive results. Higher precision levels suggest more accurate and exact results from the model. A higher precision number, then, is indicative of a well-trained architecture using the given data. Mathematically, precision is stated as in Eq. (1.3).

$$\text{Precision} = \frac{\text{Accurately identified disease pixels}}{\text{total number of pixels predicted as diseased}} = \frac{\text{TP}}{\text{TP} + \text{FP}} \tag{1.3}$$

1.4.4 Recall

Recall, also referred to as sensitivity, is the ratio of true positives to the sum of true positives and false negatives. In this context, true positive represents the accurate identification of instances from the positive class, while false negative indicates the incorrect prediction of instances from the negative class. Essentially, recall represents the fraction of true positives that are successfully detected. Similar to precision, recall is a valuable metric for evaluating prediction success, particularly when dealing with imbalanced classes. Higher values of recall signify that the model effectively captures most of the positive outcomes and correctly labels them. Mathematically, recall is stated as in Eq. (1.4).

$$\text{Recall} = \frac{\text{Accurately identified disease pixels}}{\text{total number of pixels in GT}} = \frac{\text{TP}}{\text{TP} + \text{FN}} \tag{1.4}$$

1.4.5 *F*1 Score

This metric is necessary for evaluating the accuracy of a model. It combines precision and recall into a single measure using the harmonic mean. Instead of using a conventional average, the harmonic mean restricts extreme values. This measurement is useful for striking a balance between recall and precision. The score for these metrics ranges from 0 to 1, with 1 indicating the best performance and 0 indicating the worst. Models with an $F1$ score near one are regarded as ideal, as they have a low number of false positives and false negatives. This metric is applicable to both binary and multi-class classification and segmentation problems. Mathematically, the $F1$ score is stated as in Eq. (1.5).

$$F1_{\text{score}} = 2 \times \frac{\text{Recall} \times \text{Precision}}{\text{Recall} + \text{Precision}} \tag{1.5}$$

1.4.6 Accuracy

Accuracy, also referred to as overall pixel accuracy, represents the percentage of image pixels that are correctly classified. While it is a fundamental performance metric, it has a restriction in representing segmentation performance when there is a class imbalance. When there is an imbalance between the segmentation classes, one class tends to dominate the others. There may be bias in the results if the accuracy of the dominant class is higher than that of the other class. Therefore, when there is no class imbalance in an image, accuracy should be used as a measure of segmentation performance. One alternative definition of accuracy is per-class accuracy, which averages the fraction of properly classified pixels across all classes. This statistic is especially helpful for images that have an imbalance in class. Both the average per-class accuracy and per-class accuracy should be taken into account in situations of class imbalance. However, the average per-class accuracy has a limitation in terms of reducing the confidence measurement of individual classes. Additionally, when there are fewer instances of a specific class, there may be a large variance that can affect the reliability of the results. Mathematically, accuracy is stated as in Eq. (1.6).

$$\begin{aligned} \text{Accuracy} &= \frac{\text{Accurately classified pixels}}{\text{Total number of pixels present in the image}} \\ &= \frac{\text{TP} + \text{TN}}{\text{TP} + \text{TN} + \text{FP} + \text{FN}} \end{aligned} \tag{1.6}$$

1.5 Conclusion

In conclusion, this chapter has provided a multifaceted exploration of the intricate landscape of medical image segmentation. By examining various modalities, datasets, augmentation techniques, and performance metrics, we have illuminated the breadth and depth of this essential field within healthcare. From the complexities of different imaging modalities to the nuances of dataset selection and augmentation strategies, every aspect contributes to the development of robust and accurate segmentation algorithms. Moreover, the discussion of performance metrics underscores the importance of rigorous evaluation and benchmarking in assessing the efficacy of segmentation methods.

As medical image segmentation continues to evolve, fueled by advancements in technology and methodologies, it remains at the forefront of improving diagnostic accuracy, treatment planning, and patient care. By leveraging the insights gleaned from this chapter, researchers and practitioners are poised to address the ongoing challenges and push the boundaries of medical image segmentation, ultimately enhancing our ability to unravel the intricacies of the human body and improve clinical outcomes.

References

Al-Dhabyani, W., Gomaa, M., Khaled, H., and Fahmy, A. (2020). Dataset of breast ultrasound images. *Data in Brief* 28: 104863. https://doi.org/10.1016/j.dib.2019.104863.

Armato, S.G. 3rd, McLennan, G., Bidaut, L. et al. (2011). The Lung Image Database Consortium (LIDC) and Image Database Resource Initiative (IDRI): a completed reference database of lung nodules on CT scans. *Medical Physics* 38 (2): 915–931. https://doi.org/10.1118/1.3528204.

Bernal, J., Sánchez, F.J., Fernández-Esparrach, G. et al. (2015). WM-DOVA maps for accurate polyp highlighting in colonoscopy: validation vs. saliency maps from physicians. *Computerized Medical Imaging and Graphics: The Official Journal of the Computerized Medical Imaging Society* 43: 99–111. https://doi.org/10.1016/j.compmedimag.2015.02.007.

Bilic, P., Christ, P., Li, H.B. et al. (2023). The Liver Tumor Segmentation Benchmark (LiTS). *Medical Image Analysis* 84: 102680. https://doi.org/10.1016/j.media.2022.102680.

Chambon, P., Bluethgen, C., Delbrouck, J.-B. et al. (2022). Roentgen: vision-language foundation model for chest X-ray generation. *arXiv* Available at: http://arxiv.org/abs/2211.12737.

Chatfield, K., Simonyan, K., Vedaldi, A., and Zisserman, A. (2014). Return of the devil in the details: Delving deep into convolutional nets. BMVC 2014 - Proceedings of the British Machine Vision Conference 2014, pp. 1–11. https://doi.org/10.5244/c.28.6.

Codella, N. C. F. F., Gutman, D., Celebi, M. E. et al. (2018). Skin lesion analysis toward melanoma detection: A challenge at the 2017 international symposium on biomedical imaging (ISBI), hosted by the international skin imaging collaboration (ISIC). Proceedings – International Symposium on Biomedical Imaging, April 2018, pp. 168–172. https://doi.org/10.1109/ISBI.2018.8363547.

Fernandez, V., Pinaya, W. H. L., Borges, P. et al. (2022). Can segmentation models be trained with fully synthetically generated data? International Workshop on Simulation and Synthesis in Medical Imaging. Lecture Notes in Computer Science (including subseries Lecture Notes in Artificial Intelligence and Lecture Notes in Bioinformatics), 13570 LNCS, pp. 79–90. https://doi.org/10.1007/978-3-031-16980-9_8.

Gan, M. and Wang, C. (2022). Esophageal optical coherence tomography image synthesis using an adversarially learned variational autoencoder. *Biomedical Optics Express* 13 (3): 1188–1201. https://doi.org/10.1364/BOE.449796.

Goodfellow, I., Pouget-Abadie, J., Mirza, M. et al. (2020). Generative adversarial networks. *Communications of the ACM* 63 (11): 139–144. https://doi.org/10.1145/3422622.

Guibas, J. T., Virdi, T. S. and Li, P. S. (2017). Synthetic Medical Images from Dual Generative Adversarial Networks. *arXiv* (Nips), pp. 1–9. Available at: http://arxiv.org/abs/1709.01872.

He, Y., Wang, L., Yang, F. et al. (2022). Effect of different configurations of diffusion gradient directions on accuracy of diffusion tensor estimation in cardiac DTI. International Conference on Signal Processing Proceedings, ICSP, October 2022, pp. 437–441. https://doi.org/10.1109/ICSP56322.2022.9965350.

Heller, N., Sathianathen, N., Kalapara, A. et al. (2019). The KiTS19 challenge data: 300 kidney tumor cases with clinical context, CT semantic segmentations, and surgical outcomes. *arXiv* 1–14. Available at: http://arxiv.org/abs/1904.00445.

Ho, J., Jain, A. and Abbeel, P. (2020). Denoising Diffusion Probabilistic Models. *ArXiv*, abs/2006.1. Available at: https://api.semanticscholar.org/CorpusID:219955663.

Huo, J. et al. (2022). Brain lesion synthesis via progressive adversarial variational auto-encoder. in SASHIMI@MICCAI. Available at: https://api.semanticscholar.org/CorpusID:251371486.

Jha, D., Smedsrud, P.H., Riegler, M.A. et al. (2020). Kvasir-SEG: a segmented polyp dataset. In: *MultiMedia Modeling* (ed. Y.M. Ro et al.), 451–462. Cham: Springer International Publishing.

Khader, F., Müller-Franzes, G., Arasteh, S.T. et al. (2023). Denoising diffusion probabilistic models for 3D medical image generation. *Scientific Reports* 13 (1): 1–20. https://doi.org/10.1038/s41598-023-34341-2.

Kingma, D. P. and Welling, M. (2014). Auto-encoding variational bayes. 2nd International Conference on Learning Representations, ICLR 2014 – Conference Track Proceedings, (Ml), pp. 1–14. https://doi.org/10.61603/ceas.v2i1.33.

Liang, J. and Chen, J. (2021). Data augmentation of thyroid ultrasound images using generative adversarial network. IEEE International Ultrasonics Symposium, IUS, pp. 1–4. https://doi.org/10.1109/IUS52206.2021.9593403.

Mahapatra, D., Bozorgtabar, B., and Garnavi, R. (2019). Image super-resolution using progressive generative adversarial networks for medical image analysis. *Computerized Medical Imaging and Graphics: The Official Journal of the Computerized Medical Imaging Society* 71: 30–39. https://doi.org/10.1016/j.compmedimag.2018.10.005.

Menze, B.H., Jakab, A., Bauer, S. et al. (2015). The multimodal brain tumor image segmentation benchmark (BraTS). *IEEE Transactions on Medical Imaging* 34 (10): 1993–2024. https://doi.org/10.1109/TMI.2014.2377694.

Mescheder, L., Geiger, A. and Nowozin, S. (2018) Which training methods for GANs do actually converge? 35th International Conference on Machine Learning, Stockholm, Sweden. ICML 2018, 8, pp. 5589–5626.

Nalepa, J., Marcinkiewicz, M., and Kawulok, M. (2019). Data augmentation for brain-tumor segmentation: a review. *Frontiers in Computational Neuroscience* 13 (December): 1–18. https://doi.org/10.3389/fncom.2019.00083.

Nguyen, N.-Q. and Lee, S.-W. (2019). Robust boundary segmentation in medical images using a consecutive deep encoder-decoder network. *IEEE Access* 7: 33795–33808.

Platscher, M., Zopes, J., and Federau, C. (2022). Image translation for medical image generation: Ischemic stroke lesion segmentation. *Biomedical Signal Processing and Control* 72: https://doi.org/10.1016/j.bspc.2021.103283.

Qasim, A. B., Ezhov, I., Shit, S. et al. (2020). Red-GAN: attacking class imbalance via conditioned generation. Yet another medical imaging perspective. in Arbel, T. et al. (eds) Proceedings of the Third Conference on Medical Imaging with Deep Learning. PMLR (Proceedings of Machine Learning Research), pp. 655–668. Available at: https://proceedings.mlr.press/v121/qasim20a.html.

Rahimi, S., Oktay, O., Alvarez-Valle, J., and Bharadwaj, S. (2021). Addressing the exorbitant cost of labeling medical images with active learning. in International Conference on Machine Learning in Medical Imaging and Analysis Available at: https://api.semanticscholar.org/CorpusID:237641383.

Ren, P., Xiao, Y., Chang, X. et al. (2022). A survey of deep active learning. *ACM Computing Surveys* 54 (9): https://doi.org/10.1145/3472291.

Sandfort, V., Yan, K., Pickhardt, P.J. et al. (2019). Data augmentation using generative adversarial networks (CycleGAN) to improve generalizability in CT segmentation tasks. *Scientific Reports* 9 (1): 1–9. https://doi.org/10.1038/s41598-019-52737-x.

Shen, D., Wu, G., and Suk, H.-I. (2017). Deep learning in medical image analysis. *Annual Review of Biomedical Engineering* 19: 221–248. https://doi.org/10.1146/annurev-bioeng-071516-044442.

Shi, H., Lu, J. and Zhou, Q. (2020). A Novel Data Augmentation Method Using Style-Based GAN for Robust Pulmonary Nodule Segmentation. Proceedings of the 32nd Chinese Control and Decision Conference, CCDC 2020, pp. 2486–2491. https://doi.org/10.1109/CCDC49329.2020.9164303.

Shin, H. C., Tenenholtz, N. A., Rogers, J. K. et al. (2018). Medical image synthesis for data augmentation and anonymization using generative adversarial networks. Simulation and Synthesis in Medical Imaging – Third International Workshop, SASHIMI 2018, Held in Conjunction with MICCAI 2018, Proceedings. Lecture Notes in Computer Science (including subseries Lecture Notes in Artificial Intelligence and Lecture Notes in Bioinformatics), 11037 LNCS, pp. 1–11. https://doi.org/10.1007/978-3-030-00536-8_1.

Shorten, C. and Khoshgoftaar, T.M. (2019). A survey on image data augmentation for deep learning. *Journal of Big Data* 6 (1): https://doi.org/10.1186/s40537-019-0197-0.

Sohl-Dickstein, J., Weiss, E., Maheswaranathan, N., and Ganguli, S. (2015). Deep unsupervised learning using nonequilibrium thermodynamics. in Proceedings of the 32nd International Conference on International Conference on Machine Learning, Lille, France – Volume 37. JMLR.org (ICML'15), pp. 2256–2265.

Talo, M., Baloglu, U.B., Yıldırım, O., and Acharya, U.R. (2019). Application of deep transfer learning for automated brain abnormality classification using MR images. *Cognitive Systems Research* 54: 176–188. Available at: https://api.semanticscholar.org/CorpusID:56595027.

Tschandl, P., Rosendahl, C., and Kittler, H. (2018). Data descriptor: the HAM10000 dataset, a large collection of multi-source dermatoscopic images of common pigmented skin lesions. *Scientific Data* 5: 1–9. https://doi.org/10.1038/sdata.2018.161.

Wolleb, J., Sandkühler, R., Bieder, F., and Cattin, P.C. (2022). The Swiss Army Knife for Image-to-Image Translation: Multi-Task Diffusion Models. *arXiv* 1–12. Available at: http://arxiv.org/abs/2204.02641.

2

Fundamentals of Deep Learning Models for Medical Image Segmentation

Aasia Rehman and Sajid Yousuf Bhat

Department of Computer Science, University of Kashmir, Srinagar, Jammu and Kashmir, India

2.1 Introduction

The introduction of the back-propagation learning algorithm marked a significant advancement in deep neural networks (DNNs). Although initially proposed in the 1970s, it was not until the mid-1980s that the concept was comprehensively grasped and effectively utilized in the field of neural networks. The advancement in understanding and utilization of the back-propagation algorithm facilitated the achievement of self-directed learning. What sets DNNs apart from previous machine-learning approaches is the automated extraction of features. A DNN is a specific type of neural network that takes the form of a multilayer perceptron (MLP). There is no need for laborious hand-coding of feature extractors because it is trained with algorithms that automatically learn abstractions from collections of data. The term deep learning implies the inclusion of a large number of processing layers, in contrast to shallow learning models that have fewer layers of units. The transition from shallow learning to deep learning has enabled the mapping of more intricate and nonlinear functions that cannot be efficiently mapped using shallow architectures. This development has been aided by an increasing number of inexpensive processing units, such as the general-purpose graphics processing unit (GPU), and a large volume of training data (big data). The superior abundance of parallel processing cores in GPGPUs, despite being less significant than Central Processing Unit (CPUs), makes them more suitable for the implementation of DNNs. Aside from the back-propagation algorithm and GPU, the growth of data, or "big-data," in the last 20 years has also helped machine learning (ML) and deep learning grow and be used more. ML will persist in influencing and causing significant changes in various domains, including education, finance, governance, healthcare, manufacturing, marketing, and other sectors.

Deep Learning Applications in Medical Image Segmentation: Overview, Approaches, and Challenges, First Edition. Edited by Sajid Yousuf Bhat, Aasia Rehman, and Muhammad Abulaish.

Deep learning is arguably one of the most noteworthy advancements in computer science in recent years. Its influence has permeated across numerous scientific disciplines, and it is already causing disruption and profound transformation within businesses and industries. Although significant progress has been made, there are still further advancements to be achieved in the field of deep learning. Deep learning holds the potential to enhance human lives by enabling more precise disease diagnoses, such as cancer, facilitating the discovery of new drugs, and predicting natural disasters. Many different kinds of deep architectures have been described in published works. It can be difficult to compare various designs because each has its own set of benefits that shift depending on the nature of the application and the data being processed. For instance, vision-related tasks typically favor convolutional neural networks (CNNs) (Lecun et al. 1998), while sequence and time series modeling tend to favor recurrent neural networks (RNNs) (Mikolov et al. 2010). Nonetheless, deep learning is a rapidly progressing domain. The demand for more human-like, efficient machines across a wide range of fields has led to the annual development of new architectures and learning algorithms.

Researchers have become interested in deep learning, which has demonstrated promising outcomes in a variety of applications. In this chapter, we begin by providing an overview of the many deep-learning methods currently in use for segmenting medical images. Then we explore the key applications of medical image segmentation, such as anatomy segmentation, before concluding with a discussion of the challenges of medical image segmentation.

2.2 Deep Learning Models for Medical Image Segmentation

2.2.1 Convolutional Neural Network (CNN)

CNNs are sophisticated neural network architectures designed to analyze two-dimensional (2D) images. However, it is applicable to both one-dimensional (1D) and three-dimensional (3D) data.

The core of any CNN system is the convolutional layer. Convolution, like a classic neural network, is a linear operation where weights are multiplied by the input. The data that is being input is given a linear transformation by having a 2D array of weights, also known as a mask or filter, applied to it. The size of this filter is less than that of the original data. As shown in Figure 2.1, the filter and the patch of the input that is the same size as the filter undergo an element-wise multiplication to yield a single value. This process is iteratively applied to the full input image to produce a feature map, an array of features represented in two dimensions. By continuously applying the same filter to the whole image, the approach can locate a feature submerged within the image.

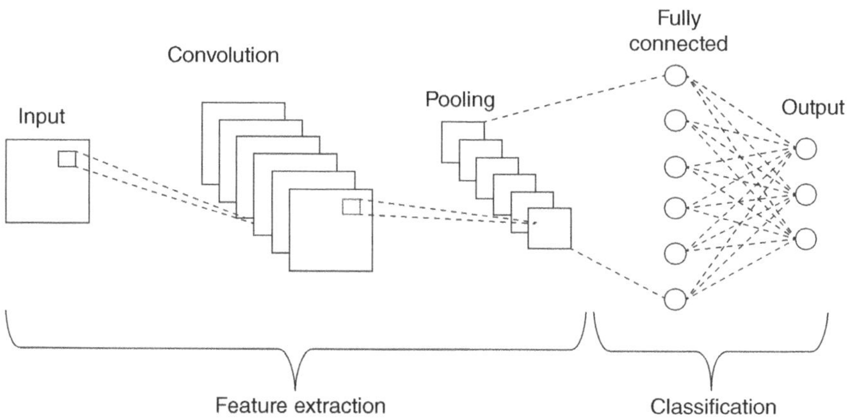

Figure 2.1 Overview of convolutional neural network.

The term "translation invariance" describes this critical quality. One of CNN's main benefits is that its filters do not have to be designed by hand. Instead, they may be learned automatically by back-propagation training, in which the reverse pass employs the convolution operation with spatially inverted filters (Litjens et al. 2017; Shi et al. 2021). Stacking CNN's convolutional layers is a highly effective technique. Simple qualities like lines and boundaries are learned by the layers closest to the input, whereas more complicated features like shapes are learned by the layers farther into the model. CNN is a regularized MLP's variant. The neurons in an MLP are all interconnected with each other. Over-fitting is possible due to the fully connected nature of these networks but can be avoided by regularization. Weights are typically added to the loss function in traditional regularization procedures. CNN, on the other hand, employs a distinct regularization method, one that makes use of the hierarchical pattern present in the data to reduce connectivity and complexity by assembling more complex patterns out of smaller and simpler patterns (Zhou et al. 2021; Kalchbrenner et al. 2014). Traditional algorithms' filters are hand engineered, but CNN can learn them. This independence from additional feature engineering knowledge is its major strength. Some of the well-known variations of CNN include Alex-Net, Inception, ResNet, VGG, Squeeze-Net, and so on.

2.2.2 Fully Convolutional Neural Network (FCN)

The final fully connected layer was swapped out for a completely convolutional layer in the fully convolutional network (FCN) created by Long et al. (Shelhamer et al. 2017), as depicted in Figure 2.2. This significant advancement enables the network to do dense pixel-wise prediction. High-resolution features are merged with up-sampled outputs and fed into convolution layers, which yield

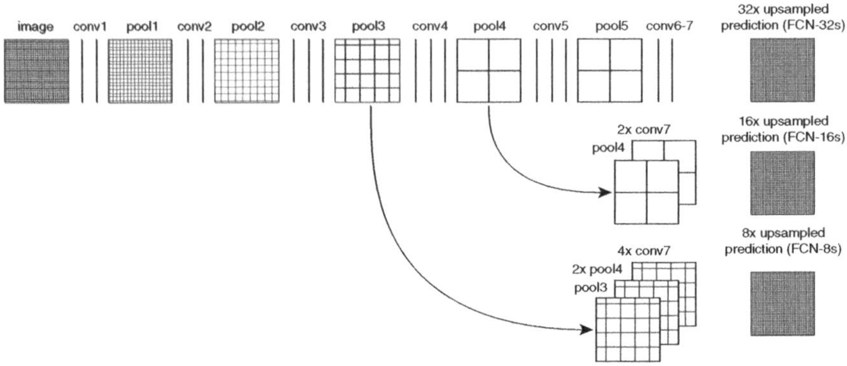

Figure 2.2 Fully convolutional neural network overview.

more accurate results, to increase localization performance. Nie et al. performed the same experiment (Zhang et al. 2015) but with the addition of FCN (Nie et al. 2016). Comparing FCN with CNN using the same modalities and dataset, the significantly higher mean Dice score (0.885 versus 0.864) demonstrates the superiority of FCN. FCN still has some significant drawbacks. The upsampled images look fuzzy and lack sensitivity to fine details. There is inadequate information from the segmentation. The idea behind segmentation is to categorize each pixel without giving them a thorough look. As a result, there is no spatial coherence among the pixels. DeepLab v1 was introduced by Chen et al. (2018b) to replace the two pooling strides that were originally used with just one. The padding size was also decreased from 100 to 1. Based on the VGG16 network, DeepLab v1 adds a full convolution layer in place of the final fully linked layer. The last two pooling layers were removed, and instead, they incorporated atrous convolution, a technique also employed for conditional random fields (Krähenbühl and Koltun 2011). DeepLab v2 (Chen et al. 2017b) introduced atrous spatial pyramid pooling (ASPP) and integrated ResNet101 for its enhanced atrous convolution capability. ASPP is able to capture the context of images at varying scales. DeepLabv3 (Chen et al. 2018b) modified the ASPP module to incorporate a second channel of global picture pooling and batch normalization after convolution and before ReLU. To further enhance the segmentation results, especially at the target border, DeepLab v3+ (Chen et al. 2018a) added an efficient decoder module to DeepLab v3. SegNet (Badrinarayanan et al. 2017) is a symmetric encoder–decoder structure that accomplishes pixel-level image segmentation by using FCN's semantic segmentation task, as depicted in Figure 2.3. The structure comprises an encoding segment and a decoding segment. The encoder, constructed atop VGG16, analyzes data and objects within the network model. Each object's label

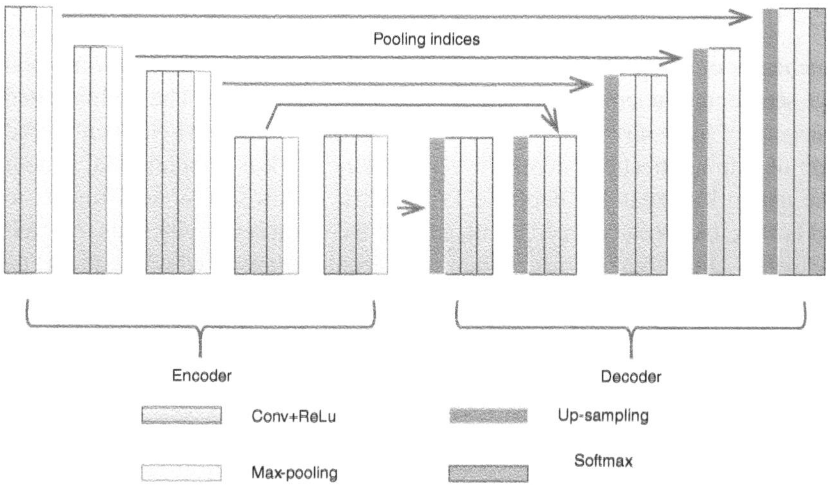

Figure 2.3 Overview of SegNet model.

is applied to its corresponding pixel as the decoder transforms the parsed data into the final image.

SegNet's decoder stands out for employing the max-pooling indices method during pooling to upsample low-resolution input features. Unlike FCN, which utilizes a deconvolution algorithm for nonlinear upsampling without learning, SegNet adopts a different approach. It utilizes a higher pooling index conveyed by the encoder, as depicted in Figure 2.4, which conserves space and yields commendable performance. Rather than storing the absolute maximum feature value, max-pooling indices record the position of the maximum feature value within the pooling window for each encoder map. By using the encoder's transferred pool indices to upsample the input, a decoder produces a sparse feature map. The feature map is then convolutioned with a trainable filter bank to increase its density. U-Net, in contrast, precedes convolution with concatenation by sending the complete feature map from the encoder to the decoder.

Figure 2.4 SegNet decoder with feature map values a, b, c, and d. SegNet first convolves with a trainable decoder filter bank using the max-pooling indices to rebuild the input image.

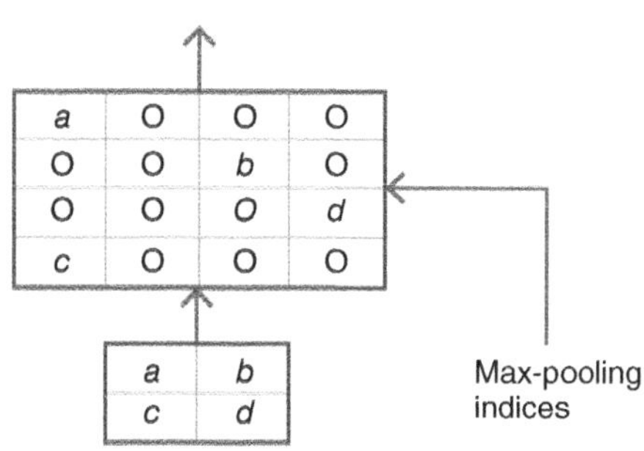

2.2.3 UNet

Ronneberger et al. (2015) introduced U-Net, a well-known structure for medical image segmentation, employing the concept of deconvolution. The sophisticated framework of FCN serves as the foundation for this concept. U-Net's enhanced design of skip connections across levels of the network is an additional benefit of the network's expanded depth to 19 layers. It makes several adjustments to avoid having to choose between localization and context sensitivity. This trade-off increases as larger regions necessitate more pooling layers, which reduces the localization precision.

Small-sized patches, on the other hand, can only see a limited amount of input context. There is a pair of paths of encoder and decoder in the suggested framework, as depicted in Figure 2.5. The encoder path is structured similarly to CNN. The decoder path consists of an upsampling layer, followed by a deconvolution layer. U-Net's primary feature is its ability to make direct connections between

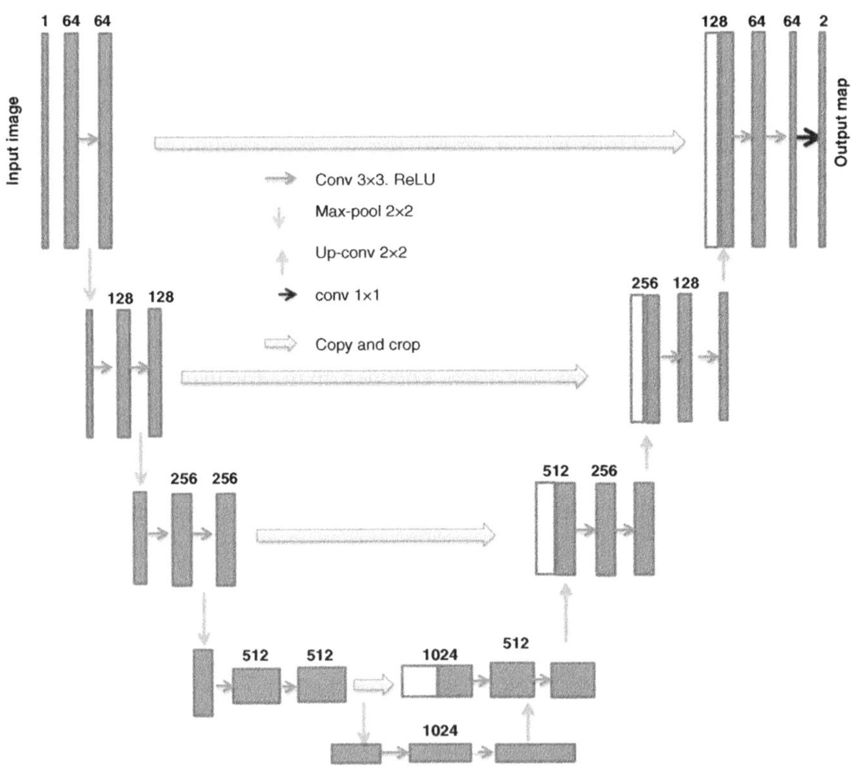

Figure 2.5 Basic U-Net architecture.

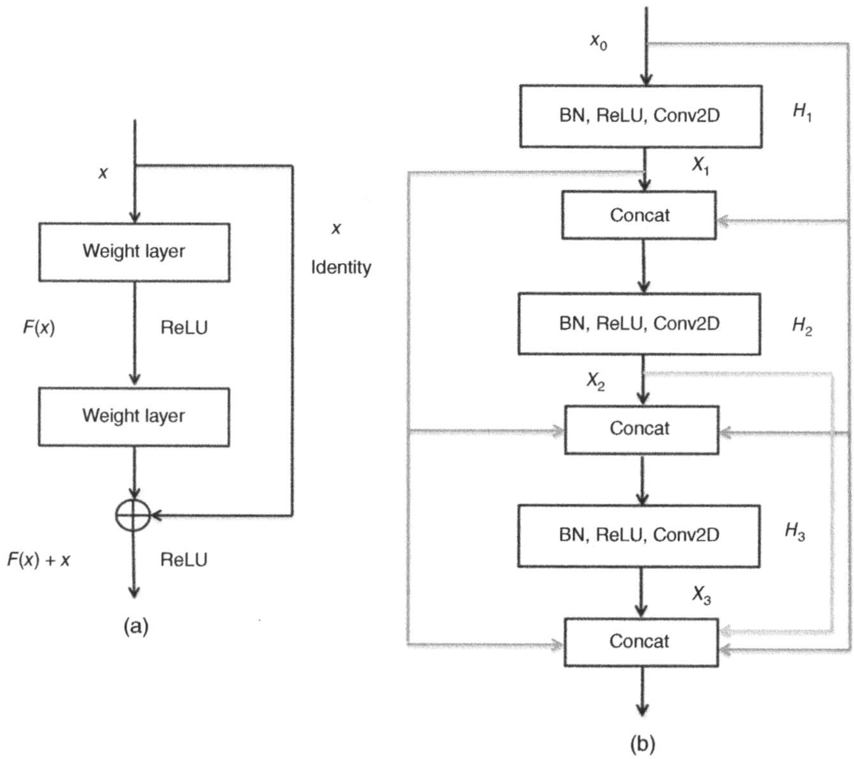

Figure 2.6 (a) Residual block. (b) Dense block.

layers with equivalent resolution along the encoder and the decoder pipelines. These links give the deconvolution layers access to crucial high-resolution characteristics. Models built on the classic U-Net (Ronneberger et al. 2015) structure can be improved by the use of other processes, such as the residual and dense blocks, as shown in Figure 2.6a,b. Cicek et al. (2016) 3D U-Net model to supplement the power of the U-Net structure with more detailed location data. From a number of 2D annotated slices, the proposed model was able to generate dense volumetric segmentation. The network could both create dense annotations from sparse examples and create dense annotations from fresh samples. The network's entire operation has been modified to support 3D operations. On top of that, a 3D structure V-Net based on the U-Net network design was also developed by Milletari et al. (2016). Residual connections can be used to avoid a vanishing gradient and hasten network convergence, allowing for the creation of more complex network architecture with better feature representation. The improved performance of V-Net is the result of its four down-sampling layers.

2.2.4 Multi-scale-Based Models

Multi-scale segmentation designs were made to deal with the fact that there are different scales in the areas of interest. By dividing an image into numerous homogenous pieces at different scales, multi-scale segmentation schemes can present information at multiple scales. These architectures improved high-level segmentation by using a mix of local and global variables to label each pixel. In 2018, researchers at Arizona State University in the United States suggested U-Net++ to address the shortcomings of U-Net, such as its reliance on same-scale feature maps. Dense-Block was employed in the architecture to boost the traditional U-Net's performance, as depicted in Figure 2.7. To bridge the gap among features across modules and boost gradient flow, this model used convolutions and dense connections on the skip-pathway, in contrast to the traditional model (U-Net) (Zhou et al. 2020). Additionally, it included the idea of deep supervision, which carries out architecture reduction. The proposed design is evaluated on multiple modalities by using four distinct medical image datasets: cell nuclei, colon polyps, liver, and lung nodules. The results show that U-Net++ outscored the basic U-Net and Wide U-Net models on the basis of the Intersection-over-Union (IoU) measure, even when deep supervision was not utilized.

2.2.5 Pyramid-Based Models

To aggregate the context, the PSPNet (Zhao et al. 2017) suggested a pyramid pooling module and employed the auxiliary loss, as depicted in Figure 2.8. The significance of global scene categories lies in the fact that they provide a hint regarding the distribution of the segmentation classes. This data is collected via the pyramid pooling module's extensive use of kernel pooling layers. Resnet is modified with dilated convolutions (DCs), and a pyramid pooling module

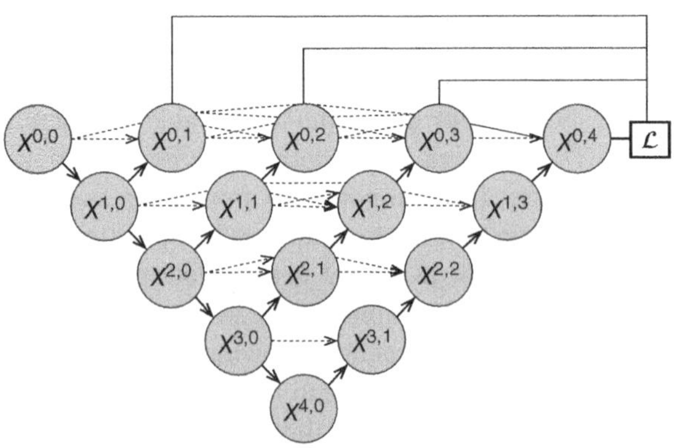

Figure 2.7 UNet++ architecture.

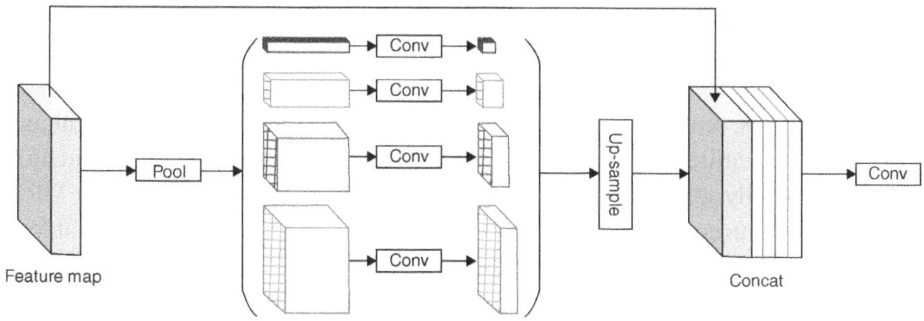

Figure 2.8 Pyramid-based architecture.

is included. This component combines the output of parallel pooling layers with kernels that cover the entire image, half of the image, and a tiny piece of the image with the feature maps generated by ResNet. After ResNet's fourth step, an auxiliary loss is imposed on top of the primary branch loss.

2.2.6 Recurrent Neural Networks (RNNs)

Processing sequential data, such as text, music, videos, and time-series, in which the data at any particular time or position is reliant on data previously observed, is a common use of the RNNs that were developed by Rumelhart et al. (1986). As can be seen in Figure 2.9, the RNN takes in an input at the present time X_i and a hidden

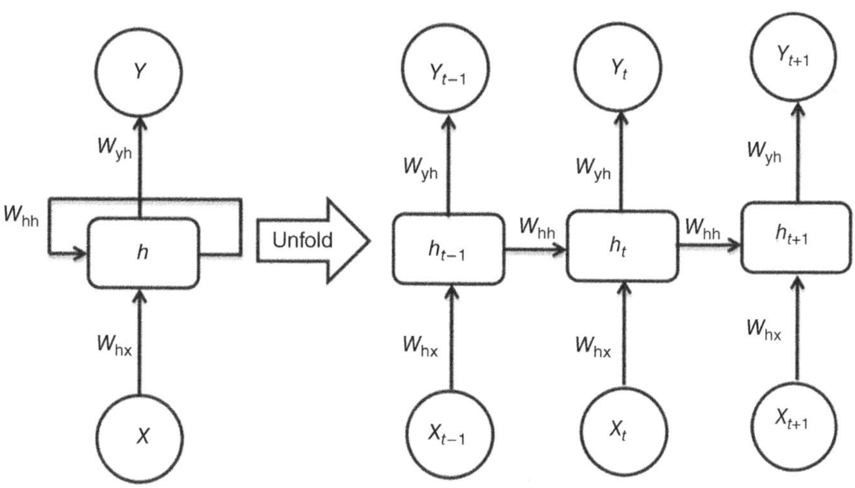

Figure 2.9 An illustration of a basic recurrent neural network with the following parameters: X as input, O as output, t as time step, h as hidden state, and U, W, and V as parameters for weights.

state at the prior step h_{i-1}, and then it generates an output at the desired value and a new hidden state. RNNs are rapidly being used for image recognition, despite having originally been designed for a 1D input. They have been put to use for segmentation issues, and their performance in the MRBrainS competition (Stollenga et al. 2015) was quite encouraging. Since the region of interest (ROI) in medical images is typically spread across numerous neighboring slices (e.g. in CT or MRI), correlations in successive slices are often observed. As a result, RNNs are able to make use of the sequential information supplied by the input slices to determine the contexts that exist between each pair. There are two main components of the RNN structure: the RNN, which handles inter-slice information extraction, and any CNN model, which handles intra-slice information extraction. Among RNNs, LSTM (Long Short-Term Memory) (Hochreiter and Schmidhuber 1997) is the most well known. The loss of spatial information that occurs in a normal LSTM network's inputs is problematic for medical image segmentation. The replacement of vector multiplication with the convolutional operation makes convolutional LSTM (Srivastava et al. 2015) (CLSTM) a promising option. By taking into account contextual information across neighboring slices, CLSTM was added to the deep CNN output layer in Armanto et al. (2011) to improve segmentation. With their strategy, the Dice Similarity Coefficient (DSC) increased to 0.8247 from 0.7976 for the well-known U-Net topology (Ronneberger et al. 2015).

2.2.7 Attention-Based Models

The human brain served as the model for the attention processes. The human brain does not fully comprehend the vast majority of the data given to the visual and auditory cortex, but it does remember the most crucial information. Both processing speed and efficiency are enhanced by the procedure. Although the RNN was where the attention mechanism first found application, it quickly spread to other areas of artificial intelligence, including image localization, speech recognition, and machine translation (Bahdanau et al. 2015; Chorowski et al. 2015; Vaswani et al. 2017). Researchers had high praise for the recurrent visual attention model proposed by Google DeepMind (Mnih et al. 2014). Similarly, the authors of Bahdanau et al. (2015) employed attention methods to address natural language processing issues. Researchers discovered that attention modules can be used in segmenting medical images, which became the primary research issue. The authors of Jin et al. (2019) applied an attention method for segmenting medical images. The method of attention was used by the authors of Jin et al. (2019) to perform semantic segmentation of medical images. It allowed the model to recover lost information. Additionally, He et al. (2016) use attention gates inside a deep network to separate the digestive tract from Computed Tomography (CT) scans. The process of attention helps the network to pick up on the variable shapes and sizes of organs. The CSAU-Net, proposed by Li et al. (2019), advocated a vessel extraction technique. Prior to producing outcomes, the model adjusted features by integrating a connection loss and an attention weight. In Oktay et al. (2018), the authors published an attention U-Net model for segmenting organs from CT images under different conditions. The use of Attention Gates allowed attention U-Net to outperform the U-Net model with higher accuracy without considerably increasing the number of parameters or necessitating post-processing.

2.2.8 Ensemble-Based Models

The ensemble mechanism is effective in decreasing overfitting through training (Maclin 2016). The ensemble module integrates the results of multiple networks running in parallel to perform the necessary segmentation (Maclin 2016). The approach is based on a concept that incorporates both pre- and post-processing modules for images. To enhance the network's ability to segment the ROI from the input image, a pre-processing unit is used, and then the result is refined in a post-processing stage. The deep learning community has discovered that ensemble mechanisms often outperform more traditional single subnetwork approaches. The training procedure benefits from the unique contributions of each subnetwork in the ensemble module (Li et al. 2018a). The authors of Kamnitsas et al. (2018), who suggested a network-of-networks ensemble to aid in tumor localization, were declared the winners of the BraTs 2016 competition. Multiple U-shaped models were defined by the authors of Li et al. (2018a) to address multiple modalities with MRI data (Han and Ye 2018). Similar to this, Feng et al. (2020) suggested two distinct U-Net-inspired algorithms for the semantic segmentation of medical images. One method involves orthogonal-wavelet frames, whereas the other captures residual signals from a low-resolution path. This strategy delivers superior outcomes compared to the traditional U-Net model.

2.2.9 Other Models

R-CNN variants like Mask R-CNN (He et al. 2017) handle the instance segmentation issue, which necessitates simultaneous object identification and segmentation. Object identification and segmentation at two distinct levels are the building blocks of mask R-CNN models. To train deep generative models, researchers have developed the generative adversarial network (GAN) (Goodfellow et al. 2020). As shown in Figure 2.10, it is made up of two networks: a generator network that finds the distribution of data, and a discriminator network that attempts to tell the difference between the genuine distribution of data and the fake data provided by the generator. Together, these models learn the data distribution. A conditional generative adversarial network (M-GAN) for segmenting retinal vessels was proposed by the authors of Park et al. (2020). M-GAN employs layered deep FCN to compensate for losses.

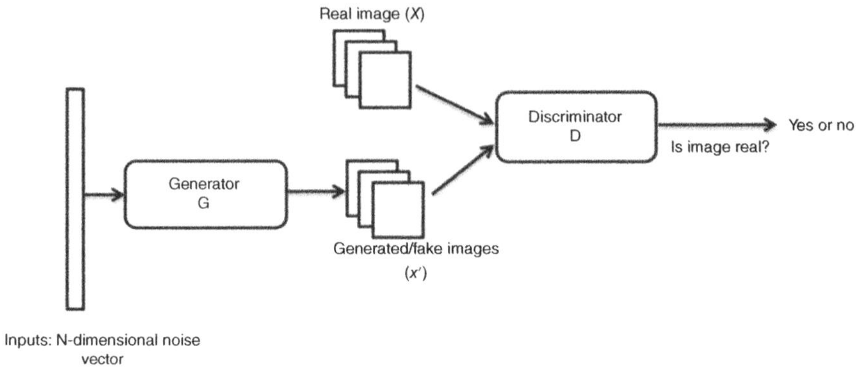

Figure 2.10 GAN architecture.

Zhou et al. (2019) presented Model Genesis, a method for segmenting 3D medical picture data using a transfer learning algorithm, in 2019. Transfer learning is essential when working with medical data, which frequently comes in 3-D formats like MRI and CT. To avoid having to train medical images from scratch, it is necessary to convert 3D images into 2D images and make the necessary adjustments. As a result of this alteration, crucial spatial information is lost, affecting the overall performance of the network. To address this issue, the authors of this work introduced Models Genesis, a set of models that can learn on their own and require no human labeling. The authors of the research used a transfer learning approach to create application-specific target architecture. They tested the paradigm on five 3D applications that faced classification and segmentation issues. Experiments showed that transfer learning from the 2D-ImageNet dataset outperformed natively trained models on 3D medical data. The relevance of the suggested framework was demonstrated by its consistent superiority in performance to any 2D technique. Furthermore, the authors have demonstrated their intent to broaden the concept beyond applications to encompass domains and modes of operation.

2.3 Applications of Medical Image Segmentation Models

Medical image analysis is the key component of the medical system dedicated to disease diagnosis. Medical imaging provides both visual and functional representations of internal human organs for the purpose of clinical study. The major goal is to categorize medical images into various classifications or to emphasize specific data within an image. Analyzing medical images is significant because it can help radiologists and clinicians accurately diagnose diseases. Medical imaging is also utilized to segment the lesions and organ anatomy.

2.3.1 Segmentation of Anatomical Organs

Medical images allow for an accurate examination of organ structure. Medical images can be more quantitatively analyzed for clinical characteristics relating to form and volume, such as brain and heart studies, by segmenting organs and anatomical features. Furthermore, it is frequently required as an initial step in Computer-Aided Detection/Diagnosis (CAD). Bones, vertebrae, blood arteries, and main organs are examples of anatomical structures of the human body. However, because 3D scans contain multiple slices, it is challenging for medical experts to extract anatomy of interest or lesions from these images, and doing so is a time-consuming operation. There are numerous DL approaches available for organ segmentation in medical image analysis. A number of bespoke models have been created to directly target segmentation tasks. Tables 2.1–2.7 summarize the segmentation procedures of the eye, brain, liver, lung, heart, kidney, and multi-organ from the literature.

2.3.1.1 Eye

The segmentation of retinal blood vessels is a difficult topic in retinal pathology research. Oversegmentation or the absence of small, fragile blood arteries is still an issue. Deep learning-based techniques for segmenting retinal vessels outperform human specialists. The first work to use a deep convolutional neural network for the segmentation of retinal blood vessels was by Liskowski and Krawiec (2016). Since then, several applications for retinal vascular segmentation have primarily used CNNs. A fully residual auto-encoder batch normalization network (PixelBNN) was presented as a quick architecture for retinal vascular segmentation by Leopold et al. (2019). U-Net and PixelCNN serve as its foundation. Within FCN, it takes advantage of both skip connections and batch normalization. The next step was to train, test, and cross-test the model on three different retinal blood vessel segmentation datasets: DRIVE (Staal et al. 2004), STARE (Hoover et al. 2000), and CHASEDB1 (Owen et al. 2009). The execution time and performance in the test were satisfactory. Wang et al. (2019a) proposed a new U-Net with two encoders, one for spatial information and one for context information, to better capture the meaning of the data. The authors created a feature fusion module at the intersection of the two roads to merge the various forms of feature representation. In addition, the authors leverage channel attention in a skip connection to pick a relevant feature map. In addition, the multi-scale prediction module combines low-level and high-level prediction for enhanced precision. The suggested DEU-Net model was able to attain higher accuracy in retinal vascular segmentation on both datasets. Yue et al. (2019) recommended an enhanced

U-net structure for vascular segmentation in the retina. Adding a multi-scale input layer and dense block to the classic U-net allows it to make use of more sophisticated spatial contextual information. The segmentation outcomes have been enhanced in particular for thin blood vessels, which are challenging to detect due to their low contrast with the surrounding pixels. To increase accuracy, Zhang et al. (Zhang and Chung 2018) employed U-Net with residual connection to spot blood vessels and implemented an edge-sensing technique to mark the boundary region with more information. Retinal blood vessel segmentation was proposed by Jaemin et al. (Son et al. 2017) using generative adversarial training. There should be less room for error in the segmentation of blood arteries with this procedure. Khan et al. (2021) efficiently segment large, medium, and thin vessels across a wide range of contrast, position, and size of the optic disc, providing a multi-scale kernel based on completely convolutional layers that are extremely lightweight. In addition, the multi-scale kernels, reduced application of pooling operations, and skip connections are all used by the presented architecture to speed up training. In terms of specificity, accuracy, Area Under the Curve (AUC), and sensitivity, the testing results demonstrated that the method consistently outperformed the control group by a considerable margin. The determination of degenerative retinal disorders relies heavily on high-fidelity segmentation of the retina's macro- and microvascular structure, yet this is a challenging task. Segmentation methods based on autoencoding encounter difficulties in extracting retinal microvascular structure due to consecutive resolution reduction during the encoding phase and the incapacity to recover this lost information in the decoding phase. In response to this issue, Kamran et al. (Kamran et al. 2021) introduced RV-GAN, an innovative multi-scale generative framework tailored for accurate retinal vascular segmentation. This proposed architecture enhanced microvessel detection and segmentation through the utilization of two generators and two multi-scale autoencoding discriminators. When compared to conventional GAN-based segmentation algorithms, the author's unique weighted feature matching loss significantly improves accuracy. The developed architecture combines reconstruction with weighted feature matching loss to obtain AUC values of 98.87, 99.14, and 98.87 in segmenting retinal vessels from three datasets, DRIVE (Staal et al. 2004), STARE (Hoover et al. 2000), and CHASE (Owen et al. 2009), respectively. Table 2.1 summarizes various deep learning-based models for retinal vessel segmentation.

2.3.1.2 Brain

MRI is typically used for the investigation of disorders that affect the brain. Alzheimer's disease, epilepsy, schizophrenia, multiple sclerosis, cancer, and neurodegenerative illnesses are only a few of the many neurological disorders that have benefited greatly from imaging studies of the brain. Several investigations have proposed deep learning techniques for brain segmentation. In particular,

Table 2.1 Summary of eye segmentation models based on deep learning.

Ref.	Modality	Model	Dataset	Performance
(Liskowski and Krawiec 2016)	Fundus	CNN	DRIVE (Staal et al. 2004), STARE (Hoover et al. 2000), CHASE (Owen et al. 2009)	Acc. – 94.9%, 95.6%, 96.2%
(Leopold et al. 2019)	Fundus	PixelBNN	DRIVE (Staal et al. 2004), STARE (Hoover et al. 2000), CHASE (Owen et al. 2009)	Acc. – 91.06%, 90.45%, 89.36%
(Staal et al. 2004)	Fundus	DEU-Net	DRIVE (Staal et al. 2004), CHASE (Hoover et al. 2000)	F1 – 82.70%, 80.37%
(Zhang and Chung 2018)	Fundus	U-Net	DRIVE (Staal et al. 2004), STARE (Hoover et al. 2000), CHASE (Owen et al. 2009)	Acc. – 95.04%, 97.12%, 97.70%
(Yue et al. 2019)	Fundus	Enhanced – UNet	DRIVE(Staal et al. 2004)	Acc. – 95.61%
(Khan et al. 2021)	Fundus	RM-FCN	DRIVE (Staal et al. 2004), STARE (Hoover et al. 2000), CHASE (Owen et al. 2009)	Acc. – 98.30%, 98.10%, 98.90%
(Kamran et al. 2021)	Fundus	RV-GAN	DRIVE(Staal et al. 2004), STARE (Hoover et al. 2000), CHASE (Owen et al. 2009)	Auc. – 98.87%, 99.14%, 98.87%

Chen et al. (2017a) created an innovative voxel-wise residual network (VoxRes-Net). When training an extremely DNN, residual units can help mitigate the degradation problem. For segmenting the brain in a 3D MRI image, Wang et al. (2019c) developed a 3D convolutional model with residual units and a pyramid pooling block. While numerous deep learning techniques have been devised for segmenting brain MR images, the majority of them neglect to integrate shape priors. This omission prevents them from leveraging the consistency of brain structures, thus hindering their ability to attain optimal performance. To solve this problem, Sun et al. (2020) presented a deep learning architecture with two subnetworks to perform ROI segmentation of the brain using anatomical attention. The first is a segmentation subnetwork, which is employed to separate ROIs from each input MR image while also extracting a discriminative picture representation. The second is a specialized subnetwork for paying attention to the brain's anatomy, which is fed by a collection of labeled atlases. The authors built two models for anatomical segmentation using this framework: the anatomically gated fully convolutional network and the anatomically gated U-Net. Experimental results on the Alzheimer's Disease Neuroimaging Initiative (ADNI) (Jack et al. 2008) and LONI-LPBA40 datasets show that the suggested algorithms provide higher performance in the ROI segmentation of brain MR images. Nie et al. (2019) took pictures of the brains of 11 healthy babies using T1, T2, and diffusion-weighted modes. The authors optimized the network by combining contextual semantic information and features with different scales. They also used 3D FCN to divide up multimodal brain MRI pictures. The brain tumor segmentation problem was broken down into two manageable tasks by Casamitjana et al. (Mangin and Rivì 2019): whole tumor segmentation and the partition of various tumor sections. When applied to completely convolutional and network topology with DCs, adversarial training improved the segmentation performance of brain MRI, as demonstrated by the work of Moeskops et al. (2017). Xue et al. (2018) inspired by traditional GAN, proposed SegAN, a novel adversarial neural network for segmenting medical images. In contrast to the extensive pixel-level labeling needed for image segmentation, the single scalar output (real or fake) from a typical GAN discriminator might not provide adequate gradient feedback for ensuring network stability. Rather than employing a conventional fully connected network for segmentation, the authors devised a novel adversarial critic network equipped with a multi-scale loss function. This approach compels both the critic and the segmentor to grasp both global and local features. This yields segmentation label maps. The authors show that a SegAN architecture beats the current U-net segmentation method, making it more effective and stable. Datasets from the Medical Image Computing and Computer-Assisted Intervention (MICCAI) BRATS brain tumor segmentation competition were used to evaluate the proposed SegAN approach. Numerous experimental findings showed that the proposed SegAN with multi-scale loss is effective. SegAN performed better than the existing models on BRATS 2015, surpassing in both dice score and precision while still providing performance comparable to the cutting-edge models on BRATS 2013 for whole tumor and tumor core segmentation. Table 2.2 summarizes various deep learning-based models for brain segmentation.

2.3.1.3 Liver

Accurate liver segmentation is crucial for a variety of computer-assisted operations, including those involving the diagnosis and development of liver disease treatments and interventions. Deep learning has been utilized in a number of studies to segment the liver in CT scans (Li et al. 2018b; (Zhou et al. 2018). Dou et al. (Dou et al. 2017) developed a unique and reliable 3D FCN with a

Table 2.2 Summary of brain segmentation models based on deep learning.

Ref.	Modality	Model	Dataset	Performance
(Wachinger et al. 2018)	MR	CNN	MICCAI BRATS (Landman and Warfield 2019)	DSC – 91.0%
(Roy et al. 2019)	MR	FCN	MALC15 (Marcus et al. 2007), ADNI-29 (Jack et al. 2008)	Acc – 88%, 83%
(Coupé et al. 2020)	MR	CNN-ensemble	Private	DSC – 73.3%
(Chen et al. 2017a)	MR	ResNet	MRBrainS	DSC – 84.3%
(Wang et al. 2019c)	MR	CNN-3D	CANDI (Kennedy et al. 2012), IBSR-18 (Frazier et al. 1910)	DSC – 90.7%, 90.4%
(Sun et al. 2020)	MR	AG – UNet, AG – FCN	ADNI-29 (Jack et al. 2008), LONILPBA40	DSC – 88.64%, 80.67%
(Xue et al. 2018)	MR	SegAN	MICCAI BRATS (Menze et al. 2015)	DSC – 85%

deep supervision method for segmenting 3D images. For liver segmentation, the 3D deeply supervised network achieved higher performance. Tran et al. (2021) proposed an alternative network architecture called $U^n\text{–}Net$ (n-fold U-Net). The $U^n\text{–}Net$ model utilizes a skip connection based on the features extracted from the convolutional unit outputs. As a result, the $U^n\text{–}Net$ network makes use of the convolution unit output features at the nodes. The authors tested a $U^2\text{–}Net$ and a $U^3\text{–}Net$ for segmentation of the liver and liver tumor in this work. Moreover, the network nodes incorporated DC and a dense structure. The proposed networks outperformed existing networks in experiments. Wang et al. (2021) proposed SAR-U-Net architecture based on the traditional U-Net. The SE block within the U-Net encoder was initially introduced to dynamically extract image features following each convolution. It achieves this by concealing less relevant areas of the image while accentuating the portions essential to the current segmentation task. Second, the ASPP was employed to gather multi-scale image details through various receptive fields, replacing both the transition layer and the output layer. Third, the conventional convolution block was substituted with residual structures to address the gradient vanishing issue, consequently enabling the network to benefit from significantly increased depth and accuracy. The proposed technique had the highest accuracy compared to similar models. Furthermore, the proposed approach attained the highest segmentation accuracy compared to other closely related models in the SLiver07 dataset trial. Fan et al. (Fan et al. 2021) proposed a Multi-Scale Nested U-Net (MSN-Net), an alternative U-Net design. Res-block and multi-scale context fusion (MSCF) blocks comprise the MSN-Net. To prevent gradient disappearance, the authors employed a deeper network constructed using the Res-block with a bottleneck layer. To address the semantic gaps, a novel skip connection was redesigned. MSCF blocks and numerous connections constitute the innovative skip connection. High-level and low-level features, as well as multi-scale semantic information, were combined in the MSCF block to produce more accurate features. Between MSCF blocks, dense connections were used. Experiment results showed that compared to other cutting-edge models, MSN-Net was more effective at closing the semantic gaps. By using innovative skip connections, the suggested strategy effectively reduced semantic gaps between the encoder and decoder paths and boosted network segmentation precision. Table 2.3 summarizes various deep learning-based models for liver segmentation.

2.3.1.4 Lung

Segmenting lung images stands as a pivotal initial stage in lung imaging analysis, playing a fundamental role in providing precise interpretations of lung CT images for the detection of lung cancer. Lung segmentation in CT and X-ray images has been thoroughly studied (Gaál et al. 2020; Pawar and Talbar 2021). For instance, Skourt et al. (Ait Skourt et al. 2018) designed a U-Net architecture for segmenting lungs from a CT image. Conventional lung segmentation methods, reliant on user-generated features, struggle to accurately segment lung parenchyma with nodules. Deep learning, proven to outperform traditional methods in image classification and object recognition, offers a more effective alternative. To alleviate the juxta pleural nodule problem, Wu et al. (Wu and Lin 2020) developed a new dilated convolutional-based weighted fully convolutional neural network for segmenting lung parenchyma. While deep learning models have improved significantly in their ability to segment anatomical structures, there is still cause for concern due to the enormous number of training parameters, which increases memory utilization and decreases generalization. To solve this problem, Yahyatabar et al. (2020) developed a Dense-UNet model. This model improved information flow by increasing the number of connections between each layer in the network. This enabled the maintenance of robust segmentation while designing a network with substantially fewer parameters. The authors claim that Dense-UNet is the most lightweight deep model put forth for segmenting lung fields in Chest X-Ray (CXR) images. In addition, one of the primary challenges of

Table 2.3 Summary of liver segmentation models based on deep learning.

Ref.	Modality	Model	Dataset	Performance
(Stollenga et al. 2015)	CT	FCN	3DIRCAD (Soler et al. 2010)	DSC – 95.7%
(Christ et al. 2017)	CT, MR	Cascaded FCN	3DIRCAD (Soler et al. 2010)	DSC – 94.3%
(Li et al. 2018b)	CT	H-Dense U-Net	LiTS (Bilic et al. 2023), 3DIRCAD (Soler et al. 2010)	DSC – 96.5%, 98.2%
(Seo et al. 2020)	CT	U-Net modified (mUNet)	LiTS (Bilic et al. 2023), 3DIRCAD (Soler et al. 2010)	DSC – 96.0%, 98.51%
(Liu et al. 2019)	CT	Cascaded UNet	LiTS (Bilic et al. 2023)	DSC – 97.16%
(Zhou et al. 2018)	CT	U-Net – Nested	LiTS (Bilic et al. 2023)	IoU – 82.9%
(Dou et al. 2017)	CT	CNN-3D	Sliver07	VOE 5.4
(Tran et al. 2021)	CT	U^n*–Net*	LiTS (Bilic et al. 2023), 3DIRCADb (Soler et al. 2010)	DSC – 96.38%, 96.45%
(Wang et al. 2021)	CT	SAR-UNet	LiTS (Bilic et al. 2023)	DSC – 95.71%
(Fan et al. 2021)	CT	MSN-Net	MICCAI2017 LiTS (Bilic et al. 2023)	DSC – 94.24%, IoU – 90.75%

segmenting lungs in chest X-rays is that the automatic lung segmentation model may be incorrectly created due to the extreme lung shape shifts and fuzzy lung regions caused by severe lung diseases. Liu et al. (2022) using the pretraining efficientnet-b4 encoder, the residual block and the *LeakyReLU* activation in the decoder enhanced the U-Net network's performance. By avoiding the gradient instability brought on by the multiplication effect in gradient back-propagation, the network was able to extract lung field features efficiently. Experiments comparing this method to others have shown that not only is it more accurate at segmenting the lung from CXR images, but it also has a lower standard deviation and is more robust. Pal et al. (2022) introduced Attention UW-Net, which links the encoder and decoder layers through a novel intermediate layer. The final encoder layer undergoes upsampling to generate the intermediate layer,

Table 2.4 Summary of lung segmentation models based on deep learning.

Ref.	Modality	Model	Dataset	Performance
(Stirenko et al. 2018)	X-ray	CNN	SH	Acc – 70%
(Gaál et al. 2020)	X-ray	Attention U-Net	JSRT (Shiraishi et al. 2000)	DSC – 97.5%
(Hofmanninger et al. 2020)	CT	U-Net, ResU-net	LTRC (Goksel and Foncubierta-Rodríguez 2017), Anatomy3 (Yang et al. 2018b)	DSC – 94%, 92%
(Pawar and Talbar 2021)	CT	GAN	ILD (Depeursinge et al. 2012)	DSC – 96%
(Ait Skourt et al. 2018)	CT	U-Net	LIDC (Armato et al. 2011)	DSC – 95.02%
(Wu and Lin 2020)	CT	Dilated – FCN	LIDC/IDRI (Armato et al. 2011)	DSC – 97.02%
(Yahyatabar et al. 2020)	X-ray	Dense-Unet	JSRT (Shiraishi et al. 2000), Montgomery	DSC – 97.6%, 97.9%
(Liu *et al.* 2022)	X-ray	Improved UNet	JSRT (Shiraishi et al. 2000), Montgomery	DSC-97.9%, 97.7%
(Pal et al. 2022)	X-ray	Attention-UWNet	NIH Chest X-ray (Wang et al. 2017)	F1 – 83.8%

comprising multiple fully connected convolutional layers. These layers establish connections with their corresponding up- and down-sampled blocks through skip connections. A down-sampling layer is employed to additionally link the intermediate layer to the decoder pipeline. UW-Net surpasses not only U-Net and its derivatives but also other traditional automatic and semiautomatic segmentation/annotation models developed in recent years. This model is optimal for the automatic annotation of organs due to the uniformity of the prediction accuracy of segmentation masks across all types (large, medium, and minor lesions). Table 2.4 summarizes various deep learning-based models for lung segmentation.

2.3.1.5 Kidney

Kidney segmentation is an essential step in analyzing images and the development of sophisticated procedures. For segmenting kidneys in CT scans,

Table 2.5 Summary of kidney segmentation models based on deep learning.

Ref.	Modality	Model	Dataset	Performance
(Couteaux et al. 2019)	CT	Ensemble UNet	COCO (Lin et al. 2014)	DSC – 86.7%
(Wang et al. 2019b)	CT	Modified U-Net	KiTS (Heller et al. 2019)	DSC – 95.4%
(Yang et al. 2018a)	CT	FCN with PPM	Private	DSC – 93.1%
(Zhang et al. 2019)	CT	3D-FCN	KiTS (Heller et al. 2019)	DSC – 90.24%
(Zhao et al. 2020)	CT	Multi-scale supervised 3D U-Net	KiTS (Heller et al. 2019)	DSC – 96.9%

several DNNs have been proposed. Couteaux et al. (2019) trained a set of fully convolutional networks and combined their predictions during testing for segmentation. The algorithm achieves highly accurate segmentation results, particularly in delineating the renal cortex. While the precision of the provided reference segmentations seems to set a modest upper limit on the numerical performance, the proposed solution offers dependable and accurate automatic segmentations of the renal cortex in CT images. Yang et al. (2018a) integrated 3D FCN-based architecture with pyramid pooling to enhance the extraction of features. Zhang et al. (2019) presented a two-phase framework based on a 3D FCN for segmenting kidney and tumor. To lessen class disparity and computation expense, the first step is locating the kidney in its preliminary stages and removing the extraneous background. The kidney and tumor on the cropped patch are then carefully segmented in the second stage. With a Composite Dice of 90.24%, the suggested technique places the fourth-place team out of 105 contending teams in the MICCAI 2019 Kidney Tumor Segmentation (KiTS) Challenge. To segment kidneys and kidney tumors from CT images, Zhao et al. (2020) presented a multi-scale supervised U-Net. Utilizing the KiTS19 dataset, the authors devised an architecture to improve the performance of the 3D U-Net by integrating deep supervision with exponential loss. Table 2.5 summarizes various deep learning-based models for kidney segmentation.

2.3.1.6 Heart

The heart is a vital organ in our bodies. However, many people's lives are also jeopardized by numerous heart problems. To tackle practical issues in the domain of cardiac medical care, automatic segmentation of the heart region must be realized. The complete heart has been segmented using DL-based neural networks, according to several studies (Wang and Smedby 2018; Payer et al. 2018). Tran et al. (Tran 2016) performed pixel categorization using a fully convolutional neural network architecture for an MRI of the heart. Short-axis cardiac MRI has never seen such sophisticated semantic segmentation as is possible with the proposed FCN architecture. Han et al. (2020) developed a volumetric FCN that is cascaded. This method employs a pair of V-Nets in series. The first network pinpoints the heart, while the second divides the heart and large vessel structures into smaller parts. To aid with heart segmentation from MR images, the authors rebuilt the V-Net into a 3D V-Net. Ye et al. (2019) provided a novel deeply supervised 3D UNET that improves upon the original network through the use of multi-depth fusion to extract context information. The authors took focus loss and extended its use to multi-category challenges in the field of picture segmentation. Finally, they coupled the focused loss with the dice loss to form the new hybrid loss function. The hybrid loss can be used to address the issue of uneven categories. Shen et al. (2019) developed a unified architecture that utilizes both deep learning and the conventional level set approach to coronary Computed Tomography Angiography (CTA) segmentation. The 3D semantic properties of coronary arteries are learned utilizing a 3D FCN, which serves as a great jumping-off point for the classical level set. Xu et al. (2020) proposed a new type of GAN called a progressive sequential causal GAN (PSCGAN).

This marks the pioneering development of a CA-free Ischemic Heart Disease (IHD) technique within cine MR imaging, capable of producing both an image akin to Late Gadolinium Enhancement (LGE) and accurately segmenting tissues relevant to diagnosis concurrently. To that goal, the PSCGAN has three very useful features:

1) An iterative framework for image synthesis and segmentation training that uses a divide-and-conquer strategy and consists of three stages (i.e. a priori generation, conditional synthesis, and enhanced segmentation).
2) A sequential causal learning network (SCLN) has been devised, featuring a multi-scale, two-stream pathway along with a multi-attention weighting unit. This architecture efficiently identifies task-specific dependencies while extracting spatial and temporal connections from cine MR images. It also incorporates the GAN architecture to use adversarial training to make it easier to understand the latent space dependencies of interest in cine MR images during the entire process.
3) Two loss concepts developed for autonomous learning: To mitigate noise during synthesis, the authors employ a synthetic regularization loss term that makes use of the spare regularization, and in segmentation, the authors employ an auxiliary loss term that makes use of the number of pixels for each tissue to compensate for discriminating.

Table 2.6 Summary of heart segmentation models based on deep learning.

Ref.	Modality	Model	Dataset	Performance
(Wang and Smedby 2018)	CT, MR	U-Net	MMWHS (Zhuang and Shen 2016)	DSC – MR 79.2%, CT 86.6%
(Dou et al. 2017)	MR	CNN-3D	MMWHS (Zhuang and Shen 2016)	DSC – 92.8%
(Payer et al. 2018)	CT	CNN	MMWHS (Zhuang and Shen 2016)	DSC – 90.8%
(Han et al. 2020)	MR	3D V-Net	HVSMR (Pace et al. 2015)	DSC – 94.2%
(Ye et al. 2019)	MRI	UNet with multidepth fusion	MICCAI 2017	DSC – 90.73%
(Shen et al. 2019)	MR	3D-FCN	Private	DSC – 90.05%
(Xu et al. 2020)	MR	GAN	Private	DSC – 91.8%

As a result, PSCGAN achieves record-breaking results while steadily training for synthesis and segmentation. These findings proved that the designed method can provide great support in the standardized assessment of heart disease. Table 2.6 summarizes various deep learning-based models for heart segmentation.

2.3.1.7 Multi-organ

To protect vital organs during radiation planning, organs at risk (OAR) must be clearly defined. Before radiation for nasopharyngeal cancer, more than 20 organs must be precisely segmented. Since then, deep learning approaches have outperformed OAR segmentation due to recent developments in deep learning. Multi-organ segmentation is notoriously challenging due to the common occurrence of organ imbalances. The U-Net architecture has shown to be highly effective at segmenting medical images, making it the de facto standard. The features learned by ordinary convolution layers, on the other hand, are not distinguishable. To solve this issue, Wang et al. (2019d) suggest a unique architecture known as the densely connected deep U-Net (DC UNet). The DC U-Net comprises three components: dense connections, selective deconvolution layers incorporating upsampling, and a trans-convolutional filling function. To segment OARs in thoracic CT scans, Vesal et al. (2019) designed a deep learning framework for the following organs and structures: heart, oesophagus, trachea, and aorta. The method suggested employed a U-Net-inspired network featuring a bottleneck comprised of DCs and aggregated residual connections, leveraging global context and dense data. Zhang et al. (2020) introduced an effective cascaded V-Net model aimed at enhancing multi-organ segmentation performance, achieved through the establishment of dense block-level skip connections within the cascaded V-Net architecture. Crespi et al. (2023) proposed exhibiting three forms of ensembles of single-organ models able to construct multi-organ masks leveraging the different specializations of their components. Positive findings indicate that this may be a viable approach to the problem of developing effective multi-organ segmentation techniques. Xing et al. (2023) proposed Diff-UNet, a unique system for segmenting volumetric images. The method efficiently captures semantic information from the input volume through a conventional U-shaped architecture, resulting in superior pixel-level representations essential for medical volumetric segmentation. The writers also create a Step Uncertainty Fusion (SUF) module for inference, merging the outputs of diffusion models at each step to enhance the stability of prediction results from the diffusion model.

The authors also performed a thorough assessment of three datasets, demonstrating that Diff-UNet significantly surpasses other current methods in classifying multimodal brain tumors in MRI scans, liver tumors, and multi-organ CT volumes. Table 2.7 summarizes various deep learning-based models for multi-organ segmentation.

2.4 Current Challenges in Segmentation of Medical Images

When employing deep learning-engineered models for medical image segmentation, various obstacles arise. In this section, we will explore some fundamental challenges encountered in medical image segmentation, as outlined below.

Deep learning models generally necessitate a substantial volume of annotated training data to attain peak performance. However, obtaining a sufficiently large and diverse dataset with accurately annotated anatomical structures can be challenging, particularly for rare or uncommon structures.

- Class imbalance occurs when certain structures or lesions are underrepresented in the training data compared to others. Imbalanced class distributions can negatively impact the performance of deep learning models, leading to biased segmentations. Additionally, medical images often exhibit high variability in terms of shape, size, and appearance, which makes it challenging to develop models that can handle such variations effectively.
- Medical images often contain structures with complex shapes, ambiguous boundaries, or overlap with neighboring structures, such as organs, vessels,

Table 2.7 Summary of multi-organ segmentation models based on deep learning.

Ref.	Modality	Model	Dataset	Performance
(Gao et al. 2019)	CT	DNN	PDDCA (Raudaschl et al. 2017)	DSC – 80.3%
(Nikolov et al. 2018)	CT	U-Net	PDDCA (Raudaschl et al. 2017)	DSC – 70.4%
(Tong et al. 2018)	CT	FCN	PDDCA (Raudaschl et al. 2017)	DSC – 67.1%
(Tang et al. 2019)	CT	Attention U-Net	PDDCA (Raudaschl et al. 2017)	DSC – 73.5%
(Agn et al. 2019)	MR, CT	Generative method	Private	DSC – 70.4%
(Wang et al. 2019d)	CT	DC U-Net	3D-IRCADb, LiTS (Bilic et al. 2023)	DSC-liver – 94.9%, Spleen-92.1%
(Vesal et al. 2019)	CT	Residual UNet	SegTHOR 2019 (Trullo et al. 2017)	DSC – 91.57%
(Zhang et al. 2020)	CT	Cascaded V-Net	SegTHOR 2019 (Trullo et al. 2017)	DSC – 88.02%
(Xing et al. 2023)	CT	Diff-UNet	BraTS2020, MSD, liver, BTCV	DSC – 85.35%, 95.72%, 83.75%

or lesions. Developing deep learning models that can handle such complex scenarios and accurately segment overlapping structures is a significant challenge.

- Anatomical structures can exhibit significant inter- and intra-patient variabilities in terms of size, shape, and appearance. Deep learning models need to be robust enough to handle such variations to generalize well across different individuals and clinical scenarios.
- Deep learning models trained on a specific dataset may struggle to generalize well to unseen medical images, especially when there are differences in imaging protocols, equipment, or patient populations. Achieving robustness and generalizability across different datasets and clinical settings is a challenging task.
- Deep learning models are frequently viewed as opaque systems, posing difficulties in interpreting and elucidating their segmentation decisions, especially in crucial medical contexts. Providing insights and explanations for the model's decisions is crucial for building trust and ensuring the clinical acceptance of deep learning-based segmentation algorithms.

- Even if a deep learning-based segmentation algorithm demonstrates promising results in research settings, its successful translation and adoption into clinical practice can be challenging. Factors such as integration with existing healthcare systems, validation in clinical trials, user friendliness, and acceptance by medical professionals need to be addressed for successful clinical adoption.
- Choosing an appropriate network architecture and optimizing its hyperparameters is a critical step in developing an effective segmentation model. Determining the optimal network depth, width, skip connections, and other architectural choices to handle anatomical structure complexity is a challenging task.

2.5 Conclusion

In this chapter, we have thoroughly detailed the application and architecture of the major cutting-edge algorithms related to deep-learning image segmentation. The Tables 2.1 to 2.7 provide a summary of the procedures and applications. There is a steady increase in the adoption of cutting-edge techniques that boost segmentation's precision and reliability. The concept of long-term medical care is realized by using artificial intelligence to diagnose various ailments. It becomes a valuable resource for clinicians. Deep learning algorithms have significantly advanced medical image segmentation. While challenges remain, they present opportunities for further exploration and innovation. By addressing these challenges, we can unlock the full potential of deep learning-based segmentation, making it an indispensable tool for clinicians and researchers in their pursuit of improved medical diagnostics and patient care.

References

Agn, M., af Rosenschöld, P.M., Puonti, O. et al. (2019). A modality-adaptive method for segmenting brain tumors and organs-at-risk in radiation therapy planning. *Medical Image Analysis* 54: 220–237. https://doi.org/10.1016/j.media.2019.03.005.

Ait Skourt, B., El Hassani, A., and Majda, A. (2018). Lung CT image segmentation using deep neural networks. *Procedia Computer Science* 127: 109–113. https://doi.org/10.1016/j.procs.2018.01.104.

Armato, S.G. 3rd, McLennan, G., Bidaut, L. et al. (2011). The Lung Image Database Consortium (LIDC) and Image Database Resource Initiative (IDRI): a completed reference database of lung nodules on CT scans. *Medical Physics* 38 (2): 915–931. https://doi.org/10.1118/1.3528204.

Badrinarayanan, V., Kendall, A. and Cipolla, R. (2017) SegNet: a deep convolutional encoder-decoder architecture for image segmentation. *IEEE Transactions on*

Pattern Analysis and Machine Intelligence, 39(12), pp. 2481–2495. doi: https://doi.org/10.1109/TPAMI.2016.2644615.

Bahdanau, D., Cho, K. H. and Bengio, Y. (2015) Neural machine translation by jointly learning to align and translate. 3rd International Conference on Learning Representations, ICLR 2015 – Conference Track Proceedings, San Diego, California, USA, pp. 1–15.

Bilic, P., Christ, P., Li, H.B. et al. (2023). The liver tumor segmentation benchmark (LiTS). *Medical Image Analysis* 84: 102680. https://doi.org/10.1016/j.media.2022.102680.

Chen, H., Dou, Q., Yu, L. et al. (2017a). VoxResNet: deep voxelwise residual networks for brain segmentation from 3D MR images. *NeuroImage* 170: 446–455.

Chen, L.-C., Papandreou, G., Schroff, F. et al. (2017b) Rethinking Atrous Convolution for Semantic Image Segmentation. *arXiv*, Available at: http://arxiv.org/abs/1706.05587.

Chen, L.-C., Zhu, Y., Papandreou, G. et al. (2018a) Encoder-decoder with atrous separable convolution for semantic image segmentation. in Ferrari, V. et al. (eds) Computer Vision – ECCV 2018, pp. 833–851. Cham: Springer International Publishing.

Chen, L.C., Papandreou, G., Kokkinos, I. et al. (2018b). DeepLab: semantic image segmentation with deep convolutional nets, atrous convolution, and fully connected CRFs. *IEEE Transactions on Pattern Analysis and Machine Intelligence* 40 (4): 834–848. https://doi.org/10.1109/TPAMI.2017.2699184.

Chorowski, J., Bahdanau, D., Serdyuk, D. et al. (2015) Attention-based models for speech recognition. Advances in Neural Information Processing Systems, 2015-Janua, pp. 577–585.

Christ, P.F., Ettlinger, F., Grün, F. et al. (2017). Automatic liver and tumor segmentation of CT and MRI volumes using cascaded fully convolutional neural networks. *arXiv* 1–20. Available at: http://arxiv.org/abs/1702.05970.

Çiçek, Ö., Abdulkadir, A., Lienkamp, S. S. et al. (2016) 3D U-net: learning dense volumetric segmentation from sparse annotation. in Medical Image Computing and Computer-Assisted Intervention–MICCAI 2016: 19th International Conference, Athens, Greece, 17–21 October 2016, Lecture Notes in Computer Science (including subseries Lecture Notes in Artificial Intelligence and Lecture Notes in Bioinformatics), 9901 LNCS, pp. 424–432. https://doi.org/10.1007/978-3-319-46723-8_49.

Coupé, P., Mansencal, B., Clément, M. et al. (2020). AssemblyNet: A large ensemble of CNNs for 3D whole brain MRI segmentation. *NeuroImage* 219: 117026. https://doi.org/10.1016/j.neuroimage.2020.117026.

Couteaux, V., Si-Mohamed, S., Renard-Penna, R. et al. (2019). Kidney cortex segmentation in 2D CT with U-Nets ensemble aggregation. *Diagnostic and Interventional Imaging* 100 (4): 211–217. https://doi.org/10.1016/j.diii.2019.03.001.

Crespi, L., Roncaglioni, P., Dei, D. et al. (2023). Ensemble methods for multi-organ segmentation in CT series. *arXiv* Available at: http://arxiv.org/abs/2303.17956.

Depeursinge, A., Vargas, A., Platon, A. et al. (2012). Building a reference multimedia database for interstitial lung diseases. *Computerized Medical Imaging and Graphics: The Official Journal of the Computerized Medical Imaging Society* 36 (3): 227–238.

Dou, Q., Yu, L., Chen, H. et al. (2017). 3D deeply supervised network for automated segmentation of volumetric medical images. *Medical Image Analysis* 41: 40–54. https://doi.org/10.1016/j.media.2017.05.001.

Fan, T., Wang, G., Wang, X. et al. (2021). MSN-Net: a multi-scale context nested U-Net for liver segmentation. *Signal, Image and Video Processing* 15 (6): 1089–1097. https://doi.org/10.1007/s11760-020-01835-9.

Feng, X., Tustison, N.J., Patel, S.H., and Meyer, C.H. (2020). Brain tumor segmentation using an ensemble of 3D U-Nets and overall survival prediction using radiomic features. *Frontiers in Computational Neuroscience* 14: 1–10. https://doi.org/10.3389/fncom.2020.00025.

Frazier, J.A., Caviness, V.S., Kennedy, D.N. et al. (1910). Internet brain segmentation repository (IBSR) 1.5 mm dataset. *Collections* 10 (C60W3M): C6RC85.

Gaál, G., Maga, B., and Lukács, A. (2020). Attention U-net based adversarial architectures for chest X-ray lung segmentation. *CEUR Workshop Proceedings* 2692: 1–7.

Gao, Y., Huang, R., Chen, M. et al. (2019) FocusNet: imbalanced large and small organ segmentation with an end-to-end deep neural network for head and neck CT images. in Shen, D. et al. (eds) Medical Image Computing and Computer Assisted Intervention – MICCAI 2019, pp. 829–838. Cham: Springer International Publishing.

Goksel, O. and Foncubierta-Rodríguez, A. (2017). VISCERAL anatomy benchmarks for organ segmentation and landmark localization: tasks and results. In: *Cloud-Based Benchmarking of Medical Image Analysis* (ed. A. Hanbury, H. Müller, and G. Langs). Springer, 107–125.

Goodfellow, I., Pouget-Abadie, J., Mirza, M. et al. (2020). Generative adversarial networks. *Communications of the ACM* 63 (11): 139–144. https://doi.org/10.1145/3422622.

Han, Y. and Ye, J.C. (2018). Framing U-Net via deep convolutional framelets: application to sparse-view CT. *IEEE Transactions on Medical Imaging* 37 (6): 1418–1429. https://doi.org/10.1109/TMI.2018.2823768.

Han, T., Ivo, R.F., Rodrigues, D.D.A. et al. (2020). Cascaded volumetric fully convolutional networks for whole-heart and great vessel 3D segmentation. *Future Generation Computer Systems* 108: 198–209. https://doi.org/10.1016/j.future.2020.02.055.

He, K., Zhang, X., Ren, S. and Sun, J. (2016) Deep residual learning for image recognition. Proceedings of the IEEE Computer Society Conference on Computer

Vision and Pattern Recognition, December 2016, pp. 770–778. https://doi.org/10.1109/CVPR.2016.90.

He, K., Gkioxari, G., Dollár, P. and Girshick, R. (2017) Mask R-CNN. in 2017 IEEE International Conference on Computer Vision (ICCV), pp. 2980–2988. https://doi.org/10.1109/ICCV.2017.322.

Heller, N., Sathianathen, N., Kalapara, A. et al. (2019). The KiTS19 challenge data: 300 kidney tumor cases with clinical context, CT semantic segmentations, and surgical outcomes. *arXiv* 1–14. Available at: http://arxiv.org/abs/1904.00445.

Hochreiter, S. and Schmidhuber, J. (1997). Long short-term memory. *Neural Computation* 9 (8): 1735–1780. https://doi.org/10.1162/neco.1997.9.8.1735.

Hofmanninger, J., Prayer, F., Pan, J. et al. (2020). Automatic lung segmentation in routine imaging is primarily a data diversity problem, not a methodology problem. *European Radiology Experimental* 4 (1): 50. https://doi.org/10.1186/s41747-020-00173-2.

Hoover, A.D., Kouznetsova, V., and Goldbaum, M. (2000). Locating blood vessels in retinal images by piecewise threshold probing of a matched filter response. *IEEE Transactions on Medical Imaging* 19 (3): 203–210. https://doi.org/10.1109/42.845178.

Jack, C.R., Bernstein, M.A., Fox, N.C. et al. (2008). The Alzheimer's disease neuroimaging initiative (ADNI): MRI methods. *Journal of Magnetic Resonance Imaging* 685–691. https://doi.org/10.1002/jmri.21049.

Jin, Q., Meng, Z., Pham, T.D. et al. (2019). DUNet: a deformable network for retinal vessel segmentation. *Knowledge-Based Systems* 178 (8): 149–162. https://doi.org/10.1016/j.knosys.2019.04.025.

Kalchbrenner, N., Grefenstette, E. and Blunsom, P. (2014) A convolutional neural network for modelling sentences. 52nd Annual Meeting of the Association for Computational Linguistics, ACL 2014 - Proceedings of the Conference, 1, pp. 655–665. https://doi.org/10.3115/v1/p14-1062.

Kamnitsas, K. et al. (2018) Ensembles of multiple models and architectures for robust brain tumour segmentation. in Brainlesion: Glioma, Multiple Sclerosis, Stroke and Traumatic Brain Injuries: Third International Workshop, BrainLes 2017, Held in Conjunction with MICCAI 2017, Quebec City, QC, Canada, 14 September 2017, Lecture Notes in Computer Science (including subseries Lecture Notes in Artificial Intelligence and Lecture Notes in Bioinformatics), 10670 LNCS, pp. 450–462. https://doi.org/10.1007/978-3-319-75238-9_38.

Kamran, S. A., Hossain, K. F., Tavakkoli, A. et al. (2021) RV-GAN: segmenting retinal vascular structure in fundus photographs using a novel multi-scale generative adversarial network. in de Bruijne, M. et al. (eds) Medical Image Computing and Computer Assisted Intervention – MICCAI 2021: 24th International Conference, Strasbourg, France, 27 September–1 October 2021, pp. 34–44. Cham: Springer International Publishing.

Kennedy, D.N., Haselgrove, C., Hodge, S.M. et al. (2012). CANDIShare: a resource for pediatric neuroimaging data. *Neuroinformatics* 10 (3): 319–322. https://doi.org/10.1007/s12021-011-9133-y.

Khan, T. M., Robles-Kelly, A., Naqvi, S. S. and Arsalan, M. (2021) Residual multiscale full convolutional network (RM-FCN) for high resolution semantic segmentation of retinal vasculature. in Torsello, A. et al. (eds) Structural, Syntactic, and Statistical Pattern Recognition: Joint IAPR International Workshops, S+ SSPR 2020, Padua, Italy, 21–22 January 2021, Proceedings, pp. 324–333. Cham: Springer International Publishing.

Krähenbühl, P. and Koltun, V. (2011) Efficient inference in fully connected crfs with Gaussian edge potentials. Advances in Neural Information Processing Systems 24: 25th Annual Conference on Neural Information Processing Systems 2011, NIPS 2011, pp. 1–9.

Landman, B. A. and Warfield, S. K. (2019) MICCAI 2012: Workshop on multi-atlas labeling. éditeur non identifié Nice, France (2012).

Lecun, Y., Bottou, L., Bengio, Y., and Haffner, P. (1998). Gradient-based learning applied to document recognition. *Proceedings of the IEEE* 86 (11): 2278–2324. https://doi.org/10.1109/5.726791.

Leopold, H.A., Orchard, J., Zelek, J.S., and Lakshminarayanan, V. (2019). PixelBNN: augmenting the PixelCNN with batch normalization and the presentation of a fast architecture for retinal vessel segmentation. *Journal of Imaging* 5 (2): https://doi.org/10.3390/jimaging5020026.

Li, H., Jiang, G., Zhang, J. et al. (2018a). Fully convolutional network ensembles for white matter hyperintensities segmentation in MR images. *NeuroImage* 183: 650–665. https://doi.org/10.1016/j.neuroimage.2018.07.005.

Li, X., Chen, H., Qi, X. et al. (2018b). H-DenseUNet: hybrid densely connected UNet for liver and tumor segmentation from CT volumes. *IEEE Transactions on Medical Imaging* 37 (12): 2663–2674. https://doi.org/10.1109/TMI.2018.2845918.

Li, R., Li, M., Li, J., and Zhou, Y. (2019) Connection sensitive attention U-NET for accurate retinal vessel segmentation. *arXiv*, Available at: http://arxiv.org/abs/1903.05558.

Lin, T.-Y., Maire, M., Belongie, S. et al. (2014) Microsoft COCO: common objects in context. in Fleet, D. et al. (eds) Computer Vision – ECCV 2014: 13th European Conference, Zurich, Switzerland, 6–12 September 2014, pp. 740–755. Cham: Springer International Publishing.

Liskowski, P. and Krawiec, K. (2016). Segmenting retinal blood vessels with deep neural networks. *IEEE Transactions on Medical Imaging* 35 (11): 2369–2380. https://doi.org/10.1109/TMI.2016.2546227.

Litjens, G., Kooi, T., Bejnordi, B.E. et al. (2017). A survey on deep learning in medical image analysis. *Medical Image Analysis* 42: 60–88. https://doi.org/10.1016/j.media.2017.07.005.

Liu, Y., Qi, N., Zhu, Q. and Li, W. (2019) 'CR-U-Net: cascaded U-Net with residual mapping for liver segmentation in CT images. in 2019 IEEE Visual Communications and Image Processing pp. 0–3. https://doi.org/10.1109/VCIP47243.2019.8966072.

Liu, W., Luo, J., Yang, Y. et al. (2022). Automatic lung segmentation in chest X-ray images using improved U-Net. *Scientific Reports* 12 (1): 1–10. https://doi.org/10.1038/s41598-022-12743-y.

Maclin, R. (2016). Popular ensemble methods: an empirical study popular ensemble methods: an empirical study. *Journal of Artificial Intelligence Research* 11 (July): 169–198.

Mangin, J.-F. and Rivì, D. (2019) Combining 3D U-Net and bottom-up geometric constraints for automatic cortical sulci recognition. Available at: www.brainvisa.info.

Marcus, D.S., Wang, T.H., Parker, J. et al. (2007). Open access series of imaging studies (OASIS): cross-sectional MRI data in young, middle aged, nondemented, and demented older adults. *Journal of Cognitive Neuroscience* 19 (9): 1498–1507. https://doi.org/10.1162/jocn.2007.19.9.1498.

Menze, B.H., Jakab, A., Bauer, S. et al. (2015). The multimodal brain tumor image segmentation benchmark (BRATS). *IEEE Transactions on Medical Imaging* 34 (10): 1993–2024. https://doi.org/10.1109/TMI.2014.2377694.

Mikolov, T., Karafiát, M., Burget, L. et al. (2010) "Recurrent Neural Network Based Language Model" was presented at the Interspeech 2010 conference held in Makuhari, Chiba, Japan, from 26–30 September 2010.

Milletari, F., Navab, N. and Ahmadi, S. A. (2016) V-Net: Fully convolutional neural networks for volumetric medical image segmentation. Proceedings – 2016 4th International Conference on 3D Vision, 3DV 2016, pp. 565–571. https://doi.org/10.1109/3DV.2016.79.

Mnih, V., Heess, N., Graves, A. et al. (2014) Recurrent models of visual attention. in Proceedings of the 27th International Conference on Neural Information Processing Systems – Volume 2, pp. 2204–2212. Cambridge, MA: MIT Press (NIPS'14).

Moeskops, P., Veta, M., Lafarge, M. W. et al. (2017) Adversarial training and dilated convolutions for brain MRI segmentation. in Deep Learning in Medical Image Analysis and Multimodal Learning for Clinical Decision Support: Third International Workshop, DLMIA 2017, and 7th International Workshop, ML-CDS 2017, Held in Conjunction with MICCAI 2017, Québec City, QC, 14 September, Proceedings 3, pp. 56–64. Lecture Notes in Computer Science (including subseries Lecture Notes in Artificial Intelligence and Lecture Notes in Bioinformatics), 10553 LNCS. https://doi.org/10.1007/978-3-319-67558-9_7.

Nie, D., Wang, L., Gao, Y., and Shen, D. (2016) Fully convolutional networks for multi-modality isointense infant brain image segmentation. Proceedings. IEEE

International Symposium on Biomedical Imaging, 2016, pp. 1342–1345. https://doi.org/10.1109/ISBI.2016.7493515.

Nie, D., Wang, L., Adeli, E. et al. (2019). 3-D fully convolutional networks for multimodal isointense infant brain image segmentation. *IEEE Transactions on Cybernetics* 49 (3): 1123–1136. https://doi.org/10.1109/TCYB.2018.2797905.

Nikolov, S., Blackwell, S., Zverovitch, A. et al. (2018). Deep learning to achieve clinically applicable segmentation of head and neck anatomy for radiotherapy. *arXiv* Available at: http://arxiv.org/abs/1809.04430.

Oktay, O., Schlemper, J., Le Folgoc, L. et al. (2018) Attention U-Net: learning where to look for the pancreas. *arXiv*, (Midl). Available at: http://arxiv.org/abs/1804.03999.

Owen, C.G., Rudnicka, A.R., Mullen, R. et al. (2009). Measuring retinal vessel tortuosity in 10-year-old children: validation of the computer-assisted image analysis of the retina (caiar) program. *Investigative Ophthalmology and Visual Science* 50 (5): 2004–2010. https://doi.org/10.1167/iovs.08-3018.

Pace, D. F., Dalca, A. V., Geva, T. et al. (2015) Interactive whole-heart segmentation in congenital heart disease. in Navab, N. et al. (eds) Medical Image Computing and Computer-Assisted Intervention – MICCAI 2015, pp. 80–88. Cham: Springer International Publishing.

Pal, D., Reddy, P.B., and Roy, S. (2022). Attention UW-Net: a fully connected model for automatic segmentation and annotation of chest X-ray. *Computers in Biology and Medicine* 150 (June): 106083. https://doi.org/10.1016/j.compbiomed.2022.106083.

Park, K.B., Choi, S.H., and Lee, J.Y. (2020). M-GAN: retinal blood vessel segmentation by balancing losses through stacked deep fully convolutional networks. *IEEE Access* 8 (M): 146308–146322. https://doi.org/10.1109/ACCESS.2020.3015108.

Pawar, S.P. and Talbar, S.N. (2021). LungSeg-Net: lung field segmentation using generative adversarial network. *Biomedical Signal Processing and Control* 64: 102296. https://doi.org/10.1016/j.bspc.2020.102296.

Payer, C., Štern, D., Bischof, H., and Urschler, M. (2018) Multi-label whole heart segmentation using CNNs and anatomical label configurations. in Pop, M. et al. (eds) Statistical Atlases and Computational Models of the Heart. ACDC and MMWHS Challenges, pp. 190–198. Cham: Springer International Publishing.

Raudaschl, P.F., Zaffino, P., Sharp, G.C. et al. (2017). Evaluation of segmentation methods on head and neck CT: auto-segmentation challenge 2015. *Medical Physics* 44 (5): 2020–2036. https://doi.org/10.1002/mp.12197.

Ronneberger, O., Fischer, P. and Brox, T. (2015) U-Net: convolutional networks for biomedical image segmentation. in Medical Image Computing and Computer-Assisted Intervention – MICCAI 2015: 18th International Conference, Munich, Germany, 5–9 October 2015, pp. 1–8. Springer International Publishing.

Roy, A.G., Conjeti, S., Navab, N. et al. (2019). Bayesian QuickNAT: model uncertainty in deep whole-brain segmentation for structure-wise quality control. *NeuroImage* 195: 11–22. https://doi.org/10.1016/j.neuroimage.2019.03.042.

Rumelhart, D.E., Hinton, G.E., and Williams, R.J. (1986). Learning representations by back-propagating errors. *Nature* 323: 533–536.

Seo, H., Huang, C., Bassenne, M. et al. (2020). Modified U-Net (mU-Net) with incorporation of object-dependent high level features for improved liver and liver-tumor segmentation in CT images. *IEEE Transactions on Medical Imaging* 39 (5): 1316–1325. https://doi.org/10.1109/TMI.2019.2948320.

Shelhamer, E., Long, J., and Darrell, T. (2017). Fully convolutional networks for semantic segmentation. *IEEE Transactions on Pattern Analysis and Machine Intelligence* 39 (4): 640–651. https://doi.org/10.1109/TPAMI.2016.2572683.

Shen, Y., Fang, Z., Gao, Y. et al. (2019). Coronary arteries segmentation based on 3D FCN with attention gate and level set function. *IEEE Access* 7: 42826–42835. https://doi.org/10.1109/ACCESS.2019.2908039.

Shi, F., Wang, J., Shi, J. et al. (2021). Review of artificial intelligence techniques in imaging data acquisition, segmentation, and diagnosis for COVID-19. *IEEE Reviews in Biomedical Engineering* 14: 4–15. https://doi.org/10.1109/RBME.2020.2987975.

Shiraishi, J., Katsuragawa, S., Ikezoe, J. et al. (2000). Development of a digital image database for chest radiographs with and without a lung nodule: receiver operating characteristic analysis of radiologists' detection of pulmonary nodules. *American Journal of Roentgenology* 174 (1): 71–74. https://doi.org/10.2214/ajr.174.1.1740071.

Soler, L., Hostettler, A., Agnus, V. et al. (2010). 3D image reconstruction for comparison of algorithm database: A patient-specific anatomical and medical image database. *IRCAD*, Strasbourg, France.

Son, J., Park, S.J., and Jung, K.-H. (2017). Retinal vessel segmentation in fundoscopic images with generative adversarial networks. *arXiv* Available at: http://arxiv.org/abs/1706.09318.

Srivastava, N., Mansimov, E. and Salakhutdinov, R. (2015) Unsupervised learning of video representations using LSTMs. 32nd International Conference on Machine Learning, ICML 2015, 1, pp. 843–852.

Staal, J., Abràmoff, M.D., Niemeijer, M. et al. (2004). Ridge-based vessel segmentation in color images of the retina. *IEEE Transactions on Medical Imaging* 23: 501–509.

Stirenko, S., Kochura, Y., Alienin, O. et al. (2018) Chest X-ray analysis of tuberculosis by deep learning with segmentation and augmentation. in 2018 IEEE 38th International Conference on Electronics and Nanotechnology, ELNANO 2018 – Proceedings, pp. 422–428. https://doi.org/10.1109/ELNANO.2018.8477564.

Stollenga, M. F., Byeon, W., Liwicki, M., and Schmidhuber, J. (2015) Parallel multi-dimensional LSTM, with application to fast biomedical volumetric image segmentation. Advances in Neural Information Processing Systems, January 2015, pp. 2998–3006.

Sun, L., Shao, W., Zhang, D., and Liu, M. (2020). Anatomical attention guided deep networks for ROI segmentation of brain MR images. *IEEE Transactions on Medical Imaging* 39 (6): 2000–2012. https://doi.org/10.1109/TMI.2019.2962792.

Tang, H., Chen, X., Liu, Y. et al. (2019). Clinically applicable deep learning framework for organs at risk delineation in CT images. *Nature Machine Intelligence* 1 (10): 480–491. https://doi.org/10.1038/s42256-019-0099-z.

Tong, N., Gou, S., Yang, S. et al. (2018). Fully automatic multi-organ segmentation for head and neck cancer radiotherapy using shape representation model constrained fully convolutional neural networks. *Medical Physics* 45 (10): 4558–4567. https://doi.org/10.1002/mp.13147.

Tran, P.V. (2016). A fully convolutional neural network for cardiac segmentation in short-axis MRI. *arXiv* 1–21. Available at: http://arxiv.org/abs/1604.00494.

Tran, S.T., Cheng, C.H., and Liu, D.G. (2021). A multiple layer U-Net, Un-Net, for liver and liver tumor segmentation in CT. *IEEE Access* 9: 3752–3764. https://doi.org/10.1109/ACCESS.2020.3047861.

Trullo, R., Petitjean, C., Ruan, S. et al. (2017) Segmentation of organs at risk in thoracic CT images using a sharpmask architecture and conditional random fields. Proceedings. IEEE International Symposium on Biomedical Imaging, 2017, pp. 1003–1006. https://doi.org/10.1109/ISBI.2017.7950685.

Vaswani, A., Shazeer, N., Parmar, N. et al. (2017) Attention is all you need. Advances in Neural Information Processing Systems, December 2017 (Nips), pp. 5999–6009.

Vesal, S., Ravikumar, N., and Maier, A. (2019). A 2D dilated residual U-net for multi-organ segmentation in thoracic CT. *CEUR Workshop Proceedings* 2349: 2–5.

Wachinger, C., Reuter, M., and Klein, T. (2018). DeepNAT: deep convolutional neural network for segmenting neuroanatomy. *NeuroImage* 170: 434–445. https://doi.org/10.1016/j.neuroimage.2017.02.035.

Wang, C. and Smedby, Ö. (2018) Automatic whole heart segmentation using deep learning and shape context. in Pop, M. et al. (eds) Statistical Atlases and Computational Models of the Heart. ACDC and MMWHS Challenges, pp. 242–249. Cham: Springer International Publishing.

Wang, X., Peng, Y., Lu, L. et al. (2017) ChestX-ray8: hospital-scale chest X-ray database and benchmarks on weakly-supervised classification and localization of common thorax diseases. Proceedings – 30th IEEE Conference on Computer Vision and Pattern Recognition, CVPR 2017, January 2017, pp. 3462–3471. https://doi.org/10.1109/CVPR.2017.369.

Wang, B., Qiu, S. and He, H. (2019a) Dual encoding U-Net for retinal vessel segmentation. in Shen, D. et al. (eds) Medical Image Computing and Computer Assisted Intervention – MICCAI 2019, pp. 84–92. Cham: Springer International Publishing.

Wang, C., He, Y., Qi, X. et al. (2019b) BiSC-UNet: A fine segmentation framework for kidney and renal tumor. Submissions to the 2019 Kidney Tumor Segmentation Challenge: KiTS19.

Wang, L., Xie, C., and Zeng, N. (2019c). RP-Net: A 3D convolutional neural network for brain segmentation from magnetic resonance imaging. *IEEE Access* 7: 39670–39679. https://doi.org/10.1109/ACCESS.2019.2906890.

Wang, Z. H., Liu, Z., Song, Y.Q. et al. (2019d) Densely connected deep U-Net for abdominal multi-organ segmentation. Proceedings – International Conference on Image Processing, ICIP, September 2019, pp. 1415–1419. https://doi.org/10.1109/ICIP.2019.8803103.

Wang, J., Lv, P., Wang, H., and Shi, C. (2021). SAR-U-Net: squeeze-and-excitation block and atrous spatial pyramid pooling based residual U-Net for automatic liver segmentation in computed tomography. *Computer Methods and Programs in Biomedicine* 208: 106268. https://doi.org/10.1016/j.cmpb.2021.106268.

Wu, Y. and Lin, L. (2020). Automatic lung segmentation in CT images using dilated convolution based weighted fully convolutional network. *Journal of Physics: Conference Series* 1646 (1): https://doi.org/10.1088/1742-6596/1646/1/012032.

Xing, Z., Wan, L., Fu, H. et al. (2023). Diff-UNet: a diffusion embedded network for volumetric segmentation. *arXiv* 1: 1–10. Available at: http://arxiv.org/abs/2303.10326.

Xu, C., Xu, L., Ohorodnyk, P. et al. (2020). Contrast agent-free synthesis and segmentation of ischemic heart disease images using progressive sequential causal GANs. *Medical Image Analysis* 62: 101668. https://doi.org/10.1016/j.media.2020.101668.

Xue, Y., Xu, T., Zhang, H. et al. (2018). SegAN: adversarial network with multi-scale L 1 loss for medical image segmentation. *Neuroinformatics* 16 (3–4): 383–392. https://doi.org/10.1007/s12021-018-9377-x.

Yahyatabar, M., Jouvet, P. and Cheriet, F. (2020) Dense-Unet: a light model for lung fields segmentation in chest X-Ray images. Proceedings of the Annual International Conference of the IEEE Engineering in Medicine and Biology Society, EMBS, July 2020, pp. 1242–1245. https://doi.org/10.1109/EMBC44109.2020.9176033.

Yang, G., Li, G., Pan, T. et al. (2018a) Automatic segmentation of kidney and renal tumor in CT images based on 3D fully convolutional neural network with pyramid pooling module. in 2018 24th International Conference on Pattern Recognition (ICPR), pp. 3790–3795. https://doi.org/10.1109/ICPR.2018.8545143.

Yang, J., Veeraraghavan, H., Armato, S.G. III, et al. (2018b). Autosegmentation for thoracic radiation treatment planning: a grand challenge at AAPM 2017. *Medical Physics* 45 (10): 4568–4581. https://doi.org/10.1002/mp.13141.

Ye, C., Wang, W., Zhang, S., and Wang, K. (2019). Multi-depth fusion network for whole-heart CT image segmentation. *IEEE Access* 7: 23421–23429. https://doi.org/10.1109/ACCESS.2019.2899635.

Yue, K., Zou, B., Chen, Z., and Liu, Q. (2019). Retinal vessel segmentation using dense U-net with multiscale inputs. *Journal of Medical Imaging* 6 (3): 34004. https://doi.org/10.1117/1.JMI.6.3.034004.

Zhang, Y. and Chung, A. C. S. (2018) Deep supervision with additional labels for retinal vessel segmentation task.in Medical Image Computing and Computer Assisted Intervention – MICCAI 2018: 21st International Conference, Granada, Spain, 16–20 September 2018, pp. 83–91. Lecture Notes in Computer Science (including subseries Lecture Notes in Artificial Intelligence and Lecture Notes in Bioinformatics), 11071 LNCS. https://doi.org/10.1007/978-3-030-00934-2_10.

Zhang, W., Li, R., Deng, H. et al. (2015). Deep convolutional neural networks for multi-modality isointense infant brain image segmentation. *NeuroImage* 108: 214–224. https://doi.org/10.1016/j.neuroimage.2014.12.061.

Zhang, Y., Wang, Y., Hou, F. et al. (2019). Cascaded volumetric convolutional network for kidney tumor segmentation from CT volumes. *arXiv* 1–7. https://doi.org/10.24926/548719.004.

Zhang, L., Zhang, J., Shen, P. et al. (2020). Block level skip connections across cascaded V-Net for multi-organ segmentation. *IEEE Transactions on Medical Imaging* 39 (9): 2782–2793. https://doi.org/10.1109/TMI.2020.2975347.

Zhao, H., Shi, J., Qi, X. et al. (2017) Pyramid scene parsing network. in 2017 IEEE Conference on Computer Vision and Pattern Recognition (CVPR), pp. 6230–6239. https://doi.org/10.1109/CVPR.2017.660.

Zhao, W., Jiang, D., Queralta, J.P., and Westerlund, T. (2020). MSS U-Net: 3D segmentation of kidneys and tumors from CT images with a multi-scale supervised U-Net. *Informatics in Medicine Unlocked* 19: 100357. https://doi.org/10.1016/j.imu.2020.100357.

Zhou, Z., Rahman Siddiquee, M.M., Tajbakhsh, N. and Liang, J. (2018) Unet++: a nested u-net architecture for medical image segmentation.in Deep Learning in Medical Image Analysis and Multimodal Learning for Clinical Decision Support: 4th International Workshop, DLMIA 2018, and 8th International Workshop, ML-CDS 2018, Held in Conjunction with MICCAI 2018, Granada, Spain, 20 September 2018, pp. 3–11. Lecture Notes in Computer Science (including subseries Lecture Notes in Artificial Intelligence and Lecture Notes in Bioinformatics), 11045 LNCS. https://doi.org/10.1007/978-3-030-00889-5_1.

Zhou, Z., Sodha, V., Rahman Siddiquee, M. M. et al. (2019) Models genesis: generic autodidactic models for 3D medical image analysis. Medical image computing and computer-assisted intervention: MICCAI … International Conference on Medical Image Computing and Computer-Assisted Intervention, 11767, pp. 384–393. https://doi.org/10.1007/978-3-030-32251-9_42.

Zhou, Z., Siddiquee, M.M.R., Tajbakhsh, N., and Liang, J. (2020). UNet++: redesigning skip connections to exploit multiscale features in image segmentation. *IEEE Transactions on Medical Imaging* 39 (6): 1856–1867. https://doi.org/10.1109/TMI.2019.2959609.

Zhou, S.K., Greenspan, H., Davatzikos, C. et al. (2021). A review of deep learning in medical imaging: imaging traits, technology trends, case studies with progress highlights, and future promises. *Proceedings of the IEEE* 109 (5): 820–838. https://doi.org/10.1109/JPROC.2021.3054390.

Zhuang, X. and Shen, J. (2016). Multi-scale patch and multi-modality atlases for whole heart segmentation of MRI. *Medical Image Analysis* 31: 77–87. https://doi.org/10.1016/j.media.2016.02.006.

3

Revealing Historical Insights: A Comprehensive Exploration of Traditional Approaches in Medical Image Segmentation

Mudasir Ashraf[1] *and Majid Zaman*[2]

[1]*School of Computer Science & IT, Univeristy of the People, CA, USA*
[2]*Scientist D, Computer Science Department, University of Kashmir, Jammu and Kashmir, India*

3.1 Introduction

Medical image segmentation, a critical facet of modern healthcare technology, underpins the precision and efficacy of diagnostic and therapeutic procedures (Sharma et al. 2018). The intricate task of delineating structures within medical images has evolved alongside advancements in imaging modalities, each step forward bringing both challenges and innovative solutions. This research embarks on a comprehensive exploration, delving into the historical tapestry of traditional approaches in medical image segmentation, aiming to illuminate their evolution, significance, and enduring impact in the landscape of healthcare.

3.1.1 Contextualizing Medical Image Segmentation

The landscape of medical image analysis has undergone a transformative journey, driven by the progression from conventional radiography to the sophistication of three-dimensional (3D) imaging modalities like magnetic resonance imaging (MRI) and computed tomography (CT). The demand for precise segmentation has grown exponentially with the expanding scope of medical imaging applications. From aiding in organ delineation for surgical planning to facilitating early detection of pathological conditions, such as tumors, accurate segmentation forms the cornerstone of effective medical image analysis (Gillies et al. 2016).

Deep Learning Applications in Medical Image Segmentation: Overview, Approaches, and Challenges, First Edition. Edited by Sajid Yousuf Bhat, Aasia Rehman, and Muhammad Abulaish.

3.1.2 The Significance of Accurate Segmentation

Accurate medical image segmentation is paramount for ensuring the reliability of subsequent analyses and treatment planning. As clinicians increasingly rely on medical imaging for decision-making, the need for robust segmentation methodologies becomes more pronounced. It is not merely a technical nuance but a critical determinant in enhancing diagnostic accuracy, guiding therapeutic interventions, and ultimately improving patient outcomes (Soni et al. 2016).

3.1.3 Traditional Approaches in Medical Image Segmentation

Against the backdrop of evolving imaging technologies, traditional approaches in medical image segmentation have played a pivotal role. Classical methodologies such as thresholding, region-based techniques, and contour-based algorithms as discussed in Table 3.1 have been the historical pillars of segmentation. These methods, although rooted in fundamental principles, have undergone significant refinements over time to meet the growing demands of clinical applications (Pham et al. 2000).

3.1.4 Evolution Over Time

The historical evolution of these traditional approaches reflects the iterative process of refinement and adaptation to technological advancements. From early heuristic methods to more sophisticated algorithmic implementations, each stage of evolution has contributed to the development of a rich tapestry in medical image segmentation. Understanding this evolution is paramount for contextualizing the historical significance of traditional methods and appreciating their continued relevance in the contemporary healthcare landscape (Sonka et al. 2014). Flowchart in Figure 3.1 illustrates the progression from traditional approaches to deep learning techniques in medical image segmentation, highlighting their respective strengths and limitations.

3.1.5 Aims of the Research

Deep learning technologies have witnessed significant advancements in recent years, revolutionizing various domains, including medical image segmentation. In the realm of cardiovascular disease prediction, cutting-edge technologies such as TensorFlow, PyTorch, and Keras have played a pivotal role (Ashraf et al. 2021). The empirical study conducted by Ashraf et al. (2021) sheds light on the predictive capabilities of these technologies, laying the groundwork for our exploration into their application in medical image segmentation.

The integration of deep learning technologies into medical analysis has been a transformative force, as evidenced by the empirical study conducted by Ashraf et al. (2021). This study not only showcases the potential of technologies like TensorFlow, PyTorch, and Keras in predicting cardiovascular diseases but also provides valuable insights into their broader applications. Moreover, the work of Ashraf et al. (2022) introduces the importance of feature selection in conjunction with these leading-edge technologies, underscoring the need for a comprehensive understanding of the tools at our disposal.

This research aims to provide a comprehensive exploration and critical analysis of traditional approaches in medical image segmentation. By tracing the historical trajectory of classical methodologies, from their inception to present-day adaptations, we seek to unravel the strengths, limitations, and enduring relevance of these methods. Through this meticulous examination, we aspire to offer valuable insights for researchers, practitioners, and developers in the field, fostering a nuanced perspective in the era of evolving computational techniques and deep learning.

3.2 Literature Review

3.2.1 Historical Evolution of Medical Image Segmentation

The history of medical image segmentation is deeply intertwined with the evolution of imaging technologies. Early attempts at segmentation were characterized by heuristic approaches, with manual interventions playing a significant role (Smith 2003). The advent of X-ray imaging marked the initiation of these heuristic methods, relying on subjective human judgment for extracting meaningful information from images. As technologies progressed, the need for automated segmentation gave rise to thresholding methods, representing one of the earliest techniques employed in medical image analysis (Gonzalez et al. 2008).

While traditional approaches, such as thresholding, region-based, and contour-based techniques, have been widely employed in medical image segmentation, they face inherent limitations as discussssed in Table 3.1. Thresholding, although simple and computationally efficient, struggles to adapt to varying intensity characteristics and complex structures (Pham et al. 2000; Zhang et al. 2019). Region-based techniques, like clustering algorithms, can handle diverse image characteristics but may encounter difficulties in defining clear boundaries, especially in the presence of noise or overlapping structures (Zhang et al. 2019; Shen et al. 2017). Contour-based algorithms, while effective in delineating precise object boundaries, are sensitive to image artifacts and often require sophisticated algorithms and preprocessing steps (Gonzalez et al. 2008; Yushkevich et al. 2006).

The integration of computational techniques, particularly deep learning, has emerged as a promising solution to overcome the limitations of traditional approaches. Deep learning models, especially convolutional neural networks (CNNs), have demonstrated exceptional performance in segmenting organs, tumors, and anatomical structures across various imaging modalities (Litjens et al. 2017; Shen et al. 2017). Their ability to automatically learn hierarchical

Table 3.1 Strengths and limitations of traditional approaches in medical image segmentation.

Approach	Strengths	Limitations
Thresholding	Simple and computationally efficient, effective for well-defined structures	Struggles with varying intensity characteristics, limited adaptability to complex structures
Region based (clustering)	Adaptable to diverse image characteristics, suitable for complex structures	Difficulty in defining clear boundaries, sensitive to noise and overlapping structures
Contour based	Effective in delineating precise object boundaries, suitable for intricate shapes	Sensitive to image artifacts, requires sophisticated algorithms and preprocessing

features from data eliminates the need for explicit feature engineering, allowing the models to adapt to the nuances present in medical images (Litjens et al. 2017; Tajbakhsh et al. 2020).

The work of Shin et al. (2016) underscores the significance of CNN architectures in computer-aided detection, showcasing their potential in automating complex tasks. The hierarchical nature of CNNs enables them to discern intricate patterns, making them well suited for medical image segmentation, where subtle details play a crucial role (Shahzad et al. 2018).

Transfer learning has become a pivotal strategy in contemporary techniques to address the challenge of limited annotated medical data (Tajbakhsh et al. 2020). By pre-training models on large datasets and fine-tuning them for specific segmentation tasks, transfer learning facilitates the development of robust models that generalize well to diverse patient populations and imaging conditions (Shin et al. 2016; Havaei et al. 2017). This methodology accelerates the deployment of effective segmentation solutions, particularly in scenarios where acquiring extensive labeled datasets is challenging.

Contemporary techniques emphasize the integration of multi-modal information to enhance the accuracy and completeness of medical image segmentation (Havaei et al. 2017; Shen et al. 2017). The fusion of data from different imaging modalities, such as MRI and CT, provides a more holistic understanding of complex anatomical structures. This integration is particularly valuable in scenarios where complementary information from multiple sources enhances the overall segmentation accuracy (Menze et al. 2015; Li et al. 2020).

Table 3.2 Comparison of deep learning architectures for medical image segmentation.

Architecture	Characteristics
U-Net	Encoder–decoder architecture with skip connections, processes entire images in a single forward pass, and effective for biomedical image segmentation
V-Net	3D variant of U-Net, incorporates 3D convolutional layers, and objective function based on the Dice coefficient
Residual U-Net	Incorporates short, residual-like skip connections, and enhances the network's capabilities

3.2.2 Thresholding Techniques and Their Applications

Thresholding, as a foundational technique, involves categorizing pixel intensities based on predefined thresholds. While simple, its effectiveness is contingent on well-defined structures in the image. Applications in radiographic images, where pixel intensities correspond to distinct anatomical features, showcase the utility of thresholding (Van Ginneken 2002). However, challenges arise in scenarios with varying intensity characteristics, necessitating careful consideration of appropriate threshold values.

3.2.3 Region-Based Techniques

Region-based techniques emerged as a response to the limitations of thresholding. Clustering algorithms, such as k-means and fuzzy c-means, gained prominence for grouping pixels with similar properties into coherent regions. These methods demonstrated adaptability to diverse image characteristics and found applications in the segmentation of complex structures, such as the brain, where clear boundaries are challenging to define using thresholding (Zhang et al. 2019).

3.2.4 Contour-Based Algorithms and Their Applications

Contour-based algorithms introduced the concept of delineating object boundaries through edge detection and tracing. While addressing challenges posed by thresholding and region-based techniques, contour-based approaches brought new complexities. Sensitivity to noise and the requirement for sophisticated algorithms were notable considerations. Applications in segmenting structures with intricate shapes, such as blood vessels or irregularly shaped tumors, showcased the potential of contour-based methods (Gonzalez et al. 2008).

3.2.5 Limitations of Traditional Approaches

Despite their historical significance, traditional approaches face inherent limitations as discussssed in Table 3.1. Thresholding struggles with adapting to variations in image intensity, making it less effective in scenarios with complex structures or varying tissue characteristics (Pham et al. 2000). Region-based techniques may encounter difficulties in defining clear boundaries, especially when faced with noisy or overlapping structures (Zhang et al. 2019). Contour-based algorithms, while effective in certain scenarios, are sensitive to image artifacts and may require intricate preprocessing steps (Gonzalez et al. 2008).

3.2.6 The Rise of Deep Learning in Medical Image Segmentation

The contemporary era of medical image segmentation is characterized by the prominent role of deep learning as discussed in Table 3.2. CNNs have demonstrated exceptional capabilities in segmenting organs, tumors, and complex anatomical structures across various imaging modalities (Litjens et al. 2017). The ability to automatically learn hierarchical features from data positions deep learning models as powerful tools in improving segmentation accuracy.

3.2.7 Transfer Learning and Multi-modal Information

Transfer learning has become a pivotal strategy in contemporary techniques. By pre-training models on large datasets and fine-tuning them for specific tasks, transfer learning facilitates the development of robust segmentation models that generalize well to diverse patient populations and imaging conditions (Shin et al. 2016). The integration of multi-modal information further enhances segmentation accuracy, providing a more holistic understanding of complex anatomical structures.

3.2.8 Real-Time Segmentation and Clinical Applications

Contemporary techniques aim for real-time segmentation capabilities crucial for applications such as intraoperative guidance and dynamic imaging scenarios. The integration of advanced computational techniques enables faster processing times, making real-time segmentation feasible in clinical settings. This development has profound implications for surgical interventions, enabling precision and efficiency in treatment procedures.

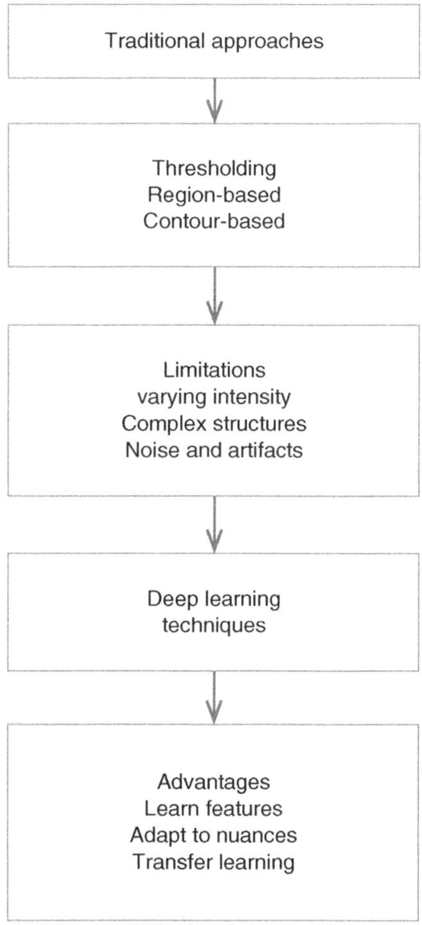

Figure 3.1 Flowchart illustrating the progression from traditional approaches to deep learning techniques in medical image segmentation, highlighting their respective strengths and limitations.

3.2.9 Challenges and Opportunities in the Modern Era

The transition to the modern era introduces new challenges and opportunities. While contemporary techniques offer superior accuracy and efficiency, challenges persist in adapting to the intricacies of modern imaging modalities. The integration of machine learning, while promising, raises considerations regarding interpretability and generalizability across diverse patient populations.

3.2.10 Future Directions and Research Implications

The literature review concludes by highlighting future directions and research implications. The integration of computational techniques opens avenues for further innovation, with a focus on addressing the challenges posed by diverse imaging scenarios. Future endeavors could explore novel approaches, advanced architectures, and methodologies that combine the strengths of traditional foundations with the adaptability of contemporary techniques.

3.3 Methodology

3.3.1 Explanation of Traditional Approaches

3.3.1.1 Thresholding

Thresholding remains a fundamental technique in medical image segmentation, involving the categorization of pixel intensities based on predefined thresholds. Despite its simplicity, adapting to variations in image intensity remains a challenge (Zhang et al. 2019).

3.3.1.2 Region-Based Techniques

Region-based techniques, such as k-means clustering and fuzzy c-means clustering, focus on grouping pixels with similar properties into coherent regions. While adaptable to diverse image characteristics, defining clear boundaries in the presence of intensity variations or overlapping structures remains a challenge (Zhang et al. 2019).

3.3.1.3 Contour-Based Algorithms

Contour-based algorithms delineate object boundaries through edge detection and tracing. Addressing some challenges of other techniques, they may be sensitive to noise and could require sophisticated algorithms for complex anatomical structures (Zhang et al. 2019).

3.3.2 Application in Medical Image Segmentation

3.3.2.1 Thresholding Applications

Thresholding finds applications where pixel intensities correspond to well-defined structures. Limitations become evident in images with varying intensity characteristics, necessitating careful consideration of appropriate threshold values (Zhang et al. 2019).

3.3.2.2 Region-Based Techniques in Practice

Clustering algorithms, as region-based techniques, prove useful in segmenting images with complex structures. Applications include brain imaging, where clear boundaries may be challenging to define using other approaches (Zhang et al. 2019).

3.3.2.3 Contour-Based Algorithm Applications

Contour-based algorithms are employed in scenarios where delineating precise object boundaries is crucial. Applications include the segmentation of structures with intricate shapes, such as blood vessels or irregularly shaped tumors. However, sensitivity to noise requires careful preprocessing steps for optimal performance (Zhang et al. 2019).

3.3.3 Datasets and Tools

To evaluate traditional approaches, diverse datasets representing various medical imaging modalities will be utilized. Established datasets like those from the Medical Image Computing and Computer Assisted Intervention (MICCAI) will be employed for benchmarking and comparison (Litjens et al. 2017).

The evaluation process will use state-of-the-art tools in the field, ensuring consistency and comparability in assessing the efficacy of traditional approaches. This includes leveraging advancements in software packages and programming environments for robust evaluations (Litjens et al. 2017).

3.3.4 Integration of Text Reports and Medical Image Data

The fusion of textual reports and medical image data has spurred research in two key directions: enhancing image classification accuracy by incorporating information from reports (Schlegl et al. 2015) and generating text reports from medical images (Kisilev et al. 2016; Shin et al. 2015, 2016; Wang et al. 2016). The latter concept draws inspiration from recent advancements in caption generation for natural images (Karpathy and Fei-Fei 2015). Notably, the pioneering work of Schlegl et al. (2015) took the initial step in leveraging reports by addressing the challenge of acquiring large annotated datasets. Their approach involved augmenting image datasets with semantic descriptions extracted from textual reports, training the system to predict semantic class labels during test time. Results demonstrated improved classification accuracy across various pathologies in optical coherence tomography (OCT) images.

Building on this foundation, Shin et al. (2015) and Wang et al. (2016) explored semantic interactions between radiology reports and images using a vast dataset extracted from a picture archiving and communication system (PACS). Their methodology incorporated latent Dirichlet allocation (LDA), a stochastic model generating topic distributions based on document words. Subsequently, Shin et al. (2016) introduced a system for generating descriptions from chest X-rays. Employing a CNN, they generated image representations label by label, subsequently training a recurrent neural network (RNN) to produce sequences of MeSH keywords. In a different approach, Kisilev et al. (2016) predicted BI-RADS descriptors for breast lesions, focusing on mammography descriptors such as shape, margin, and density.

3.4 Historical Context

3.4.1 Early Heuristic Approaches

In the nascent stages of medical image analysis, segmentation relied heavily on heuristic methods that lacked systematic algorithms. The advent of X-ray imaging witnessed the application of manual interventions for image interpretation (Smith 2003). This era was characterized by subjective human judgment, marking the early attempts to extract meaningful information from medical images.

3.4.2 Emergence of Thresholding

As imaging technologies advanced, the need for automation led to the emergence of thresholding as one of the earliest segmentation techniques (Gonzalez et al. 2008). By categorizing pixel intensities based on predefined thresholds, thresholding provided a rudimentary yet automated method for segmenting images. However, its simplicity limits its adaptability to variations in image intensity.

3.4.3 Rise of Region-Based Techniques

The historical evolution continued with the rise of region-based techniques, addressing the limitations of thresholding. Algorithms such as k-means clustering and fuzzy c-means clustering aim to group pixels with similar properties into coherent regions, providing adaptability to diverse image characteristics (Zhang et al. 2019). Region-based techniques found applications in complex structures such as the brain, where clear boundaries were challenging to define using earlier methods.

3.4.4 Introduction of Contour-Based Algorithms

Another milestone in the historical context was the introduction of contour-based algorithms. These methods focused on delineating object boundaries through edge detection and tracing, offering a more nuanced approach to segmentation (Zhang et al. 2019). While contour-based algorithms addressed challenges posed by earlier techniques, they introduced new complexities, requiring sophisticated preprocessing steps and advanced computational capabilities.

3.4.5 Computational Advancements and Modern Era

The historical trajectory from heuristic methods to algorithmic precision aligned with the computational advancements of the late 20th and early 21st centuries. As computational capabilities expanded, traditional segmentation methodologies underwent refinement, enabling more precise delineation of anatomical structures (Litjens et al. 2017). This period marks the bridge to the modern era of medical image segmentation, where the integration of computational techniques and the advent of deep learning applications have reshaped the landscape.

3.5 Segmentation

Segmentation of organs and substructures in medical images is crucial for quantitative analysis of clinical parameters related to volume and shape. This process is foundational for various medical analyses, including cardiac or brain analysis, and serves as a vital initial step in computer-aided detection pipelines. The segmentation task involves identifying voxels constituting the contour or interior of the object of interest. Within the realm of deep learning applications to medical imaging, segmentation emerges as a predominant theme, showcasing diverse methodologies, including unique CNN architectures and the broader application of RNNs.

One notable CNN architecture in medical image analysis is U-net, introduced by Ronneberger et al. in 2015. U-net incorporates equal amounts of upsampling and downsampling layers, along with skip connections between opposing convolution and deconvolution layers. These skip connections concatenate features from the contracting and expanding paths, allowing U-net to process entire images or scans in a single forward pass. This unique architecture considers the full context of the image, offering advantages over patch-based CNNs (Ronneberger et al. 2015).

Several derivative architectures based on U-net have been proposed. Milletari et al. (2016) introduced V-net, a 3D variant of U-net, employing 3D convolutional layers and an objective function based on the Dice coefficient for 3D image segmentation. Drozdzal et al. (2016) explored short ResNet-like skip connections in addition to the long skip connections in a regular U-net, enhancing the network's capabilities.

In parallel, RNNs have gained popularity for segmentation tasks. Xie et al. (2016) utilized a spatial clockwork RNN to segment perimysium in H&E-histopathology images. The incorporation of bidirectional information from both left/top and right/bottom neighbors was achieved through applying the RNN four times in different orientations. Similarly, Stollenga et al. (2015) introduced a 3D LSTM-RNN with convolutional layers in six directions. Other studies, such as

Andermatt et al. (2016) and Chen et al. (2016), explored 3D RNNs with gated recurrent units for segmenting gray and white matter in brain MRI and structures in anisotropic 3D electron microscopy images, respectively.

While these specific segmentation architectures exhibit advantages, patch-trained neural networks have also demonstrated excellent results. Ciresan et al. (2012) applied pixel-wise segmentation of membranes in electron microscopy imagery using a sliding window strategy. More recent approaches favor fully convolutional neural networks (fCNNs) over sliding-window-based classification to reduce redundant computation.

Extensions of fCNNs to 3D have been explored, addressing multiple targets simultaneously. Korez et al. (2016) utilized 3D fCNNs to generate vertebral body likelihood maps, driving deformable models for vertebral body segmentation in MR images. Zhou et al. (2016) segmented 19 targets in the human torso, while Moeskops et al. (2016) trained a single fCNN to segment brain MRI, the pectoral muscle in breast MRI, and the coronary arteries in cardiac CT angiography (CTA).

Despite the success of voxel classification approaches, spurious responses can occur. To address this, researchers have combined fCNNs with graphical models, such as Markov random fields (MRFs) and conditional random fields (CRFs), to refine segmentation outputs (Shakeri et al. 2016; Christ et al. 2016; Fu et al. 2016). Graphical models act as label regularizers, enhancing the overall segmentation performance.

The field of medical imaging segmentation has witnessed a surge in deep learning methodologies. Unique architectures specifically designed for segmentation tasks have demonstrated promising results, often outperforming traditional fCNNs.

3.6 Challenges and Opportunities

3.6.1 Challenges in Traditional Approaches

Despite their historical significance, traditional approaches in medical image segmentation face inherent challenges. Thresholding methods, while simple, struggle with adapting to variations in image intensity, making them less effective in scenarios with complex structures or varying tissue characteristics (Pham et al. 2000). Region-based techniques, such as clustering algorithms, may encounter difficulties in defining clear boundaries, especially when faced with noisy or overlapping structures (Zhang et al. 2019). Contour-based algorithms, though effective in certain scenarios, are sensitive to image artifacts and may require intricate preprocessing steps (Gonzalez et al. 2008).

3.6.2 Limitations in Handling Modern Imaging Modalities

As medical imaging modalities continue to advance, traditional approaches find limitations in handling the complexity and richness of modern image data. The intricacies introduced by 3D imaging, dynamic imaging, and multi-modal imaging pose challenges to methodologies rooted in two-dimensional, static assumptions. Traditional techniques may struggle to capture the spatial and temporal nuances inherent in these advanced modalities.

3.6.3 Bridging the Gap: Integrating Computational Techniques

One opportunity lies in bridging the gap between traditional approaches and modern computational techniques. The integration of machine learning, particularly deep learning, presents an avenue for addressing the limitations of classical methodologies. By leveraging the power of neural networks, deep learning models can automatically learn intricate features and adapt to the complexities of diverse medical imaging scenarios (Litjens et al. 2017). This fusion of classical foundations with contemporary computational advancements holds promise for enhancing the accuracy and robustness of medical image segmentation.

3.6.4 Leveraging Big Data and Real-World Applications

The era of big data presents an opportunity to enhance the capabilities of medical image segmentation. Large-scale datasets, encompassing diverse patient populations and imaging conditions, offer the potential for training more robust and generalizable models. Real-world applications, such as computer-aided diagnosis and personalized treatment planning, can benefit from segmentation methodologies that are trained on extensive and representative datasets.

3.7 Case Studies

3.7.1 Application of Traditional Approaches in Clinical Settings

Several case studies illustrate the practical application of traditional approaches in diverse clinical settings. In oncology, thresholding methods have been employed for tumor segmentation in positron emission tomography (PET) images (Hatt et al. 2010). Region-based techniques, such as clustering algorithms, have found utility in segmenting brain structures for neurosurgical planning (Menze et al. 2015). Contour-based algorithms have been applied in cardiac imaging for delineating myocardial boundaries (Lorenz et al. 2000). These case studies provide insights into the strengths and limitations of traditional approaches across different medical domains.

3.7.2 Challenges Encountered in Real-World Scenarios

Despite their historical relevance, traditional approaches face challenges when applied to real-world scenarios. In cases where pathology introduces variations in tissue characteristics, thresholding methods may struggle to adapt. The presence of noise and artifacts in medical images poses challenges for region-based techniques, impacting the accuracy of segmentation. Contour-based algorithms may encounter difficulties in scenarios with irregular shapes or overlapping structures. These challenges underscore the need for innovative solutions and pave the way for exploring the integration of computational techniques.

3.7.3 Integration of Computational Techniques

Recent case studies highlight the integration of computational techniques, particularly deep learning, to enhance the accuracy and robustness of medical image segmentation. Deep learning models have demonstrated superior performance in segmenting organs, tumors, and anatomical structures across various imaging modalities (Litjens et al. 2017). The adaptability of deep learning to complex image characteristics positions it as a promising solution to overcome the limitations of traditional approaches.

3.7.4 Leveraging Big Data for Improved Segmentation

Case studies exploring the use of large-scale datasets showcase the potential of big data in improving the capabilities of medical image segmentation. The availability of extensive and diverse datasets enables the training of models that generalize well to different patient populations and imaging conditions. Real-world applications, such as automated diagnosis and treatment planning, benefit from segmentation methodologies trained on comprehensive datasets.

3.8 Modern Era and Contemporary Techniques

3.8.1 Evolution Beyond Traditional Approaches

The landscape of medical image segmentation has undergone a profound transformation with the advent of the modern era, marked by a departure from traditional approaches toward more sophisticated and data-driven methodologies. The transition signifies a paradigm shift from heuristic and manual methods to computational precision, propelled by the integration of contemporary techniques.

The evolution beyond traditional approaches is epitomized by the rise of deep learning, a subfield of machine learning that leverages neural networks to automatically learn hierarchical features from data. Deep learning has become a cornerstone in contemporary medical image segmentation, offering unparalleled capabilities in capturing intricate patterns and adapting to the complexities of diverse imaging scenarios (Litjens et al. 2017).

3.8.2 Role of Deep Learning in Medical Image Segmentation

Deep learning, especially CNNs, has emerged as a powerful tool in medical image segmentation. CNNs demonstrate exceptional performance in segmenting organs, tumors, and anatomical structures across various imaging modalities. The ability to automatically learn features from data eliminates the need for explicit feature engineering, allowing the model to adapt to the nuances present in medical images (Litjens et al. 2017).

The work of Shin et al. (2016) emphasizes the importance of CNN architectures in computer-aided detection, showcasing the significance of neural networks in automating complex tasks. The hierarchical nature of CNNs enables them to discern intricate patterns, making them well suited for medical image segmentation where subtle details play a crucial role.

3.8.3 Transfer Learning and Generalization

Transfer learning has become a pivotal strategy in contemporary techniques to overcome challenges associated with limited annotated medical data. The approach involves pre-training models on large datasets and fine-tuning them for specific segmentation tasks. Transfer learning facilitates the development of robust segmentation models that generalize well to diverse patient populations and imaging conditions (Shin et al. 2016). This methodology accelerates the deployment of effective segmentation solutions, particularly in scenarios where acquiring extensive labeled datasets is challenging.

The study by Shin et al. (2016) provides insights into the characteristics of CNN architectures, dataset characteristics, and the principles of transfer learning. The work underscores the importance of transfer learning in achieving high performance with limited labeled data, a common challenge in medical image segmentation.

3.8.4 Integration of Multi-modal Information

Contemporary techniques emphasize the integration of multi-modal information to enhance the accuracy and completeness of medical image segmentation. The fusion of data from different imaging modalities, such as MRI and CT, provides a more holistic understanding of complex anatomical structures. This integration is particularly valuable in scenarios where complementary information from multiple sources enhances the overall segmentation accuracy (Litjens et al. 2017).

Studies such as Menze et al.'s (2015) work on the Multi-modal Brain Tumor Image Segmentation Benchmark (BRATS) exemplify the importance of multi-modal data in achieving accurate segmentation results. The comprehensive analysis of various modalities contributes to a more nuanced understanding of brain tumor characteristics and aids in treatment planning.

3.8.5 Real-Time Segmentation and Clinical Applications

Contemporary techniques aim to achieve real-time segmentation capabilities, a crucial requirement for applications such as intraoperative guidance and dynamic imaging scenarios. The integration of advanced computational techniques enables faster processing times, making real-time segmentation feasible in clinical settings. This development has profound implications for surgical interventions, enabling precision and efficiency in treatment procedures (Litjens et al. 2017).

The real-time segmentation capabilities are exemplified in studies such as the work by Lorenz et al. (2000) , where automatic segmentation of the left ventricle in 3D echocardiography data was achieved. The application of real-time segmentation in cardiac imaging demonstrates the potential for immediate clinical impact, especially in scenarios where timely decision-making is crucial.

3.8.6 Challenges and Ongoing Research

Despite the remarkable progress in contemporary techniques, challenges persist in the field of medical image segmentation. The interpretability of deep learning models remains an ongoing concern, particularly in medical contexts where decisions have direct implications for patient care. The need for robustness to diverse imaging conditions, including variations in resolution, noise, and artifacts, continues to be a focus of research.

Ongoing research endeavors are exploring innovative solutions to address these challenges. Architectural modifications to neural networks, ensemble learning approaches, and the integration of attention mechanisms are among the strategies being investigated. The exploration of unsupervised and self-supervised learning techniques aims to reduce dependence on annotated datasets, providing avenues for more scalable and generalizable segmentation models.

3.9 Conclusion

In conclusion, this comprehensive exploration has delved into the historical foundations of medical image segmentation, focusing on traditional approaches. From heuristic methods to thresholding, region-based techniques, and contour-based algorithms, we traced the evolution of methodologies that laid the groundwork for contemporary techniques. The strengths and limitations of each approach were critically analyzed, providing valuable insights into their historical significance.

Challenges faced by traditional approaches, including adaptability to modern imaging modalities and limitations in handling real-world scenarios, were highlighted. These challenges underscored the need for innovation and paved the way for opportunities in the integration of computational techniques. The role of big data, real-world applications, and the potential of leveraging machine learning, especially deep learning, were explored as avenues for overcoming the limitations of classical methodologies.

The transition to the modern era of medical image segmentation showcased the pivotal role of contemporary techniques. The integration of deep learning, transfer learning, and the emphasis on multi-modal information demonstrated a paradigm shift in the field. Real-time segmentation capabilities and applications in clinical settings underscored the transformative impact of these advanced methodologies.

As we conclude, the insights gained from this exploration provide a roadmap for future research in medical image segmentation. The integration of computational techniques opens avenues for further innovation, with a focus on addressing the challenges posed by diverse imaging scenarios. Future endeavors could explore novel approaches, advanced architectures, and methodologies that combine the strengths of traditional foundations with the adaptability of contemporary techniques.

In closing, this comprehensive review serves as a valuable resource for researchers, practitioners, and developers in the field of medical image segmentation. By understanding the historical context, challenges, and opportunities, we pave the way for innovative solutions that push the boundaries of medical image analysis. The continuous evolution from traditional approaches to contemporary techniques represents a dynamic journey, with each milestone contributing to the ongoing quest for precision and efficiency in medical image segmentation.

References

Andermatt, S., et al. (2016). 3D RNNs with gated recurrent units for segmenting gray and white matter in brain MRI. In Proceedings of the 13th International Symposium on Biomedical Imaging (ISBI 2016), pp. 143–146.

Ashraf, M., Ahmad, S. M., Ganai, N. A. et al. (2021). Prediction of cardiovascular disease through cutting-edge deep learning technologies: an empirical study based on TENSORFLOW, PYTORCH, and KERAS. In International Conference on Innovative Computing and Communications: Proceedings of ICICC 2020, Volume 1, pp. 239–255. Springer Singapore.

Ashraf, M., Salal, Y. K., Abdullaev, S. M. et al. (2022). Introduction of feature selection and leading-edge technologies viz. TENSORFLOW, PYTORCH, and KERAS: an empirical study to improve prediction accuracy of cardiovascular disease. In International Conference on Innovative Computing and Communications: Proceedings of ICICC 2021, Volume 3, pp. 19–31. Springer Singapore.

Chen, X., et al. (2016). Segmentation of structures in anisotropic 3D electron microscopy images using deep learning techniques. In Proceedings of the 29th Annual Meeting of the IEEE Engineering in Medicine and Biology Society (EMBC 2016), pp. 1387–1390.

Christ, P.F., Elshaer M. E. A., Ettlinger F. et al. (2016). Automatic Liver and Lesion Segmentation in CT Using Cascaded Fully Convolutional Neural Networks and 3D Conditional Random Fields. In: Ourselin, S., Joskowicz, L., Sabuncu, M., Unal, G., Wells, W. (eds) Medical Image Computing and Computer-Assisted Intervention – MICCAI 2016. MICCAI 2016. Lecture Notes in Computer Science, vol 9901. Springer, Cham. https:/doi.org/10.1007/978-3-319-46723-8_48

Ciresan, D., Giusti, A., Gambardella, L.M., and Schmidhuber, J. (2012). Deep neural networks segment neuronal membranes in electron microscopy images. In: *Advances in Neural Information Processing Systems*, 2843–2851.

Drozdzal, M., Vorontsov, E., Chartrand, G. et al. (2016). The importance of skip connections in biomedical image segmentation. In: *Deep Learning and Data Labeling for Medical Applications*, 179–187. Springer.

Fu H., Xu Y., Wong D. W. K. and Liu J. (2016), "Retinal vessel segmentation via deep learning network and fully-connected conditional random fields," IEEE 13th International Symposium on Biomedical Imaging (ISBI), Prague, Czech Republic, 2016, pp. 698–701, doi: 10.1109/ISBI.2016.7493362.

Gillies, R.J., Kinahan, P.E., and Hricak, H. (2016). Radiomics: images are more than pictures, they are data. *Radiology* 278 (2): 563–577.

Gonzalez, R.C. and Woods, R.E. (2008). *Digital Iimage Processing*, 3rde. Upper Saddle River, NJ: Prentice Hall.

Gonzalez, R.C. and Woods, R.E. (2008). *Digital image processing*. Pearson Education.

Hatt, M., le Rest, C.C., Turzo, A. et al. (2010). Fuzzy locally adaptive bayesian segmentation of positron emission tomography images. *European Journal of Nuclear Medicine and Molecular Imaging* 37 (1): 77–89.

Havaei, M., Davy, A., Warde-Farley, D. et al. (2017). Brain tumor segmentation with deep neural networks. *Medical Image Analysis* 35: 18–31.

Karpathy, A. and Fei-Fei, L. (2015). Deep visual-semantic alignments for generating image descriptions. Proceedings of the IEEE Conference on Computer Vision and Pattern Recognition (CVPR), 3128–3137.

Kisilev, P. et al. (2016). Predicting BI-RADS descriptors in mammography from region descriptors. Proceedings of the IEEE Conference on Computer Vision and Pattern Recognition (CVPR), 546–554.

Korez, R., Ibragimov, B., Likar, B., and Pernuš, F. (2016). Vertebral body segmentation with a 3D probabilistic atlas from a small training dataset. *Physics in Medicine & Biology* 61 (14): 5084.

Li, X., Chen, H., Qi, X. et al. (2020). H-DenseUNet: hybrid densely connected UNet for liver and liver tumor segmentation from CT volumes. *IEEE Transactions on Medical Imaging* 39 (12): 4047–4057.

Litjens, G., Kooi, T., Bejnordi, B.E. et al. (2017). A survey on deep learning in medical image analysis. *Medical Image Analysis* 42: 60–88.

Lorenz, C. et al. (2000). Automatic segmentation of the left ventricle in 3D echocardiography data. *IEEE Transactions on Medical Imaging* 19 (7): 713–725.

Menze, B.H., Jakab, A., Bauer, S. et al. (2015). The multimodal brain tumor image segmentation benchmark (BRATS). *IEEE Transactions on Medical Imaging* 34 (10): 1993–2024.

Milletari, F., Navab, N., and Ahmadi, S. A. (2016). V-net: fully convolutional neural networks for volumetric medical image segmentation. In 3D Vision (3DV), 2016 Fourth International Conference on, pp. 565–571. IEEE.

Menze, B.H., Jakab, A., Bauer, S. et al. (2015). The multimodal brain tumor image segmentation benchmark (BRATS). *IEEE Transactions on Medical Imaging* 34 (10): 1993–2024.

Moeskops, P., Wolterink J. M., van der Velden. H.M.B. et al. (2016). Deep Learning for Multi-task Medical Image Segmentation in Multiple Modalities. In: Ourselin, S., Joskowicz, L., Sabuncu, M., Unal, G., Wells, W. (eds) Medical Image Computing and Computer-Assisted Intervention – MICCAI 2016. MICCAI 2016. Lecture Notes in Computer Science, vol 9901. Springer, Cham. https:/doi.org/10.1007/978-3-319-46723-8_55

Pham, D.L., Xu, C., and Prince, J.L. (2000). Current methods in medical image segmentation. *Annual Review of Biomedical Engineering* 2 (1): 315–337.

Pham, D.L. et al. (2000). Current methods in medical image segmentation. *Annual Review of Biomedical Engineering* 2 (1).

Ronneberger, O., Fischer, P., and Brox, T. (2015). U-net: convolutional networks for biomedical image segmentation. In International Conference on Medical Image Computing and Computer-Assisted Intervention, pp. 234–241. Springer.

Schlegl, T., Seeböck, P., Waldstein, S.M. et al. (2015). Unsupervised anomaly detection with generative adversarial networks to guide marker discovery. *Medical Image Analysis* 63–72.

Shahzad, R., Lohinger, U., Stöttinger, J., and Uhl, A. (2018). Convolutional neural networks for computer-aided diagnosis from medical imaging: a review. In International Conference in Central Europe on Computer Graphics, Visualization and Computer Vision, June 2018, pp. 295–302.

Shakeri, M., Tsogkas, S., Ferrante, E. et al (2016). Sub-cortical brain structure segmentation using F-CNN'S. 2016 IEEE 13th International Symposium on Biomedical Imaging (ISBI), 269–272.

Sharma, P. et al. (2018). Medical image segmentation: a brief review. *Journal of Biomedical Science and Engineering* 11 (12): 590–607.

Shen, D., Wu, G., and Suk, H.I. (2017). Deep learning in medical image analysis. *Annual Review of Biomedical Engineering* 19: 221–248.

Shin, H. C., Roberts, K., Lu, L. et al. (2015). Learning to read chest X-rays: recurrent neural cascade model for automated image annotation. IEEE Conference on Computer Vision and Pattern Recognition (CVPR), 2497–2506.

Shin, H.C., Roth, H.R., Gao, M. et al. (2016). Deep convolutional neural networks for computer-aided detection: CNN architectures, dataset characteristics and transfer learning. *IEEE Transactions on Medical Imaging* 35 (5): 1285–1298.

Smith, T.G. (2003). Heuristic methods in medical image analysis. *Journal of Medical Imaging* 10 (2): 123–136.

Soni, S.U. et al. (2016). Application of image processing in medicine. *Journal of Evolution of Medical and Dental Sciences* 5 (68): 5009–5013.

Sonka, M., Hlavac, V., Boyle, R. et al. (2014). *Image processing, analysis, and machine vision*. Cengage Learning.

Stollenga, M.F., Byeon, W., and Liwicki, M. (2015). Parallel multi-dimensional LSTM, with application to fast biomedical volumetric image segmentation. In: *Advances in Neural Information Processing Systems*, 2998–3006.

Tajbakhsh, N., Jeyaseelan, L., Li, Q. et al. (2020). Embracing imperfect datasets: a review of deep learning solutions for medical image segmentation. *Medical Image Analysis* 63: 101693.

Van Ginneken, B. (2002). Computer-aided diagnosis in chest radiography. Proceedings of the American Thoracic Society, 1(1), 66–75.

Wang, X., Peng, Y., Lu, L. et al. (2016). ChestX-ray8: hospital-scale chest X-ray database and benchmarks on weakly-supervised classification and localization of common thorax diseases. Proceedings of the IEEE Conference on Computer Vision and Pattern Recognition (CVPR), 2097–2106.

Xie, S., Girshick, R., Dollar, P., and Tu, Z. (2016). Aggregated residual transformations for deep neural networks. In Proceedings of the IEEE Conference on Computer Vision and Pattern Recognition, pp. 1492–1500.

Yushkevich, P.A., Piven, J., Hazlett, H.C. et al. (2006). User-guided 3D active contour segmentation of anatomical structures: significantly improved efficiency and reliability. *NeuroImage* 31 (3): 1116–1128.

Zhang, Y., Luo, Y., Zhang, Y. et al. (2019). Challenges, methodologies, and opportunities in medical image analysis. *Frontiers in Medicine* 6: 74.

Zhang, L. et al. (2019). Challenges, methodologies, and opportunities in medical image analysis. *Frontiers in Medicine* 6: 74.

Zhou, Y., Lu, H., Chen, W. et al. (2016). Multi-target deep learning for real-time 3D multi-modality cardiac data segmentation. *Medical Image Analysis* 30: 74–86.

4

Segmentation and Quantitative Analysis of Myelinated White Matter Tissue in Pediatric Brain Magnetic Resonance Images

Chelli N. Devi[1], *Anupama Chandrasekharan*[2], *V. K. Sundararaman*[3], *and Zachariah C. Alex*[4]

[1] *Department of Biomedical Engineering, Kalasalingam Academy of Research and Education, Srivilliputhur*
[2] *Department of Radiology, Sri Ramachandra University, Chennai, India*
[3] *Independent Consultant, MR Imaging and Former Adjunct Professor, VIT University, Vellore, India*
[4] *School of Electronics Engineering, VIT University, Vellore, India*

4.1 Introduction

The pediatric brain represents the growing and maturational stage of overall brain development. The phase from birth to 2 years is very important in a child's brain growth and is characterized by an increase in brain size, volume, nerve maturation, and impulse transmission. Particularly, the stage from birth to the first 28 days is called neonatal period, while the duration from 29 days to 1 year is early infancy, and the second year of life is called late infancy. These three phases are crucial in brain development and are marked by extensive maturation of brain tissues.

The human brain comprises three major tissues: grey matter (GM), white matter (WM) and cerebrospinal fluid (CSF) (Devi et al. 2016b). Each component has a distinct functionality. The GM is composed of several elevations and grooves that play a major role in human cognition, sensory perception, and learning. WM is located in the interior of the brain and aids nerve impulse transmission. This is enabled by the myelin sheaths in the WM that speed up the conduction of nerve signals. The CSF surrounds the brain in the cranial cavity and protects the brain from injuries and shocks. Although each brain tissue has a unique physiological role in brain development, the maturation of WM (especially, its myelination) is considered clinically significant.

Myelination denotes the formation of a protective myelin sheath around the neuronal axon. This sheath has many junctions called the nodes of Ranvier that enable faster impulse transmission. In fact, this myelination is a unique aspect of

Deep Learning Applications in Medical Image Segmentation: Overview, Approaches, and Challenges, First Edition. Edited by Sajid Yousuf Bhat, Aasia Rehman, and Muhammad Abulaish.

higher animals or vertebrates that enables them to recognize and respond faster to stimuli. The characteristics of normal human myelination are as follows:

- Myelination begins in the prenatal stage of the baby (i.e. before birth). The WM of the brain is not completely myelinated at birth. It progresses during the neonatal and infancy stages and continues into the early pediatric phase (Cowan 2002). Most of the myelination is completed during the initial 2 years of the child, making its study in the pediatric brain a clinically relevant area.
- Besides, myelination progresses in a predefined and orderly fashion. To understand this, three simple neuroanatomic axioms were laid down: myelin formation proceeds from the caudal to rostral, posterior to anterior, and central to peripheral areas (Welker and Patton 2012). Nevertheless, there are a few exceptions to this general rule.
- In addition, the development of myelin is not uniform across all human beings. A certain degree of variation between babies in the myelination process is normal and expected (Knaap and Valk 2005).

Furthermore, the reduced incidence of malformation of myelin results in various disorders such as hypomyelination (indicates a lack or deficiency of myelin formation), dysmyelination (represents irregular or abnormal myelination), and retarded myelination (i.e. delayed myelin deposition) (Knaap and Valk 2005). Thus, it is imperative to closely study, monitor, and analyze myelin progress in babies.

The segmentation and analysis of myelinated WM (MWM) was initially based on manual and histological tissue analyses. However, this process is cumbersome and time-intensive. The usage of magnetic resonance imaging (MRI) enables the visualization and quantification of brain tissues in greater detail (Devi et al. 2016a; Devi et al. 2016c). Several qualitative works based on MRI are currently available for the study of MWM in the human brain. These involve a mere description of the appearance and progression of age-specific myelination (Knaap and Valk 2005; Welker and Patton 2012). The quantitative studies on myelination entail various advanced techniques such as relaxation time mapping and myelin water fraction (MWF) imaging. For instance, Deoni et al. utilized a novel multi-component driven equilibrium single pulse observation (mcDESPOT) to map myelin deposition (Deoni et al. 2011). Subsequently, they used relaxation time mapping and MWF imaging to evaluate cortical myelination in young children (Deoni et al. 2012; Deoni et al. 2015). Likewise, Chonka et al. investigated the interdependency between cortical maturation and WM myelin formation based on MWF imaging (Chonka et al. 2016). Dean et al. analyzed WM and myelin growth in male babies using MWF maps (Dean et al. 2014). In their follow-up work, the age of healthy pediatric cases was estimated with quantitative MWF maps (Dean et al. 2015) and myelin g-ratio was computed by mcDESPOT and neurite orientation dispersion and density imaging (Dean et al. 2016). Recently, Travis et al. coupled diffusion MRI and quantitative T1 relaxometry to examine premature and term-birth myelination in older children (Travis et al. 2019). Conversely, magnetization prepared rapid acquisition gradient echo (MPRAGE) technique was utilized to map relaxation and myelination rates in subjects aged between 3 months and 6 years (Kuhne et al. 2021). The latest works in the literature deploy T1/T2 mapping to quantify myelination in young infants (Filimonova et al. 2023) and early adolescents (Dipnall et al. 2023).

Despite the availability of many such quantitative studies to map ongoing myelination in the pediatric brain, they are fraught with several shortcomings:

- Primarily, these works entail additional quantitative scanning techniques other than the usual diagnostic scan employed in clinics and hospitals. This increases the time, effort, and monetary cost associated with the MRI scan. The longer time also makes it difficult to image the young babies who are usually restless and uncooperative.
- Further, the current studies often focus more on older babies, such as 3-month-olds, (Deoni et al. 2011; Deoni et al. 2012; Dean et al. 2014; Dean et al. 2015; Dean et al. 2016) 1-year olds, (Deoni et al. 2015) older infants, (Kuhne et al. 2021) 8-year-olds (Travis et al. 2019), and young adolescents (Dipnall et al. 2023). There is a paucity of work dealing with the myelination of neonates and very young infants.
- Apart from this, various myelination-related challenges make the imaging and segmentation of MWM a daunting task (Devi et al. 2014a; Devi et al. 2015). This includes the apparent myelination on Magnetic Resonance (MR) images, that is, myelination as it appears on T1 and T2 scans. A time delay is observed between the visualization of myelin tissue on T1 and T2 scans (MWM is viewed later on T2 images). Besides, the age-specific process of myelin deposition necessitates numerous atlases and training images for accurately mapping myelination throughout early childhood (Barkovich et al. 1988). Moreover, myelin formation is not an all-or-none process; the myelination of WM is a slow and gradual phenomenon that cannot be fully detected on MR images (Knaap and Valk 2005). Coupled with this, there are vast differences in the myelination progress between premature babies and full-term births.

To address the above limitations, we put forth a new and automated method for the segmentation, study, and quantitative analysis of MWM in the pediatric brain. The contributions of our work are listed below:

1) We propose a novel automated approach for brain extraction and myelin segmentation using the weighted localized Tsallis entropy thresholding technique. We also develop a unique three-dimensional (3D) model for the visualization of WM myelination.

2) Further, a quantitative "myelin index" (MI) is introduced to measure the ratio of WM that is myelinated. To our knowledge, this is the first study to objectively quantify the extent of myelination by a reproducible metric based on MWM segmentation from T1 to T2 MR images.
3) Growth model fitting is used to analyze the differences in myelination between the right and left hemispheres of the brain.
4) The myelination pattern in preterm babies is closely monitored and compared with regular-term-born babies.

This chapter is structured as follows. Section 2 presents an overview of the recent publications in myelin segmentation and analysis. While Section 3 elucidates the proposed methodology, Section 4 details the results and outcomes of the study. Section 5 discusses and compares the findings with state-of-the-art methods. Finally, Section 6 summarizes the salient aspects of this research work.

4.2 Literature Review

4.2.1 Segmentation of MWM in the Pediatric Brain

Although several techniques are available in the literature to segment the pediatric brain, (Prastawa et al. 2005; Xue et al. 2007; Weisenfeld and Warfield 2009; Melbourne et al. 2012; Gui et al. 2012; Gousias et al. 2013; Anbeek et al. 2013; Egekher et al. 2013; Makropoulos et al. 2014; Wang et al. 2015) only very few approaches detect the MWM tissue separately (Prastawa et al. 2005; Weisenfeld and Warfield 2009; Melbourne et al. 2012; Gui et al. 2012; Anbeek et al. 2013; Egekher et al. 2013). This is attributed to the various difficulties in imaging and segmenting myelin tissue along with the pertinent problems of limited dataset availability, anatomic differences in the pediatric brain, and variations caused by brain anomalies. In this section, we elaborate on the recent methods available for myelin delineation.

Initially, Prastawa et al. proposed a segmentation technique using probabilistic brain templates and graph clustering (Prastawa et al. 2005). The neonatal brain was classified into MWM, unmyelinated WM (UWM), GM, and CSF. The approach yielded an average Dice ratio of 0.61–0.77 for myelin demarcation. Likewise, Weisenfeld and Warfield postulated an algorithm for detecting the cortical and subcortical GM, MWM, UWM, and CSF based on T1 and T2 scans (Weisenfeld and Warfield 2009). The study entailed spatial atlas priors and tissue prototypes for precise delineation. The work achieved a mean Dice coefficient of 0.72 for myelin tissue.

Similarly, Melbourne et al. implemented an adaptive segmentation with manual tissue priors as atlases (Melbourne et al. 2012). The method detected eight tissues, namely, MWM, WM, deep and cortical GM, cerebellum, brainstem, CSF, and ventricles on the NeoBrainS12 database. The separate segregation of ventricles and myelin tissue is an important aspect of this approach. Conversely, Gui et al. put forward a completely atlas-free technique for pediatric brain segmentation based on morphology and tissue structure (Gui et al. 2012). Both global and tissue-specific classification was attained, that is, intracranial cavity, brainstem, cerebellum, right and left hemispheres, MWM, UWM, cortical and subcortical GM, and CSF. The algorithm was found effective in anomalous cases such as ventriculomegaly.

Anbeek et al. formulated probabilistic atlas segmentation on a large cohort of 108 newborn babies (Anbeek et al. 2013). The cortical and central GM, UWM, MWM, and CSF in ventricles and extracerebral space, brainstem, and cerebellum were identified. However, the study recorded lower accuracy values for MWM delineation with an average Dice score of 0.47. Similarly, Egekher et al. entailed multiple atlases combined with supervised classification (i.e. k-nearest neighbors and Bayes classifier) and extensive post-processing (Egekher et al. 2013). The pediatric brain was divided into the cortical GM, UWM, MWM, and basal ganglia and thalami (BGT), cerebellum, brainstem, ventricles, and CSF. Despite obtaining mean Dice ratios between 0.77 and 0.93 for the other tissues, myelin detection attains a low segmentation accuracy of 0.55.

Recently, Moeskops et al. performed an all-inclusive brain segmentation study targeting young children, early adults, and aged people (Moeskops et al. 2015). The following tissue classes were demarcated using deep learning networks: MWM, UWM, cortical GM, cerebellum, brainstem, and BGT. The salient aspect of the work is the use of single-modality images (either T1 or T2). This approach reported good performance for MWM with a Dice coefficient of 0.69 and 0.56 on babies at 30 weeks and 40 weeks, respectively. Alternatively, McAllister utilized synthetic MR scans to map the age-dependent increase in GM, WM, CSF, and MWM volumes (McAllister et al. 2017). A pediatric database with normal subjects aged between 0.1 and 21.5 years was created. The analysis revealed a rapid linear increase of MWM in the initial 18 months and a subsequent gradual rise during early childhood.

4.2.2 Qualitative and Quantitative Study of Myelination

Various methods and imaging techniques are available for both qualitative and quantitative mapping of the myelination process of the pediatric brain. The most basic of these is the anatomical MR imaging based on T1 and T2 weighted images. The myelination cycle is viewed as three different contrasts on the MRI scans (Wang et al. 2015):

- neonatal phase (birth – 28 days): inverted tissue contrast compared to adult brain, that is, hypointensity of WM on T1 scans and hyperintensity on T2 images);
- isointense stage (around 6 months): marked by poor WM – GM contrast;
- adult-like appearance (more than 1 year): hyperintensity of WM on T1 images and hypointensity on T2 scans (similar to the adult brain).

Apart from this, diffusion MRI and diffusion tensor imaging (DTI) are also utilized to assess WM connectivity and maturation. Recently, high angular resolution diffusion imaging has been employed to estimate the orientation and distribution of WM tracts and fibers (Dubois et al. 2021). Besides, many other quantitative techniques, such as magnetization transfer, susceptibility-weighted MRI, and perfusion imaging, are entailed to study WM myelination in the pediatric brain.

Particularly, Travis et al. combined diffusion MRI and quantitative relaxometry to analyze WM differences, especially in the corpus callosum (Travis et al. 2019). The corpus callosum was divided into four zones based on its location in the brain and the growth trajectory of each zone was compared between premature and full-term babies. Similarly, Grotheer et al. also integrated diffusion and quantitative MRI to validate the various developmental hypotheses of myelination in the child's brain (Grotheer et al. 2022). The results of the work revealed that myelination pattern is not uniform and increases in the inferior-superior and anterior–posterior directions.

In contrast, Kuhne et al. utilized MPRAGE and MP2RAGE sequences to evaluate myelination in brain anomalies and pathologies (Kuhne et al. 2021). Rapid myelination progress was observed in the corpus callosum, while reduced myelin deposition was found in cases of hypomyelination and dysmyelination. Thus, a reference model to gauge atypical myelination and brain abnormalities was developed. Recently, many researchers have involved T1/T2 mapping to obtain specific information on WM myelination. The major merit of this technique is the widespread availability of T1 and T2 images, coupled with their faster acquisition. Dipnall et al. carried out a detailed examination of myelination tracts from late childhood to the early adolescent stage (Dipnall et al. 2023). They also studied the myelination differences between male and female children. The research work concluded that while there was a significant change in brain microstructure and WM myelination between childhood and adolescent phases, no notable variation was found based on the subject's sex. Likewise, T1/T2 mapping was implemented in 94 neonates and infants with normal brain scans by Filimonova (Filimonova et al. 2023). The results showed an initial rapid rise in WM myelination during the early months, followed by a gradual reduction subsequently. The relationship between the baby's age and the extent of myelination was perceived to be nonlinear in this study.

4.3 Methodology

The proposed methodology is divided into four sections, namely, extraction of the brain from pediatric MRI scans along with MWM delineation, computation of MI and model fitting, study of myelination differences between the right and left brain hemispheres, and analysis of myelination in preterm born babies. The technical details of each phase are elucidated below.

4.3.1 Input Datasets

The sample consists of pediatric brain MR images of 40 babies acquired from the Department of Radiology, Sri Ramachandra University, Chennai, India. The babies were aged between 1 day and 2 years at the time of scan. Their age distribution is as follows:

- 30 babies born preterm (with gestational age between 30 and 33 weeks) and scanned at 40 weeks term-corrected age.
- 10 older babies aged 7 weeks, 9.6 weeks, 10 weeks, 2.9 months, 5.5 months, 10 months, 11 months, 16.3 months, 18.1 months, and 21.5 months.

The MR parameters used for imaging are presented below:

- Scanner: Signa HDxt MR machine with field strength 1.5 Tesla.
- T1 images: Repetition time (TR) – 500 ms, echo time (TE) – 12 ms, flip angle – 75°, voxel size – $0.3516 \times 0.3516 \times 4\,mm^3$.
- T2 images: TR – 5400 ms, TE – 117.488 ms, flip angle – 90°, voxel size – $0.3516 \times 0.3516 \times 4\,mm^3$.

4.3.2 Pediatric Brain Extraction and Myelin Segmentation

The proposed flow for brain extraction and demarcation of MWM is shown in Figure 4.1. Primarily, the acquired MR images are pre-processed and skull-stripped. Pre-processing is based on contrast-limited adaptive histogram equalization technique. Whereas, we propose a new automatic histogram valley-based thresholding approach for skull stripping. This involves obtaining the MR scan's histogram, followed by smoothing and removal of spurious peaks. The smoothed histogram houses two peaks; the lower peak corresponds to brain tissue, while

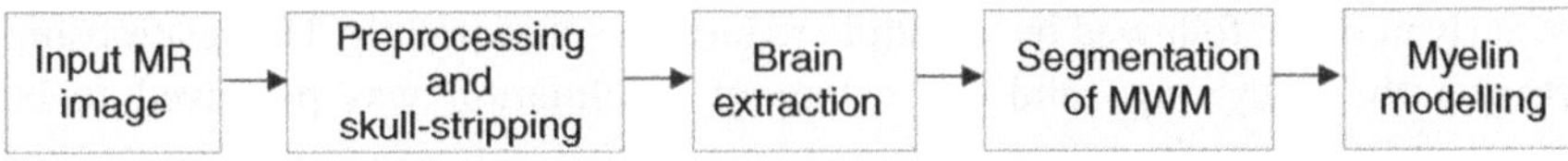

Figure 4.1 Flow chart of the proposed method.

the higher intensity peak indicates the skull. The valley between these two peaks is determined and used as intensity threshold in skull stripping.

The next stage entails brain extraction. Initially, the CSF is detected by the Chan-Vese active contour model (Chan and Vese 2001). Subsequently, the brain is identified by a series of two steps, that is, single largest component analysis and gray level co-occurrence matrix (GLCM) based approach (Devi et al. 2014b). The largest component of the brain is obtained by equation 4.1:

$$I_{\text{brain}} = C(\text{argmax}\, A(i)), \quad 1 \leq i \leq n \tag{4.1}$$

where $A(i)$ denotes the area of each component $C(i)$, $i = 1, 2 \ldots n$.

For extracting the total brain volume, the GLCM matrix is computed for each component with offset $d = 1$ and $\theta = 0^{\circ}$. Using this matrix, the textural features are derived. Of these, the inverse difference moment (IDM) is given in equation 4.2:

$$\text{IDM} = \sum_{u}\sum_{v} \frac{1}{1 + (u - v)^2} p(u, v) \tag{4.2}$$

where $p(u, v)$ is the GLCM matric element at location (u, v). IDM is a measure of the component's homogeneity in the brain image. Based on experimental investigation, a homogeneity threshold of 80% is set for total brain extraction.

Subsequently, the MWM tissue is segmented from the extracted brain. For this, a novel weighted localized Tsallis entropy thresholding technique is proposed. The traditional Tsallis entropy method entails global threshold. We introduce a patch-based local thresholding approach. The brain image is first divided into many uniform blocks of equal dimension (in increments of 5 pixels). Tsallis entropy threshold is applied to each individual block and the final output is concatenated. In addition, a majority voting mechanism is utilized for detecting MWM tissue. This ensures that spurious detections and outliers are eliminated from the result (Devi et al. 2017).

To further improve segmentation performance, especially in the peripheral areas, we incorporate a new weighting mechanism. The entropy output at each block is weighed according to its similarity with the ground truth of myelin segmentation. For this, two sets of weights are obtained. While weights $w1$ are computed from all datasets, weights $w2$ are acquired after age-based segregation of the input datasets.

The total 40 input datasets are randomly split in the ratio 75 : 25 for training and testing, respectively. The leave-one-out cross-validation is used for training

(Wang et al. 2015). Based on this cross-validation, weights $w1$ are derived as follows. For every training dataset $d_t(t = 1, 2\ldots29)$, the corresponding entropy result at each block size s is obtained as $e_{ts}(t = 1, 2\ldots29), (s = 5, 10\ldots50)$. Given that the manual reference segmentation for myelin in each dataset d_t is denoted by ref_t, the similarity value is represented by equation 4.3:

$$\text{simval}_{ts} = \frac{2\,|e_{ts} \cap \text{ref}_t|}{|e_{ts}| + |\text{ref}_t|} \tag{4.3}$$

Weights $w_1(s)$ are calculated based on these similarity values as given in equation 4.4:

$$w_1(s) = \frac{1}{29}\left(\sum_t \text{simval}_{ts}\right) \tag{4.4}$$

Thus, the final result E is computed based on the individual entropy outcomes $e_s(s = 5, 10\ldots50)$ as given in equation 4.5:

$$E = \sum_s w_1(s) * e_s \tag{4.5}$$

On the other hand, weights $w2$ are age specific. They are designed to take into account the age-based changes in myelination of WM. The input datasets are split into two groups, that is, neonates (less than 28 days) and infants (older than one month). In each group, the leave-one-out cross-validation approach is used in weight calculation as in equations 4.6 and 4.7. Therefore:

$$w2_{\text{neonate}}(s) = \frac{1}{29}\left(\sum_t \text{simval}_{ts}\right), \quad t \in \text{neonates} \tag{4.6}$$

$$E = \sum_s w2_{\text{neonate}}(s) * e_s \tag{4.7}$$

Likewise, in older infants, the weights and final MWM segmentation are given by equations 4.8 and 4.9:

$$w2_{\text{infant}}(s) = \frac{1}{9}\left(\sum_t \text{simval}_{ts}\right), \quad t \in \text{infants} \tag{4.8}$$

$$E = \sum_s w2_{\text{infant}}(s) * e_s \tag{4.9}$$

As the weights $w_2(s)$ closely match the specific age range of the input dataset, they achieve more accurate delineation of myelin in the pediatric brain.

4.3.3 Myelin Visualization, Computation of Myelin Index, and Growth Model Fitting

The segmentation of myelinated regions (elucidated in Section 3.2) yields a two-dimensional (2D) view of myelination. In addition, we acquire a 3D visualization of myelin maturation using the marching cubes algorithm (Lorensen 2020).

This 3D view offers a complete visualization of myelin development in the baby's brain from birth up to 2 years. Such a qualitative view of myelin progress also helps reinforce the neuroanatomic axioms of myelination (Welker and Patton 2012).

However, the above 3D visualization of myelination provides only a qualitative and subjective view. To attain a reliable, objective, and quantitative metric for myelin maturation, we propose a novel MI. The MI is obtained as the ratio of myelin present to the total brain. This index is age specific and increases as the baby grows from the neonatal to infancy and pediatric stages. The MI values for normal term-born babies are used in growth model fitting.

Various growth models are investigated to recognize the model that is best suited to represent the myelination of WM in children. Here, MI values are modeled as a continuous function of age (t days). It is ensured that the proposed model has biologically meaningful parameters that facilitate the interpretation of myelin progress with age. We consider the following twelve growth models that satisfy the above requirements:

- Basic models: Linear, quadratic, logarithmic, exponential, and negative exponential.
- Advanced models: Gompertz, logistic, Weibull, Richards, and three hyperbolastic models (Tabatabai et al. 2005).

Table 4.1 shows the equations for the different growth models. The parameters for these models (c_0–c_4) are adapted from Narinc (Narinc et al. 2010). Their biological significance is given below:

- c_0 – maximum MI value at 2 years
- c_1 – scale parameter (related to MI value at birth)
- c_2 – growth rate
- c_3 – shape parameter
- c_4 – parameter specific to hyperbolastic models

The growth models in Table 4.1 are fitted to the MI values. The best-suited model is obtained using Akaike information criterion (AIC) and Bayesian information criterion (BIC). Mathematically represented by equation 4.10:

$$\text{AIC} = n_d \ln \frac{\text{RSS}}{n_d} + 2n_p \tag{4.10}$$

Here, n_d represents the number of data points, RSS signifies the residual sum of squares and n_p indicates the number of estimated parameters. Nevertheless, this expression is suitable only for large datasets. When the ratio of n_d and n_p is less than 40, finite sample correction is done as in equation 4.11 (Wagenmakers and Farrell 2004):

$$\text{AIC}_{\text{corrected}} = n_d \ln \frac{\text{RSS}}{n_d} + 2n_p + \frac{2n_p(n_p + 1)}{(n_d - n_p - 1)} \tag{4.11}$$

Table 4.1 Different growth models.

Model	Equation
Linear	$\mathrm{MI}(t) = \mathrm{at} + b$
Quadratic	$\mathrm{MI}(t) = \mathrm{at}^2 + \mathrm{bt} + c$
Logarithmic	$\mathrm{MI}(t) = a \log t + b$
Exponential	$\mathrm{MI}(t) = c_1\, e^{c_2 t}$
Negative exponential	$\mathrm{MI}(t) = c_0\left(1 - e^{-c_2 t}\right)$
Gompertz	$\mathrm{MI}(t) = c_0\, e^{-c_1 e^{-c_2 t}}$
Logistic	$\mathrm{MI}(t) = \dfrac{c_0}{1 + c_1 e^{-c_2 t}}$
Weibull	$\mathrm{MI}(t) = c_0 - c_1\, e^{-c_2 t^{c_3}}$
Richards	$\mathrm{MI}(t) = \dfrac{c_0}{\left(1 + c_1 e^{-c_2 t}\right)^{1/c_3}}$
Hyperbolastic model H1	$\mathrm{MI}(t) = c_0\left(1 + c_1 e^{-c_0 c_2 t - c_4 \operatorname{arcsinh}(t)}\right)$
Hyperbolastic model H2	$\mathrm{MI}(t) = \dfrac{c_0}{\left(1 + c_1 \operatorname{arcsinh}\left(e^{-c_0 c_2 t^{c_3}}\right)\right)}$
Hyperbolastic model H3	$\mathrm{MI}(t) = c_0 - c_1 e^{-c_2 t^{c_3} - \operatorname{arcsinh}(c_4 t)}$

The corrected AIC metric is used in our work and simply denoted by AIC for convenience. In addition using equation 4.12,

$$\mathrm{BIC} = n_d \ln \frac{\mathrm{RSS}}{n_d} + n_p \ln(n_d) \tag{4.12}$$

Note that AIC and BIC have completely different frameworks with BIC housing a higher penalty term when $n_d > e^2$.

The optimal growth model is the one that achieves the lowest AIC and BIC metrics. For better analysis and interpretation of results, the Akaike and Bayesian weights are computed from the Akaike and Bayesian information criteria, respectively. For each model, the difference in AIC value is calculated as in equation 4.13:

$$\Delta_{\mathrm{AIC}_k} = \mathrm{AIC}_k - \mathrm{AIC}_{\min}, \quad k = 1, 2 \ldots 12 \tag{4.13}$$

where $\mathrm{AIC}_{\min}$ is the lowest AIC value of the twelve models. Further, the Akaike weights are represented as given in equation 4.14:

$$w_{\mathrm{AIC}_k} = \frac{e^{-0.5\Delta_{\mathrm{AIC}_k}}}{\sum_{m=1}^{12} e^{-0.5\Delta_{\mathrm{AIC}_m}}} \tag{4.14}$$

Using these weights, the evidence ratio (ER) between models M_1 and M_2 is given by equation 4.15:

$$\mathrm{ER}_{\mathrm{AIC}} = \frac{w_{\mathrm{AIC}_{\mathrm{M1}}}}{w_{\mathrm{AIC}_{\mathrm{M2}}}} \tag{4.15}$$

Thus, the model M_1 is ER times likely to be the optimal growth model compared to M_2. Likewise, the Bayesian weights and corresponding ER_{BIC} are also computed as given in equation 4.16 and 4.17:

$$w_{BIC_k} = \frac{e^{-0.5\Delta_{BIC_k}}}{\sum_{m=1}^{12} e^{-0.5\Delta_{BIC_m}}}, \quad k = 1, 2 \dots 12 \tag{4.16}$$

$$ER_{BIC} = \frac{w_{BIC_{M1}}}{w_{BIC_{M2}}} \tag{4.17}$$

Therefore, the ER is an essential metric to assess the relative likelihood of a model with respect to other models. This enables better decision-making in model selection.

4.3.4 Study of Hemispheric Differences in Myelination

The growth model fitting is expanded to evaluate potential hemispheric differences in myelination. There are several changes in the pediatric brain including developmental and maturational aspects, such as increase in brain size and cortical folding patterns. In this context, it is interesting to investigate the differences in myelination progress between the right and left hemispheres of the developing brain.

Primarily, we segment the hemispheres based on the inter-hemispheric fissure (IHF). The IHF is a deep groove that separates the right and left hemispheres. However, the IHF is not always oriented vertically to the image axis. There is a certain degree of rotational and translational offset. To identify the IHF, we propose a novel approach based on a pseudo midline (PML). For this, a horizontal projection of the extracted brain image (obtained in Section 3.2) is derived and its minimum is computed. The PML is designated as an imaginary line passing through this minimum point. This line is then rotated in small angular increments of 0.1° over the entire image. The rotated PML with zero or near-zero brain crossovers is considered the line of IHF. Using this IHF, the brain is split into its right and left hemispheres along with the myelinated regions, as shown in Figure 4.2.

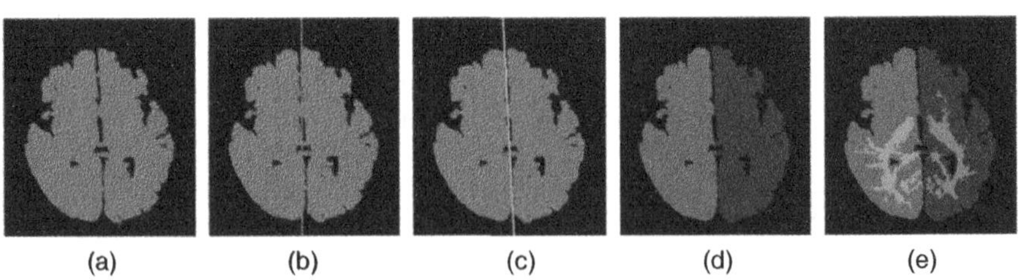

Figure 4.2 Inter-hemispheric separation: (a) extracted brain image, (b) pseudo midline superimposed on the brain, (c) inter-hemispheric fissure superimposed on the brain, (d) separated hemispheres, and (e) demarcated MWM.

After hemispheric separation, the MI values are obtained individually for the two hemispheres to study the inherent difference in myelin progress. The optimal growth model (obtained in Section 3.3) is fit in two ways:

- Simple model based on combined right and left hemispheric MI values.
- Complex model with two different curves for the right and left hemispheres.

The statistical F test is utilized to compare the above models and identify the model of best fit. The F ratio is calculated as in equation 4.18:

$$F\text{ ratio} = \frac{(SS_{\text{simple}} - SS_{\text{complex}})/(\text{dof}_{\text{simple}} - \text{dof}_{\text{complex}})}{SS_{\text{complex}}/\text{dof}_{\text{complex}}} \tag{4.18}$$

Here, SS_{simple} and SS_{complex} refer to the sum of squares values for the two models, whereas $\text{dof}_{\text{simple}}$ and $\text{dof}_{\text{complex}}$ indicate their degrees of freedom. Subsequently, the p value is derived and compared with the significance level ($\alpha = 0.05$), such that:

- If $p < \alpha$, the complex model is the best suited to describe myelination progress in the individual hemispheres of the brain.
- If $p \geq \alpha$, the simple model fits significantly better than the proposed complex model (Motulsky and Christopoulos 2003).

4.3.5 Study of Myelination in Premature Babies

As mentioned in Section 3.3, the computation of MI values and growth model fitting was done for full-term born babies. Nevertheless, there is considerable variation between the myelination patterns between premature and full-term births. This is attributed to the lower gestational time of preterm babies in the mother's womb. Usually, term-born babies have a gestational age (GA) of 37–42 weeks, whereas premature babies have a much smaller GA and are segregated as follows:

- extremely preterm (GA <28 weeks)
- very preterm (GA: 28–32 weeks)
- moderate/late preterm (GA: 32–37 weeks)

The problem with premature births is that brain development is not completed at birth owing to its reduced intrauterine period. Once born, there are several physiological changes and variations in the external environment that affect brain maturation, especially WM myelination. Thus, it is essential to study preterm myelin progress and its relation to full-term myelination.

We calculate the MI values for premature babies (MI_{preterm}). Using the optimal growth model for myelination of full-term babies (obtained in Section 3.3), the corresponding MI values for term births at equivalent age are computed ($\widehat{MI}_{\text{term}}$).

Based on these metrics, the percentage lag in myelination ($plag_{MI}$) of premature babies is given by equation 4.19:

$$plag_{MI} = \frac{\widehat{MI}_{term} - MI_{preterm}}{\widehat{MI}_{term}} * 100 \tag{4.19}$$

The advantages of the proposed $plag_{MI}$ index are as follows:

- The metric enables a quantitative assessment of the delay or retardation in preterm myelination against full-term births.
- It is useful in longitudinal studies of premature children to demarcate the age at which the myelination gap closes.
- Given that preterm myelination is affected by various prenatal and postnatal conditions, such as birth complications, congenital anomalies, and environmental aspects, it is clinically significant to closely monitor myelin progress and detect anomalies early.

4.4 Results

4.4.1 Brain Extraction, Myelin Segmentation, and 3D Visualization

The primary step in the segmentation of myelin is brain extraction. Figure 4.3 depicts the various stages involved in MWM segmentation, namely, pre-processing and skull stripping, extraction of brain and CSF, and finally segmentation of myelinated tissue. The obtained segmentation results are validated against the ground truth, that is, reference manual annotation. The major strength of our algorithm is its capacity to handle a wide age range (0–2 years) of subjects and its ability to segment without using any brain atlases or templates.

Furthermore, we perform a 3D visualization of myelin progress as shown in Figure 4.4. This is a salient aspect of myelin study as it enables a holistic overview of brain development and myelin maturation across three important pediatric phases, namely, neonatal (<28 days), early infancy (1 month to 1 year), and late infancy (1 to 2 years) stages.

4.4.2 Growth Model Fitting

The growth model that is best suited to represent myelination progress in the pediatric brain is obtained. We examined twelve growth models for this purpose: linear, quadratic, logarithmic, exponential, negative exponential, Gompertz, logistic, Weibull, Richards, and hyperbolastic models H1–H3. While Figure 4.5 portrays these models fitted to the actual MI values, their AIC and BIC metrics are tabulated in Table 4.2.

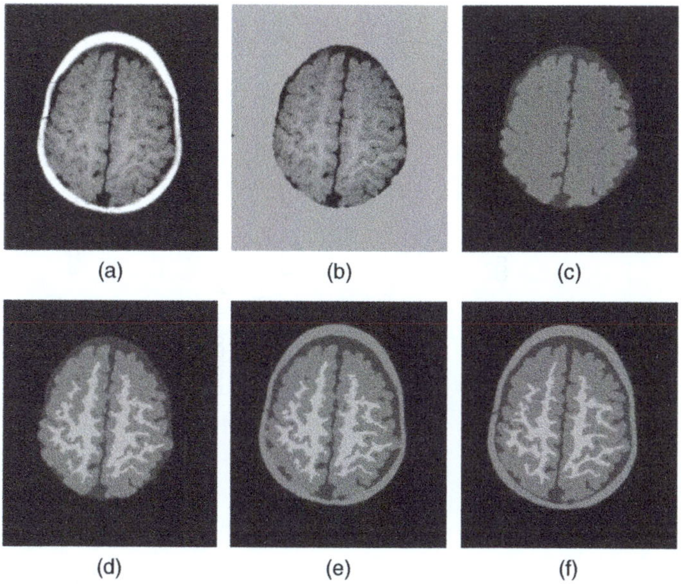

Figure 4.3 Segmentation results: (a) input T1 image, (b) pre-processed and skull-stripped image, (c) extracted brain and CSF, (d) segmented MWM, (e) final segmentation result, and (f) ground truth image (legend: pink – skull, blue – CSF, green – brain, yellow – MWM) (For colour representation, refer online version).

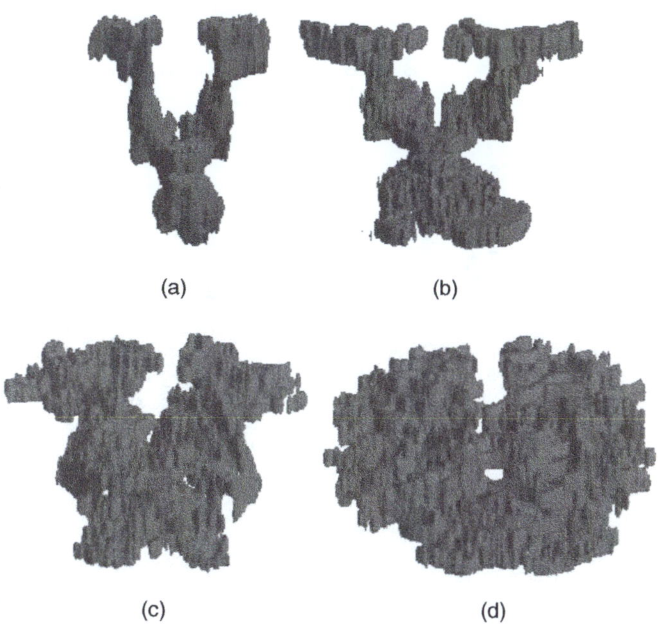

Figure 4.4 3D visualization of MWM in the pediatric brain (babies are aged: (a) 1 day, (b) 97 days, (c) 325 days, and (d) 690 days).

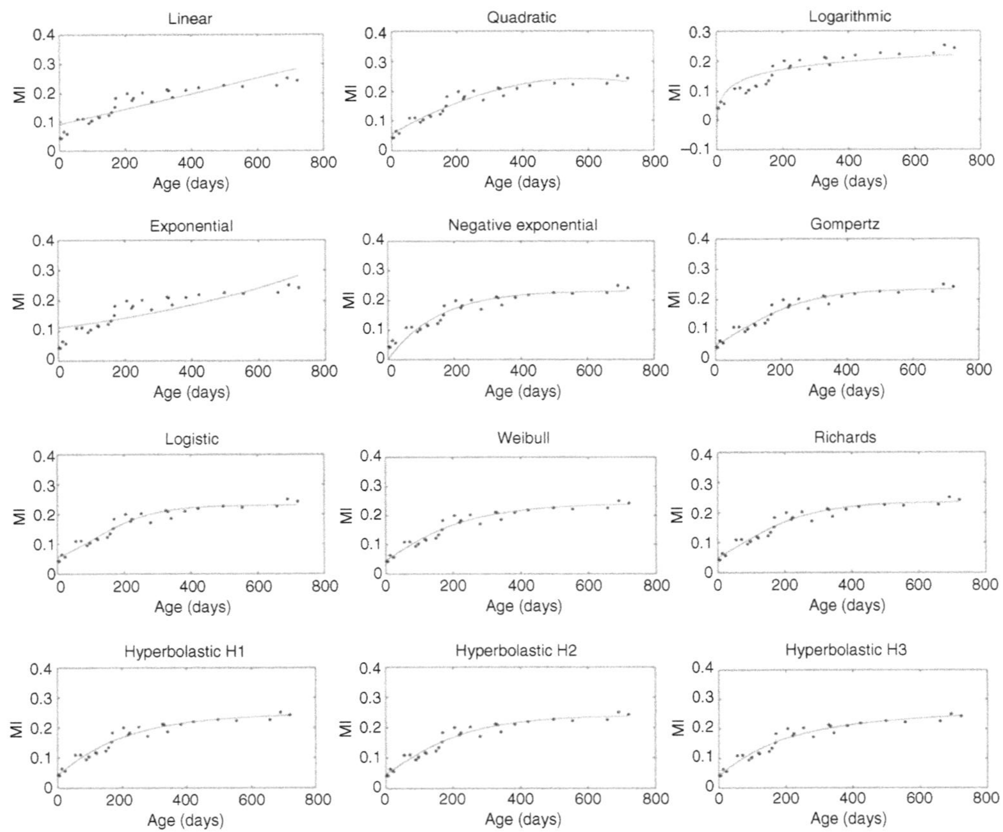

Figure 4.5 Growth models for myelination.

Table 4.2 AIC and BIC values.

Model	AIC	BIC
Linear	−206.786	−203.505
Quadratic	−239.940	−235.935
Logarithmic	−208.607	−205.327
Exponential	−194.948	−191.667
Negative exponential	−226.009	−222.729
Gompertz	**−246.204**	**−242.199**
Logistic	−244.018	−240.013
Weibull	−243.503	−238.997
Richards	−243.274	−238.768
Hyperbolastic H1	−243.190	−238.684
Hyperbolastic H2	−244.011	−239.505
Hyperbolastic H3	−239.758	−235.003

Based on Table 4.2, the Gompertz model yields the lowest value for both AIC and BIC metrics. The negative sign (i.e. AIC, BIC <0) implies lesser information loss and thus signifies a better model. The Gompertz model is given by equation 4.20:

$$\mathrm{MI}(t) = c_0\, e^{-c_1 e^{-c_2 t}} \tag{4.20}$$

Here, the estimated parameter values with a 95% confidence interval are as follows:

- $c_0 = 0.2366\ (0.2219, 0.2512)$
- $c_1 = 1.554\ (1.314, 1.793)$
- $c_2 = 0.007592\ (0.005909, 0.009275)$

Using the above values, the MI metric at full-term birth is calculated by equation 4.21:

$$\mathrm{MI}(0) = c_0\, e^{-c_1} = 0.05 \tag{4.21}$$

The clinical significance of the Gompertz model in understanding myelin progress, its role in assessing overall brain development, and the biological relevance of parameters c_0, c_1 and c_2 are discussed in Section 5.2.

Additionally, Akaike and Bayesian weights and corresponding ER values are obtained (Table 4.3). As the Gompertz model achieves the lowest AIC and BIC metrics, it is considered the optimal growth model to describe myelin progress in pediatric cases. Thus, ER values are derived based on the Gompertz model. The ER metric offers an overview of the relative likelihood of the Gompertz model. In other

Table 4.3 Akaike and Bayesian weights and ERs.

Model	Akaike weights	Akaike ER	Bayesian weights	Bayesian ER
Linear	1.12×10^{-9}	3.63×10^{8}	1.78×10^{-9}	2.53×10^{8}
Quadratic	0.0177	22.92	0.0197	22.92
Logarithmic	2.78×10^{-9}	1.46×10^{8}	4.44×10^{-9}	1.02×10^{8}
Exponential	3.01×10^{-12}	1.35×10^{11}	4.79×10^{-12}	9.39×10^{10}
Negative exponential	1.67×10^{-5}	2.43×10^{4}	2.67×10^{-5}	1.69×10^{4}
Gompertz	0.4058	1.00	0.4504	1.00
Logistic	0.1360	2.98	0.1510	2.98
Weibull	0.1051	3.86	0.0908	4.96
Richards	0.0938	4.33	0.0810	5.56
Hyperbolastic H1	0.0899	4.51	0.0777	5.80
Hyperbolastic H2	0.1355	2.99	0.1171	3.85
Hyperbolastic H3	0.0162	25.1	0.0123	36.53

words, it reflects the possibility of the Gompertz model being the optimal choice compared to other growth models. Table 4.3 reveals that the Gompertz model is 2.98 times more likely than the logistic model (the second best model for myelination) and 10 billion times more likely compared to the exponential model (the least optimal model). Likewise, the Gompertz model is a hundred million times more likely to best suit myelin development than the linear and logarithmic models.

4.4.3 Myelination in Right and Left Hemispheres

The myelin progress is assessed separately in the right and left hemispheres to identify possible variations in the normal myelination pattern. As shown in Section 4.2, Gompertz model is considered the model of best fit for whole myelination. To analyze hemispheric changes in myelination, two sub-models (namely, simple and complex models) are proposed based on the Gompertz growth model. The equations and parameters for these models are illustrated in Table 4.4. The F ratio between the models is 3.2705 and their p value 0.0280. As α is set as 0.05, $p < \alpha$ is true. We conclude that the complex model for hemispheric myelination fits significantly better. Thus, modeling the MI values separately for the two hemispheres is justified. Our results suggest significant differences between the myelination patterns in the right and left hemispheres of the pediatric brain. Specific information on the conspicuous differences in myelin progress and a comparison with the findings of other works are presented in Section 5.3.

Table 4.4 Simple and complex models for hemispheric myelination.

	Simple model	Complex model
Equation	$MI_{rl}(t) = c_{rl0}\, e^{-c_{rl1} e^{-c_{rl2} t}}$	Right hemisphere: $MI_r(t) = c_{r0}\, e^{-c_{r1} e^{-c_{r2} t}}$ Left hemisphere: $MI_l(t) = c_{l0}\, e^{-c_{l1} e^{-c_{l2} t}}$
Parameters (95% confidence interval)	c_{rl0}: 0.2367 (0.2246, 0.2488) c_{rl1}: 1.551 (1.354, 1.748) c_{rl2}: 0.007,574 (0.006,186, 0.008,963)	Right hemisphere c_{r0}: 0.2282 (0.2111, 0.2452) c_{r1}: 1.560 (1.274, 1.845) c_{r2}: 0.007,498 (0.005,513, 0.009,483) Left hemisphere c_{l0}: 0.2453 (0.2291, 0.2615) c_{l1}: 1.543 (1.287, 1.798) c_{l2}: 0.007,636 (0.005,816, 0.009,457)

4.4.4 Myelination in Premature Babies

The results reported in Sections 4.2 and 4.3 are for normal full-term myelination. However, we should closely monitor and analyze preterm myelination to record its inherent differences with myelin progress in term-born neonates and infants. We have obtained the percentage lag in myelination ($plag_{MI}$) index of premature babies compared to term births. To our knowledge, this is the first-ever quantitative metric to accurately map the delay or retardation in preterm myelination. In our study, we measure a $plag_{MI}$ value between 27.97% and 46.65% in premature children relative to their term-equivalent controls. Nevertheless, it should be noted that the above $plag_{MI}$ value holds good for the pediatric subjects considered in this work. Extension of the results to an unknown and heterogeneous population can be done only after ensuring compatibility with the study population in the following aspects: gestational age of the preterm baby at birth, presence of birth complications, brain anomalies, congenital malformations, injuries, etc. More information on premature myelination and the associated challenges are elucidated in Section 5.4.

4.5 Discussion

4.5.1 Clinical Significance of the Study of Myelination

Myelination of WM is a unique aspect of vertebral myelination that is not found in lower animals. The process of myelination happens around the neuronal axons and ensures faster conduction of nerve impulses. Another interesting feature of myelination is that the child's brain is not completely myelinated at birth. It progresses in the early pediatric stages to reach full maturity. Coupled with this, there is vast variation in myelin development between subjects. This is particularly true in anomalous cases and premature births. However, despite all these concerns, it is clinically important to study myelin progression in the pediatric brain because:

1) Myelin formation mirrors brain maturation in the child. Age-appropriate myelination indicates that the growth and development of the brain are normal.
2) Abnormal myelination in the form of less-than-normal (hypomyelination), perceived delay (retarded myelination), or abnormality (dysmyelination) points to serious underlying brain disorders that must be detected and treated early.
3) Sometimes, even normal myelination (such as preterm births) needs close monitoring to diagnose potential developmental anomalies in the future.

In this light, we have proposed a qualitative and quantitative study of myelination. The major contributions of our work are:

- The research entails only structural brain MR images (T1 and T2 scans). We do not involve functional or quantitative MRI like other recent studies (Deoni et al. 2015; Chonka et al. 2016; Dean et al. 2016; Travis et al. 2019; Kuhne et al. 2021, Filimonova et al. 2023).
- Our approach acquires both 2D image segmentation and 3D visualization of MWM across a wide age range of babies (0–2 years).
- We introduce a novel MI to quantify the amount of WM that is myelinated at any given age. To the best of our knowledge, this is the first method to quantify the extent of WM myelination based on structural MRI scans.
- Further, an optimal growth model to accurately represent myelin progress in the pediatric brain is identified. Using this model, potential differences in hemispheric myelination are analyzed.
- We also study myelin maturation in premature babies to compare their developmental milestones with normal term-born children.

4.5.2 Modeling Myelination in Neonates, Infants, and Children

We have proposed a method for automated segmentation and visualization of the MWM in the pediatric brain. The salient feature of our work is that it performs well on different age groups having varying levels of brain maturity and image contrasts. For instance, the neonatal scans have an inverted image contrast compared to the adult brain. Early infantile images (around 6 months) have an

Table 4.5 Comparison with other myelination models.

Publication	No. of models	Growth models	Optimal model	Measure of best fit
Deoni et al. (2011)	—	Not mentioned	Power curves	Minimal residual
Deoni et al. (2012)	—	Not mentioned	Logarithmic	—
Dean et al. (2014)	8	Gompertz, modified Gompertz, Bleasdale and Nelder, Richards, Stannard, hyperbolic tangent, logistic, general logistic	Modified Gompertz	BIC
Deoni et al. (2015)	3	Linear, logarithmic, quadratic	Logarithmic	BIC
Dean et al. (2016)	—	Not mentioned	Logarithmic	—
Siying Wang et al. (2019)	2	Linear, exponential	Linear in brainstem, exponential in deep brain	Coefficient of determination
Grotheer et al. (2023)	—	Not mentioned	Linear	AIC
Proposed work	12	Linear, quadratic, logarithmic, exponential, negative exponential, Gompertz, logistic, Weibull, Richards, three hyperbolastic models	Gompertz model	AIC, BIC

isointense contrast and later infantile scans (beyond 1 year) have a near adult-like appearance. Our approach accurately segments and models the myelin tissue in all three age ranges.

Moreover, our study determines a model of best fit for myelination based on the obtained MI values. We present an overview of other recent works that have modeled myelination in Table 4.5. The table shows that various publications have considered different growth models and measures of best fit. Nevertheless, there is no consensus on the optimal growth model. This may be attributed to the following reasons:

- Varied research groups have evaluated diverse growth models. Often, there is no preliminary information on how these models were chosen for comparison.

- Besides, the age range of the pediatric population is vastly different. While our method can visualize myelination even in 1-day-old babies, several approaches start with a minimum age of 3 months (Deoni et al. 2011; Deoni et al. 2012; Dean et al. 2014; Dean et al. 2016) or 1 year (Deoni et al. 2015).
- Likewise, there are widespread changes in the myelin visualization techniques employed. These techniques have varying sensitivities to myelin, particularly, at different age groups.

Therefore, we conclude that the optimal growth model obtained by work is highly specific to the samples and conditions of the study.

In our research, we evaluate twelve growth models and the Gompertz model ($MI(t) = c_0 e^{-c_1 e^{-c_2 t}}$) best describes myelin progress. The biological significance of these parameters is given below:

- c_0 depicts the MI value at 2 years ($c_0 = 0.2366$)
- c_1 identifies the scale parameter based on initial MI value ($c_1 = 1.554$)
- c_2 shows the growth rate ($c_2 = 0.007{,}592$)

The MI value at term birth (MI(0)) is calculated as 0.05. Thus, we infer from the Gompertz model that 5% of the pediatric brain is myelinated at term birth and 23.66% is myelinated by 2 years. The growth rate is approximately 0.76%.

4.5.3 Hemispheric Differences in Myelination

The potential differences in the rate and progress of myelination between the right and left hemispheres are analyzed using the simple and complex models. The complex model fits significantly better, thereby indicating the presence of hemispheric variations. The growth rate parameters ($c_{r2} = 0.007498$, $c_{l2} = 0.007636$) symbolize a myelination rate of 0.75% in the right hemisphere and 0.76% in the left hemisphere. The myelination achieved at 2 years (c_{r0} and c_{l0}) is higher for the left hemisphere compared to the right hemisphere. Therefore, we conclude that the left hemisphere myelinates rapidly relative to the right hemisphere.

A comparison with other recent publications reveals diverse results on hemispheric myelination. Some works report asymmetric myelin maturation and substantial hemispheric differences (left hemisphere myelinates faster), similar to our findings (Deoni et al. 2011). Structural asymmetries in WM pathways are also identified (Dubois et al. 2009). Whereas other studies perceive region-specific and age-specific cortical asymmetry, for example, asymmetry in the occipital lobe at 1 year and precentral/lingual gyri in later years (Deoni et al. 2015). Yet other researchers recognize no significant differences in hemispheric myelination (Deoni et al. 2012; Dean et al. 2016). Such a vast variation in the results is due to diversity in the age range of pediatric subjects, uneven sampling density, and dissimilarity in MRI techniques to study myelination between different methods.

4.5.4 Preterm Myelination

Currently, there is a paucity of works that quantify myelination progress in prematurely born babies. This can be attributed to the problems in segmenting and modeling preterm myelination such as high variability in premature brain development, lack of atlases and models for preterm births, and lack of availability of dedicated datasets. Thus, it is not practical to fit generic growth models for premature myelination, unlike term-born children. We obtain a percentage lag in the myelination index for preterm births to gauge their extent and level of myelination relative to equivalent-term babies. Our results reveal a myelination lag of 27.97–46.65%. A continuous monitoring and analysis of the lag in myelination is necessary to determine the age at which the myelination gap between premature and full-term babies closes. This will help determine the degree and duration of specialized medical care required for preterm neonates and infants.

4.6 Conclusion

The segmentation, visualization, and analysis of the myelinated regions of the pediatric brain are important from the clinical and research perspectives as they help detect normal brain maturation and growth. However, the study of MWM in pediatric subjects (including neonates, early, and late infants) is fraught with many challenges such as large variability in normal myelination, lack of uniform myelination in all areas, scarcity of specific datasets and myelin atlases, and need for additional quantitative MRI techniques. We propose a novel myelin segmentation and visualization method based only on clinical T1 and T2 MRI scans. The segmentation approach introduces a new weighted localized Tsallis entropy threshold to detect MWM. Using the myelin segmentation maps, we put forth a novel MI to quantify the extent of myelination. Furthermore, the Gompertz growth model is identified as the model of best fit to describe myelin progress in the pediatric brain based on AIC and BIC metrics. In addition, we investigate the hemispheric differences in myelination along with a close analysis of myelin development in premature babies. The results obtained show a clear demarcation in the myelination patterns of the right and left hemispheres, with the left hemisphere myelinating rapidly. Besides, we observe a 27.97–46.65% lag in the myelination of preterm children. On the whole, our study performs a qualitative and quantitative analysis of MWM that will aid clinicians to objectively identify various myelin disorders and anomalies such as hypomyelination, retarded myelination, and dysmyelination.

References

Anbeek, P., Isgum, I., Kooij, B.J.M. et al. (2013). Automatic segmentation of eight tissue classes in neonatal brain MRI. *PLoS One* 8 (12): 1–9.

Barkovich, A.J., Kjos, B.O., Jackson, D.E., and Norman, D. (1988). Normal maturation of the neonatal and infant brain: MR imaging at 1.5 T. *Radiology* 166: 173–180.

Chan, T.F. and Vese, L.A. (2001). Active contours without edges. *IEEE Transactions on Image Processing* 10 (2): 266–277.

Cowan, F.M. (2002). Magnetic resonance imaging of the normal infant brain: term to 2 years. In: *MRI of the Neonatal Brain* (ed. M.A. Rutherford). Saunders Limited.

Croteau-Chonka, E.C., Dean, D.C., Remer, J. et al. (2016). Examining the relationships between cortical maturation and white matter myelination throughout early childhood. *NeuroImage* 125: 413–421.

Dean, D.C., Muircheartaigha, J.O., Dirks, H. et al. (2014). Modeling healthy male white matter and myelin development: 3 through 60 months of age. *NeuroImage* 84: 742–752.

Dean, D.C., Muircheartaigh, J.O., Dirks, H. et al. (2015). Estimating the age of healthy infants from quantitative myelin water fraction maps. *Human Brain Mapping* 36: 1233–1244.

Dean, D.C., Muircheartaigha, J.O., Dirks, H. et al. (2016). Mapping an index of the myelin G-ratio in infants using magnetic resonance imaging. *NeuroImage* 132: 225–237.

Deoni, S.C.L., Mercure, E., Blasi, A. et al. (2011). Mapping infant brain myelination with magnetic resonance imaging. *Journal of Neuroscience* 31 (2): 784–791.

Deoni, S.C.L., Dean, D.C., Muircheartaigh, J.O. et al. (2012). Investigating white matter development in infancy and early childhood using myelin water faction and relaxation time mapping. *NeuroImage* 63: 1038–1053.

Deoni, S.C.L., Dean, D.C., Remer, J. et al. (2015). Cortical maturation and myelination in healthy toddlers and young children. *NeuroImage* 115: 147–161.

Devi C.N., Chandrasekharan A., Sundararaman V.K., and Alex Z.C. 2014a. Automatic segmentation of neonatal brain magnetic resonance images. In Proceedings of the International Conference on Communications and Signal Processing, April 2014, 640–643. IEEE.

Devi C.N., Chandrasekharan A., Sundararaman V.K., and Alex Z.C. 2014b. Segmentation of myelinated white matter in pediatric brain magnetic resonance images. In Proceedings of the International Conference on Computational Intelligence and Computing Research, December 2014, 726–729. IEEE.

Devi, C.N., Chandrasekharan, A., Sundararaman, V.K., and Alex, Z.C. (2015). Neonatal brain MRI segmentation: a review. *Computers in Biology and Medicine* 64: 163–178.

Devi C.N., Chandrasekharan A., Sundararaman V.K., and Alex Z.C. 2016a. Automatic brain segmentation in pediatric MRI without the use of atlas priors. In Proceedings of the International Conference on Wireless Communications, Signal Processing and Networking, March 2016, 1525–1528. IEEE.

Devi, C.N., Chandrasekharan, A., Sundararaman, V.K., and Alex, Z.C. (2016b). Hybrid method for brain tissue classification in magnetic resonance images of children. *Indian Journal of Science and Technology* 9 (28): 1–5.

Devi C.N., Chandrasekharan A., Sundararaman V.K., and Alex Z.C. 2016c. Automatic ventricle segmentation in brain MRI of young children. In Proceedings of the International Conference on Computational Intelligence and Computing Research, December 2016, 31–34. IEEE.

Devi, C.N., Chandrasekharan, A., Sundararaman, V.K., and Alex, Z.C. (2017). Automatic segmentation of infant brain MR images: with special reference to myelinated white matter. *Biocybernetics and Biomedical Engineering* 37: 143–158.

Dipnall, L.M., Yang, J.Y.M., Chen, J. et al. (2023). Childhood development of brain white matter myelin: a longitudinal T1w/T2w ratio study. *Brain Structure and Function* 229 (1): 151–159.

Dubois, J., Hertz-Pannier, L., Cachia, A. et al. (2009). Structural asymmetries in the infant language and sensori-motor networks. *Cerebral Cortex* 19: 414–424.

Dubois, J., Alison, M., Counsell, S.J. et al. (2021). MRI of the neonatal brain: a review of methodological challenges and neuroscientific advances. *Journal of Magnetic Resonance Imaging* 53: 1318–1343.

Egekher V.S., Benders M.J.N.L., Viergever M.A., and Isgum I. 2013. Automatic neonatal brain tissue segmentation with MRI. In Proceedings of Medical Imaging: Image Processing, 86691. SPIE.

Filimonova, E., Amelina, E., Sazonova, A. et al. (2023). Assessment of normal myelination in infants and young children using the T1w/T2w mapping technique. *Frontiers in Neuroscience* 17: 1102691.

Gousias, I.S., Hammers, A., Counsell, S.J. et al. (2013). Magnetic resonance imaging of the newborn brain: automatic segmentation of brain images into 50 anatomical regions. *PLoS One* 8 (4): 1–16.

Grotheer, M., Rosenke, M., Wu, H. et al. (2022). White matter myelination during early infancy is linked to spatial gradients and myelin content at birth. *Nature Communications* 13: 997.

Grotheera, M., Bloom, D., Kruper, J. et al. (2023). Human white matter myelination rate slows down at birth. *BioRxiv Preprint.* https://doi.org/10.1101/2023.03.02.530800.

Gui, L., Lisowski, R., Faundez, T. et al. (2012). Morphology-driven automatic segmentation of MR images of the neonatal brain. *Medical Image Analysis* 16: 1565–1579.

Knaap, M.S. and Valk, J. (2005). *Magnetic Resonance of Myelination and Myelin Disorders*. Springer-Verlag.

Kuhne, F., Neumann, W.J., Hofmann, P. et al. (2021). Assessment of myelination in infants and young children by T1 relaxation time measurements using the magnetization-prepared 2 rapid acquisition gradient echoes sequence. *Pediatric Radiology* 51: 2058–2068.

Lorensen, W.E. (2020). History of the marching cubes algorithm. *IEEE Computer Graphics and Applications* 40 (2): 8–15.

Makropoulos, A., Gousias, I.S., Ledig, C. et al. (2014). Automatic whole brain MRI segmentation of the developing neonatal brain. *IEEE Transactions on Medical Imaging* 33 (9): 1818–1831.

McAllister, A., Leach, J., West, H. et al. (2017). Quantitative synthetic MRI in children: normative intracranial tissue segmentation values during development. *American Journal of Neuroradiology* 38 (12): 2364–2372.

Melbourne A., Cardoso M.J., Kendall G.S. et al. 2012. NeoBrainS12 challenge: adaptive neonatal MRI brain segmentation with myelinated white matter class and automated extraction of ventricles I-IV. In Proceedings of MICCAI Grand Challenge: Neonatal Brain Segmentation (NeoBrainS12), 16–21. MICCAI.

Moeskops, P., Benders, M.J.N.L., Chita, S.M. et al. (2015). Automatic segmentation of MR brain images of preterm infants using supervised classification. *NeuroImage* 118: 628–641.

Motulsky, H.J. and Christopoulos, A. (2003). *Fitting Models to Biological Data using Linear and Nonlinear Regression: A Practical Guide to Curve Fitting*. GraphPad Software.

Narinc, D., Karaman, E., Firat, M.Z., and Aksoy, T. (2010). Comparison of non-linear growth models to describe the growth in Japanese quail. *Journal of Animal and Veterinary Advances* 9 (14): 1961–1966.

Prastawa, M., Gilmore, J.H., Lin, W., and Gerig, G. (2005). Automatic segmentation of MR images of the developing newborn brain. *Medical Image Analysis* 9: 457–466.

Tabatabai, M., Williams, D.K., and Bursac, Z. (2005). Hyperbolastic growth models: theory and application. *Theoretical Biology and Medical Modelling* 2 (14): 1–13.

Travis, K.E., Castro, M.R.H., Berman, S. et al. (2019). More than myelin: probing white matter differences in prematurity with quantitative T1 and diffusion MRI. *NeuroImage: Clinical* 22: 101756.

Wagenmakers, E.J. and Farrell, S. (2004). AIC model selection using Akaike weights. *Psychonomic Bulletin and Review* 11 (1): 192–196.

Wang, L., Gao, Y., Shi, F. et al. (2015). LINKS: learning-based multi-source integration framework for segmentation of infant brain images. *NeuroImage* 108: 160–172.

Wang, S., Ledig, C., Hajnal, J.V. et al. (2019). Quantitative assessment of myelination patterns in preterm neonates using T2-weighted MRI. *Scientific Reports* 9: 12938.

Weisenfeld, N.I. and Warfield, S.K. (2009). Automatic segmentation of newborn brain MRI. *NeuroImage* 47 (2): 564–572.

Welker, K.M. and Patton, A. (2012). Assessment of normal myelination with magnetic resonance imaging. *Seminars in Neurology* 32: 15–28.

Xue, H., Srinivasan, L., Jiang, S. et al. (2007). Automatic segmentation and reconstruction of the cortex from neonatal MRI. *NeuroImage* 38: 461–477.

5

Deep Learning Transformations in Medical Imaging: Advancements in Brain Tumor, Retinal Vessel, and Inner Ear Segmentation

Rejaul Karim Barbhuiya[1] *and Chayan Paul*[2]

[1]*Central Institute of Educational Technology (CIET), National Council of Educational Research and Training (NCERT), New Delhi, India*
[2]*Department of Computer Science and Engineering, Swami Vivekananda University, Barakpore, West Bengal, India*

5.1 Introduction

Image segmentation, also known as segmentation, is one of the fundamental tasks in computer vision. It is the process of separating an image into different parts or segments based on factors such as color, brightness, texture, and motion. Image segmentation is used for a variety of purposes such as medical imaging, autonomous driving vehicles, robots, processing images captured through satellites, and more. To ensure the accuracy of the segmented image, it is necessary to maintain homogeneity, which means that pixels in the same segment should share similar properties, such as intensity, color, texture, or motion. Additionally, the segments should have logical boundaries and be uniform, with smooth transitions between them. The primary objective while segmenting an image is to split it into meaningful areas and, during this process, each pixel or group of pixels is assigned a label based on their similarity to the surrounding pixels.

The fundamental concepts that underpin image segmentation are as follows:

1) Smoothness: To prevent over- or under-segmentation, the segments should exhibit smooth transitions at their boundaries.
2) Completeness: Every pixel in the image must be segmented, leaving no unassigned pixels.
3) Efficiency: In real-time applications, segmentation algorithms must be computationally efficient to handle large-scale images.

Several methods exist for image segmentation, each with its own advantages, disadvantages, and applicability in specific situations. The most commonly used methods include:

Deep Learning Applications in Medical Image Segmentation: Overview, Approaches, and Challenges, First Edition. Edited by Sajid Yousuf Bhat, Aasia Rehman, and Muhammad Abulaish.

1) Thresholding: Thresholding is a process of dividing an image based on pixel intensity values. Pixels with intensities above or below a selected threshold are allocated to distinct segments based on the threshold value.
2) Region growing: This bottom-up method divides pixels into segments based on similarity standards. If nearby pixels satisfy certain similarity requirements, they are iteratively added to the segment starting from the seed points.
3) Clustering: Algorithms for image segmentation, such as K-means or Gaussian mixture models (GMMs), group pixels based on the similarity of features, including color or texture. Each cluster represents a portion of the image.
4) Edge detection: Techniques for edge-based segmentation, such as the Canny edge detector and Sobel operator, aim to identify abrupt changes in gradient magnitude or intensity to identify object boundaries.
5) Contour-based segmentation: This method uses the edges or contours of an image to determine object boundaries, dividing the images into regions based on these outlines.
6) Deep learning methods: Deep learning has revolutionized the image segmentation industry by directly learning hierarchical representations from data. Convolutional neural networks (CNNs) are commonly used for semantic and instance segmentation tasks, with architectures such as U-Net, fully convolutional networks (FCNs), and DeepLab being frequently employed (Khan et al. 2020).

Image segmentation has numerous applications across various domains, including medical imaging for organ delineation, tumor identification, and illness diagnosis; autonomous driving for video feed recognition of items such as cars, people, and road markings; and object detection and recognition systems for identifying and locating objects within pictures or videos (Ma et al. 2024). Additionally, satellite imagery segmentation is utilized in remote sensing applications for the classification of land cover and land use, precision-agriculture, disaster response and management, monitoring of infrastructure and water resources, urban planning, and climate change. Facial recognition systems also use segmentation to identify and locate facial characteristics such as the mouth, nose, and eyes. Despite advances in image segmentation, complex scenes with overlapping or occluded objects, or with ambiguous object borders, remain a challenge. Future research directions include developing segmentation methods that can effectively handle such complex scenes.

The commonly used medical imaging techniques are computed tomography (CT), positron emission tomography (PET), and magnetic resonance imaging (MRI).

In the field of medical imaging, many techniques assist in visualizing the internal organs and aid in diagnosing various health conditions. The common techniques include:

- CT utilizes X-ray technology to produce detailed cross-sectional images of the body, which are checked by medical professionals for identification of fractures, tumors, and internal injuries.
- MRI uses magnets and radio waves to generate high-resolution images of soft tissues, organs, and joints. MRI is very useful for diagnosing medical conditions involving the brain and spinal cord, injuries of joints, and bone tumors.
- PET imaging is based on radioactive materials that help in identifying the metabolic activity in tissues. This is essential to diagnose various types of cancers as well as neurological disorders.

However, manual evaluation of a large number of images generated by these imaging techniques is time-taking and error-prone for medical practitioners such as doctors and radiologists. Therefore, there is a serious need to design a computer-based diagnosing system. The development of any computer-based mechanism for diagnosis, planning, and monitoring of diseases through image processing starts with the fundamental task of segmentation.

In medical image segmentation, the goal is to identify features or abnormalities of interest by separating an image into distinct regions or segments. This process helps with accurate diagnosis and treatment planning and allows professionals to extract quantitative data (Lei and Nandi 2022). Examples of segmentation tasks include organ delineation, tumor detection, lesion localization, and anatomical structure extraction.

Despite being extensively utilized, conventional segmentation approaches can be imprecise, labor-intensive, and frequently necessitate human involvement. The development of deep learning techniques, particularly CNNs, has revolutionized medical image segmentation, automating the process and achieving impressive results (Barbhuiya et al. 2022; Mall et al. 2023).

Deep learning algorithms, including CNNs, are useful for segmenting images because they can automatically learn the hierarchical characteristics of the input images. Initially, conventional machine learning methods such as support vector machines (SVMs) and random forests were used for feature extraction and classification in medical image segmentation tasks. However, the introduction of CNNs, particularly the U-Net architecture by Ronneberger et al. (2015), led to a significant improvement in segmentation accuracy. The U-Net architecture is based on the encoder-decoder concept along with skip links, which allows for accurate structure segmentation and localization even with limited annotated data.

Subsequent architectures, including DeepLab, fully convolutional networks (FCNs), and SegNet, have introduced modifications to address specific challenges in medical imaging, such as class imbalance, small dataset sizes, and fine-grained structure segmentation.

5.2 Classical Image Segmentation Techniques

Traditional image segmentation methods, often referred to as classical techniques, are employed to partition images into distinct sections or objects depending on specific features such as color, brightness, texture, or motion. These methods have been extensively studied and implemented in various industries, including medical imaging and industrial quality control. The list of classical image segmentation tasks includes thresholding, region growing, edge detection, clustering, and watershed (Figure 5.1). In this section, we will elaborate on the fundamental concepts and operational procedures of classical image segmentation techniques.

5.2.1 Thresholding

Thresholding is a widely used and straightforward image segmentation approach that involves selecting a threshold value and classifying image pixels based on whether their intensity values are higher or lower than the threshold. There are several thresholding methods available, including global thresholding, adaptive

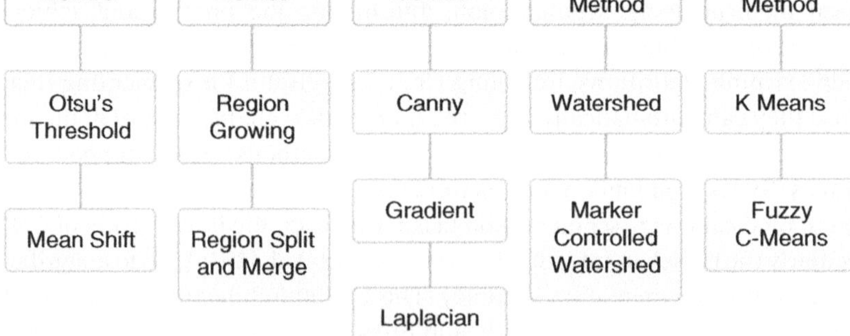

Figure 5.1 A taxonomy of classical image segmentation techniques. Source: With permission of Hmrishav Bandyopadhyay (2023).

thresholding, and Otsu's method. Global thresholding assigns a single threshold value to the entire image, while adaptive thresholding calculates threshold values locally based on the characteristics of small regions within an image. Otsu's method automatically selects an optimal threshold by maximizing the between-class variance, effectively separating foreground and background pixels. This method is useful in situations where the histogram of pixel intensities contains two or more distributions.

5.2.2 Region Growing

Region growing is a bottom-up segmentation approach that groups pixels into regions based on similarity criteria. The process typically starts with seed points that can be manually selected or automatically generated. Neighboring pixels are then iteratively added to the region if they meet predefined similarity conditions, such as having similar intensity values or gradients. Region-growing algorithms continue expanding regions until no more pixels can be added, resulting in coherent and homogeneous segments.

5.2.3 Edge Detection

Edge detection techniques focus on identifying abrupt changes or discontinuities in pixel intensity, which often correspond to object boundaries in the image. Two popular edge detection algorithms are (i) the Sobel operator which is named after Irwin Sobel, and (ii) the Canny edge detector named after John Canny. The former detects edges by calculating the gradient magnitude of an image, highlighting regions with high-intensity gradients. The latter, in contrast, is a multistage method that combines gradient computation, noise reduction, non-maximum suppression, and hysteresis thresholding to detect edges while minimizing false positives.

5.2.4 Clustering

Clustering-based segmentation methods involve grouping pixels together based on their similar features, such as color, intensity, or texture. One commonly used clustering technique is the K-means algorithm, which iteratively assigns pixels to clusters based on their proximity to the mean value of the cluster. GMMs extend the K-means algorithm by modeling the distribution of pixel intensities as a mixture of Gaussian distributions, allowing for more flexible cluster shapes.

5.2.5 Watershed Transform

The watershed transform is a morphological segmentation method inspired by hydrology, where pixel intensities are treated as elevation values and flooding is simulated from immersion points (markers) to delineate regions based on watershed basins. This technique is particularly useful for segmenting objects with distinct boundaries and has applications in medical imaging, remote sensing, and industrial inspection.

Classical image segmentation techniques also present numerous challenges, such as over-segmentation and under-segmentation, which can occur in images with complex backgrounds or uneven lighting conditions. In addition, classical segmentation algorithms often involve manual tuning of parameters, which is often time-taking and may be prone to human error, leading to suboptimal results. Moreover, classical techniques may find it difficult to segment images with a lot of noise or artifacts, resulting in inaccurate segmentation results. Finally, some classical segmentation algorithms may not scale well to large images or datasets, limiting their applicability in real-world scenarios.

5.3 Deep Learning-Based Image Segmentation Methods for Medical Images

In recent years, deep learning techniques such as CNNs have revolutionized the area of image segmentation, particularly in the context of medical imaging. The architecture of CNNs is well suited for learning hierarchical representations of visual data, making them particularly effective for tasks such as medical image segmentation. In medical image segmentation, CNNs are used to automatically extract and learn key features from raw image data without requiring a manual or handcrafted feature extraction. They can effectively capture complex patterns and spatial relationships in medical images, allowing for more accurate segmentation of anatomical structures, lesions, and abnormalities. Several CNN architectures have been developed or adapted specifically for medical image segmentation tasks (Kayalibay et al. 2017; Malhotra et al. 2022). One popular architecture is U-Net, which has a symmetric expanding path for accurate localization and a contracting path for recording context (Ronneberger et al. 2015; Siddique et al. 2021). U-Net has been widely used in biomedical image segmentation because of its capability to generate high-quality segmentation masks.

Another common approach is the use of FCNs, which uses convolutional layers in place of fully connected layers (Dai et al. 2016). This allows FCNs to process images of arbitrary sizes and produce dense pixel-wise predictions. FCNs have been effectively used in medical imaging segmentation tasks, allowing for precise delineation of anomalies and structures from a variety of imaging modalities. Deep learning techniques that are used for medical image segmentation also often incorporate advanced techniques such as attention mechanisms, conditional random fields (CRFs), and multi-scale architectures to improve segmentation accuracy and robustness (Guo et al. 2020).

Despite all these advantages of deep learning methods, there are still several challenges to be addressed while applying them for medical image segmentation. These include the requirement of large annotated datasets, high-end computational resources such as graphics processing unit (GPU), and the interpretability of results. But the recent progress in deep learning-based approaches and the availability of large-scale medical imaging datasets provide hope for further improving the accuracy and applicability of DL-based segmentation methods in processing medical images (Bhattacharya et al. 2021).

Deep learning methods, particularly CNNs and their variants, have brought significant advancement to the field of medical image segmentation by allowing for automated and accurate delineation of structures and abnormalities from medical images. These methods have the potential to revolutionize medical diagnostics, treatment planning, and patient care by providing valuable insights from imaging data to clinicians.

The following section presents elaborate discussions on some deep learning algorithms in the area of medical image segmentation.

5.3.1 Convolutional Neural Network (CNN)

O'Shea and Nash (2015), proposed CNNs, a benchmark algorithm in the domain of image classification. CNNs are specifically designed to handle structured grid-like data, such as images (Khan et al. 2020). A CNN architecture typically consists of alternate layers of convolution and pooling, and one or more fully connected layers at the end. Sometimes, a global average pooling is used in place of a fully connected layer (Khan et al. 2020). CNNs are frequently used for tasks such as object identification, image classification, and segmentation. They have had a significant impact on the field of computer vision. The simplified architecture of CNN is given in Figure 5.2.

5.3.1.1 Convolutional Layer

A core component of CNNs is the convolutional layer, where a set of special filters called convolutional kernels are applied to the input image as shown in Figure 5.3. These kernels slide over the image, computing the dot product between its weights and the values in the receptive field. This way, it checks every small part of the image to see how much it matches the pattern the kernel is looking for (Khan et al. 2020). If the kernel is symmetrical, the operation becomes a correlation operation. This convolutional kernel divides the image into small receptive fields, starts extraction of feature motifs, and convolves with the image using specific weights to capture relevant information.

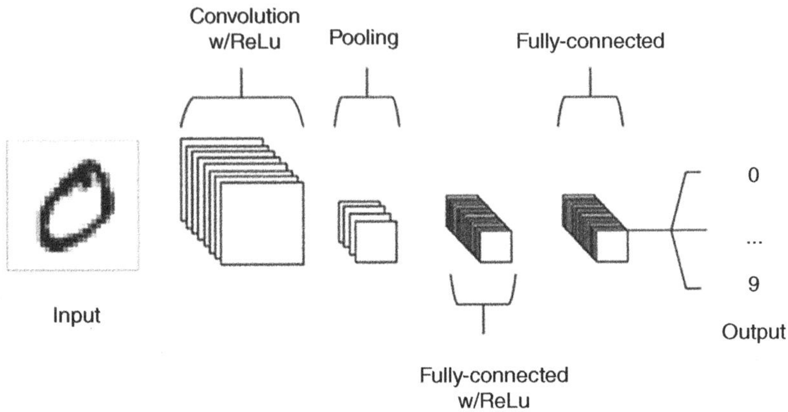

Figure 5.2 A CNN architecture having five layers. Source: O'Shea and Nash (2015)/with permission of Keiron O'Shea.

5.3.1.2 Activation Function

After the convolution operation, an activation function such as Rectified Linear Unit (ReLU), is applied to each element. The activation function brings nonlinearity into the neural network, enabling CNNs to learn complex and non-linear relationships among input features. Apart from ReLU, there are many other activation functions such as sigmoid, tanh, maxout, SWISH, and variants of ReLU – such as leaky ReLU, ELU, and PReLU – that are used to introduce nonlinearity (Gu et al. 2018). This step is important as it helps the model learn complex patterns and features from the data.

5.3.1.3 Pooling Layers

Pooling layers are commonly inserted between successive convolutional layers to reduce the spatial dimensions of the feature maps while retaining important information. Common pooling operations include max pooling and average pooling, which downsample the feature maps by taking the maximum or average value within each pooling window.

5.3.1.4 Fully Connected Layers

In the final stages of the network, one or more fully connected layers are typically added to perform high-level reasoning and decision-making. These layers connect every neuron in one layer to every neuron in the next layer, allowing the network to learn intricate relationships between features extracted by the convolutional layers.

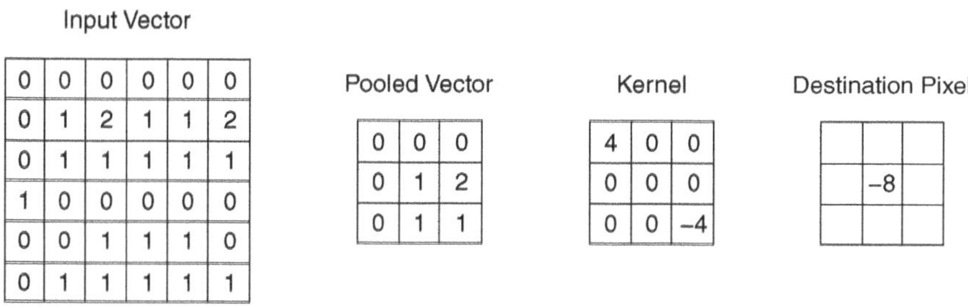

Figure 5.3 A visual representation of a convolutional layer. Source: O'Shea and Nash (2015)/with permission of Keiron O'Shea.

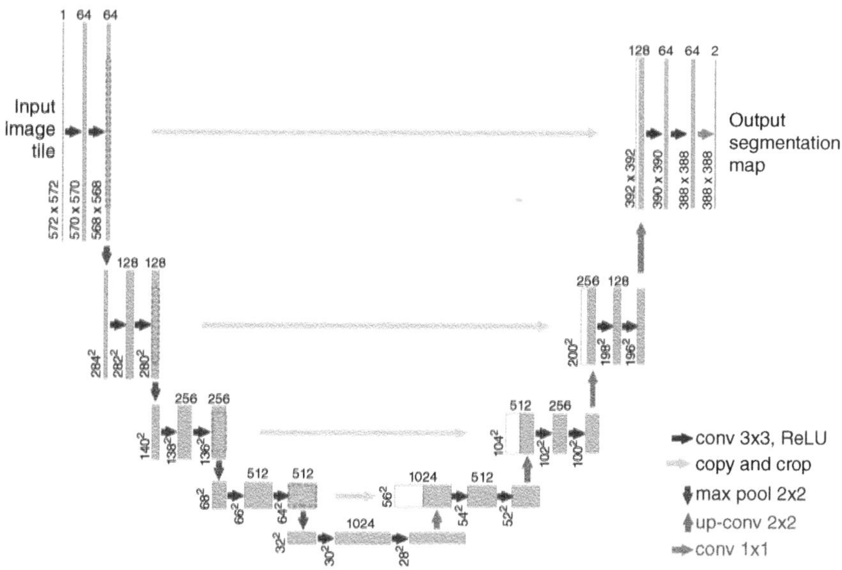

Figure 5.4 U-Net architecture. Source: Ronneberger et al. (2015)/Springer Nature.

5.3.1.5 Softmax Activation

For classification tasks, the output layer of the CNN often utilizes a softmax activation function, which normalizes the output scores across classes into a probability distribution. This enables the network to output probabilities indicating the likelihood of each class.

5.3.1.6 Loss Function and Optimization

During the training phase, the neural network is optimized to minimize a loss function, which assesses the discrepancy between the predicted outputs and the ground truth labels. Commonly used loss functions for classification tasks include

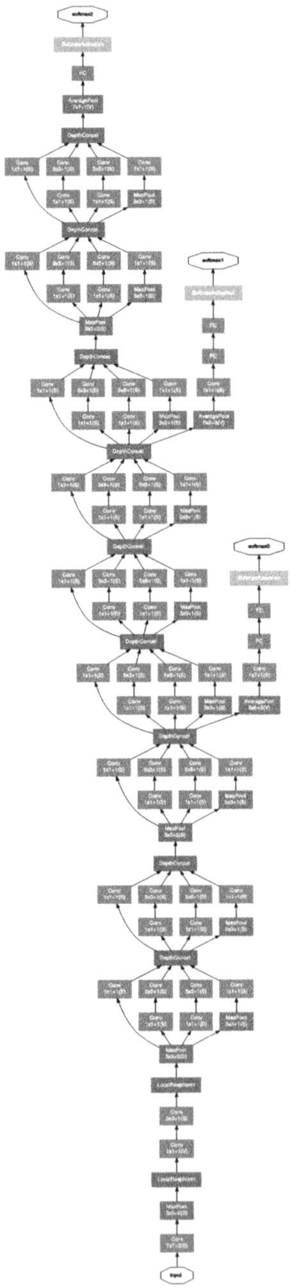

Figure 5.5 GoogleNet with all its bells and whistles. Source: Szegedy et al. (2015)/with permission of IEEE.

cross-entropy loss. To minimize the loss function, optimization algorithms such as stochastic gradient descent (SGD) or its variants are employed.

5.3.1.7 Backpropagation

The computation of gradients with respect to the network parameters is performed using backpropagation, which efficiently propagates errors backward through the network. These gradients are then utilized to update the weights of the network through the chosen optimization algorithm.

CNNs achieve state-of-the-art performance on various computer vision tasks by learning hierarchical representations of input data through the repeated application of convolution, activation, pooling, and fully connected layers. This process enables CNNs to capture increasingly complex features and patterns, allowing them to excel in tasks such as image classification, object detection, and semantic segmentation.

As the domain of deep learning is continuously evolving, the classical version of CNN has gone through a number of modifications and upgrades. Some of the variations widely used in medical image segmentation are AlexNet (Chen et al. 2021b; Priya and Vasudevan 2024).

5.3.2 U-Net

U-Net is a CNN architecture developed by Ronneberger et al. (2015) as depicted in figure 5.4. It is a widely used architecture for biomedical image segmentation and semantic segmentation tasks. U-Net is based on the FCN.

U-Net has an encoder–decoder network architecture in the shape of a U. It has four encoder and decoder blocks joined by a bridge. The encoder and decoder networks' information flow is completed by the bridge. At every block, the encoder network doubles feature channels and cuts spatial dimensions in half, functioning as a feature extractor by activating convolutional layers before ReLU. The skip connections improve gradient flow and conserve information for improved semantic features, and the max-pooling lowers computing costs. By upscaling and concatenating skip connection feature maps, the decoder network creates segmentation masks. Convolutions and sigmoid activation are then used for pixel-wise classification. The researcher found U-Net. U-Net found a wide range of applications in the domain of brain tumor detection. Akter et al. proposed a deep CNN and U-Net for image classification and segmentation of brain tumor images and they could achieve accuracy of 90.8% (Akter et al. 2024). Cheng et al. proposed a deep network incorporating VGG-19 network in the coding stage of U-Net for edge detection in brain tumor images. They also added an edge detection module to enhance the performance of the proposed model. The experimental result shows that the proposed model could achieve promising results across different standard datasets (Cheng et al.).

In the field of ever-evolving deep learning techniques, U-Net has gained wide acceptance in the domain of medical image segmentation.

5.3.3 GoogleNet or Inception

GoogleNet, also known as Inception-v1, marks a significant development in the evolution of CNN architectures, particularly in the realm of image classification as shown in figure 5.5. Introduced by researchers at Google in 2014, GoogleNet revolutionized deep learning by offering an efficient and scalable solution for processing large-scale image datasets.

At the core of GoogleNet lies the groundbreaking concept of the Inception module, which fundamentally altered the way CNNs process information. Unlike traditional convolutional layers that utilize fixed-size filters, Inception modules incorporate multiple parallel convolutional branches with varying filter sizes. This configuration empowers the network to capture features at different spatial scales concurrently, heightening its capacity to identify intricate patterns and objects within images.

A key design principle underpinning GoogleNet is its commitment to computational efficiency without compromising performance. To achieve this, GoogleNet incorporates dimensionality reduction techniques, such as 1×1 convolutions, prior to applying larger convolutions. By diminishing the number of input channels, these convolutions alleviate the computational burden while preserving informative content.

Furthermore, GoogleNet adopts a novel architectural structure that fosters both depth and width in the network. Instead of merely stacking layers upon layers, the architecture features multiple levels of abstraction, with deeper layers capturing more abstract and elevated features. This hierarchical representation empowers the network to discern increasingly intricate patterns, resulting in enhanced classification accuracy.

Another noteworthy aspect of GoogleNet is its utilization of global average pooling instead of conventional fully connected layers at the conclusion of the network. Global average pooling computes the average value of each feature map, significantly reducing the number of parameters in the network and mitigating the risk of overfitting. This refined solution not only simplifies the model but also fortifies its generalization capability.

GoogleNet has emerged as a trailblazer in the domain of deep learning, providing an exemplary instance of innovative architectural design in CNNs. Its exceptional performance on standard benchmark datasets has positioned it as a leading model in the field, and its broad range of applications across various domains makes it invaluable in healthcare, autonomous vehicles, security, and e-commerce. GoogleNet has made significant strides in optimizing computational resources, organizing feature representation hierarchically, and implementing auxiliary supervision methods. These innovations have positioned it as a fundamental building block in the creation of advanced neural network architectures not only for image classification but also for other applications.

5.4 Deep Learning Algorithms Employed in the Segmentation of Brain Tumor Images

Brain tumor segmentation refers to a process in medical image processing where algorithms are applied to delineate and identify regions of interest (tumor tissues) within brain images, typically acquired through techniques such as MRI or CT. Segmentation involves partitioning the brain image into multiple regions or classes, such as tumor tissue, healthy tissue, edema, and necrosis. This is important for various medical applications, including diagnosis, treatment planning, and monitoring of brain tumors. The rising popularity of machine learning and deep learning methods, notably CNNs, for brain tumor segmentation stems from their capacity to grasp intricate patterns from extensive datasets and their adeptness in processing high-dimensional medical images. These algorithms are trained on annotated datasets containing manually outlined tumor regions by experts. Subsequently, they can autonomously segment tumors in previously unseen images.

Deepak and Ameer (2019) presented a deep transfer learning approach for classifying glioma, meningioma, and pituitary tumors from brain MRI images, achieving a mean classification accuracy of 98% and outperforming existing methods. Transfer learning proves effective even with limited medical image data, with insights into misclassifications provided for further analysis. Cheng et al. (2015) proposed a method for improving brain tumor classification in T1-weighted contrast-enhanced MRI images by augmenting the tumor region and splitting it into ring-form subregions. This approach significantly enhanced classification accuracy compared to traditional methods, demonstrating its feasibility and effectiveness for computer-aided diagnosis. Cheng et al. (2016) introduced a novel content-based image retrieval (CBIR) for classifying brain tumors in T1-weighted contrast-enhanced MRI images, achieving a mean average precision of 94.68% by augmenting tumor regions, employing adaptive spatial division for feature extraction, and applying Fisher kernel framework for similarity measurement. The new system outperformed related state-of-the-art methods, showcasing its effectiveness in supporting clinical decisions through image retrieval in the medical field. Pereira et al. (2016) proposed an automatic brain tumor segmentation method using CNNs with small kernels and intensity normalization, achieving top performance in the BRATS 2013 Challenge and second place in the BRATS 2015 Challenge. The method demonstrated effectiveness in accurately segmenting brain tumors from MRI images, offering the potential for improved treatment planning and clinical practice. Biratu et al. (2021) provided a comprehensive survey of recent advancements in brain tumor segmentation and classification methods, including region growth, shallow machine learning, and deep learning techniques. They compared their strengths, weaknesses, technical aspects, and performance metrics to offer insights into the current state-of-the-art in this field. Cheng et al. (2023) introduced EAV-U-Net, a novel system for accurately detecting brain tumor lesion regions by incorporating a VGG-19 network structure, attention mechanism module, and edge detection module into the U-Net architecture. EAV-U-Net significantly improves segmentation performance, particularly in cases with hazy tumor margins, achieving impressive results across multiple performance metrics on various standard datasets. Priya and Vasudevan (2024) introduced a hybrid model combining AlexNet and GRU neural networks for brain tumor classification using MRI data, achieving high accuracy, precision, recall rate, and F1-Score, showcasing the potential for improved patient outcomes and healthcare environment in brain tumor detection. The model demonstrated effectiveness in distinguishing between different types of brain tumors, contributing to early detection and characterization of malignancies.

5.5 Deep Learning Models for Retinal Vessel Segmentation

Retinal vessel segmentation, integral in medical image analysis within ophthalmology, involves identifying blood vessels in retinal images for diagnosing conditions such as diabetic retinopathy. Accurate segmentation aids in disease detection and progression tracking, and facilitates the development of computer-aided diagnosis systems, playing a pivotal role in managing ocular pathologies.

Jiang et al. (2018) presented a supervised method utilizing pretrained fully convolutional networks and transfer learning for accurate retinal blood vessel segmentation, achieving state-of-the-art accuracy across multiple databases. Additional unsupervised post-processing techniques are applied to refine segmentation results, showcasing the effectiveness of transfer learning in medical imaging applications. Zhao et al. (2020) introduced a retinal vessel segmentation technique employing generative adversarial learning with an extensive receptive field. This approach attained remarkable segmentation accuracy rates, surpassing current leading methods. By effectively capturing both intricate small blood vessels and broad, high-level semantic vessel features, the proposed algorithm showcases promise in aiding the diagnosis of ophthalmological conditions. Guo et al. (2020) introduced a Dense U-Net architecture using inception modules for retinal vessel segmentation, incorporating generative adversarial networks (GANs) in training for improved performance. Evaluation of the DRIVE dataset demonstrates high segmentation accuracy with a Dice rate of 82.15% and AU-ROC and AU-PR values of 0.9772 and 0.9058, respectively, indicating effectiveness in automated retinal vessel segmentation. Atli and Gedik (2021) proposed Sine-Net, a novel deep learning architecture for retinal blood vessel segmentation, achieving high accuracy and robustness. Experimental validation on three publicly available databases (STARE, CHASE_DB1, and DRIVE) shows Sine-Net outperforms existing methods in certain metrics, demonstrating its potential for clinical applications. Chen et al. (2021a) proposed a comprehensive review of deep learning-based retinal blood vessel segmentation, emphasizing its importance in diagnosing diseases such as diabetes and hypertension to prevent blindness. It surveyed recent publications, identified trends in network architectures, outlined challenges, and suggested future research directions to advance and enhance models in this domain. Gegundez-Arias et al. (2021) introduced a deep learning-based method for retinal blood vessel segmentation using a simplified U-Net architecture with novel loss function and batch normalization, achieving robust and accurate results across diverse fundus image datasets. Evaluation against manual segmentations in DRIVE, STARE, and CHASE_Db1 databases demonstrates superior performance compared to existing methods, suggesting its potential for integration into clinical tools for vascular structure segmentation. Liu et al. (2022) introduced an improved U-Net algorithm for retinal vessel segmentation, employing global convolutional networks, attention modules, and multi-scale feature extraction to accurately delineate vessel boundaries. Evaluation of DRIVE and CHASE_DB1 datasets demonstrates superior accuracy, outperforming existing algorithms with an average performance enhancement. Abbasi et al. (2023) have created LMBiS-Net, a lightweight pixel-level CNN with a very small number of learnable parameters (only 0.172 M), for the purpose of segmenting retinal capillaries. In order to facilitate information flow between the encoder and the decoder, the network includes bidirectional skip links in addition to multipath feature extraction blocks. Ilesanmi et al. (2023) presented a systematic review of CNN algorithms for retinal fundus image segmentation and classification, highlighting their potential to aid early detection and treatment of eye problems. Analysis of 62 studies reveals CNNs' effectiveness in enhancing segmentation precision and reducing reliance on human expertise, with consistently high accuracies observed despite some limitations.

5.6 Deep Learning Models for Inner Ear Segmentation

Inner ear segmentation involves recognizing and outlining the anatomical elements within the inner ear from medical imaging data, such as MRI or CT scans. The inner ear, a multifaceted structure responsible for both hearing and balance, comprises interconnected components such as the cochlea, vestibule, and semicircular canals.

Segmentation is essential for understanding the morphology and spatial relationships of these structures, aiding in the diagnosis and treatment of inner ear disorders and pathologies. Accurate segmentation allows clinicians to quantify and analyze the volume, shape, and abnormalities of inner ear structures, which can inform treatment decisions, surgical planning, and disease monitoring.

Expert manual segmentation is both time-intensive and subjective, resulting in inconsistencies between different observers. Therefore, automated segmentation methods, particularly those based on deep learning algorithms, have gained traction for their ability to efficiently and accurately delineate inner ear structures from medical imaging data. These automated methods streamline the segmentation process, reduce human error, and enable consistent and reproducible results across different patients and imaging modalities.

Wang et al. (2019) proposed the challenge of metal artifact reduction in post-implantation CT images for accurate segmentation of intra-cochlear anatomy (ICA) crucial for cochlear implant programming. They introduced a 3D conditional GAN-based approach, demonstrating significant improvement over prior 2D methods by synthesizing preoperative images, enhancing segmentation accuracy without requiring pre-implantation CT scans. Jeevakala et al.(2020) proposed a Mask R-CNN approach driven with U-Net for the detection and segmentation of inner auditory canal and its nerves. On experimenting with the clinical dataset of over 50 different patients of different age groups, they found the model outperforms the state-of-the-art models. Zeng et al. (2021) proposed an ensemble deep learning method for the effective and precise identification of a range of ear diseases utilizing otoscope images, attaining an impressive average accuracy of 95.59% across eight distinct disease categories. The real-time classifier showcased its potential in clinical settings, offering promise for early detection and treatment of ear diseases, particularly in the absence of expert diagnosis. A 3-D U-Net was trained by Vaidyanathan et al. (2021) utilizing 944 MRI scans that had the inner ears manually segmented as reference standards. The model was found to perform equivalent to human experts. The result of the research work also suggests the model was efficient, consistent, and reliable for inner ear segmentation. Atebani proposed a model where a single, dual-headed volumetric 3D U-Net was implemented in a completely automated workflow, trained using manually labeled internal datasets from clinical practice (N = 43) and cadaveric specimens (N = 43), and subsequently evaluated. The robustness of the model was further scrutinized through the use of three independent open-source datasets (N = 23+7+17), which comprised scans from cadaveric specimens.

5.7 Conclusion

In this chapter, an in-depth examination of the profound effects of deep learning techniques on the medical imaging domain was conducted, with a specific focus on advancements in brain tumor, retinal vessel, and inner ear segmentation. The investigation has revealed a paradigm shift in medical image processing, driven by the exceptional capabilities of deep learning algorithms. The advent of deep learning techniques, notably CNNs, has revolutionized the domain of medical imaging, allowing for the automated and accurate segmentation of anatomical structures and pathological irregularities.

Within the domain of brain tumor segmentation, deep learning models have reached unparalleled levels of precision and efficacy, enabling timely detection, accurate delineation of tumor borders, and tailored strategies for treatment planning. These advancements hold the promise of enhancing patient outcomes through prompt interventions and tailored therapeutic approaches. Similarly, in retinal vessel segmentation, deep learning algorithms have demonstrated remarkable effectiveness in extracting vascular structures from fundus images with high accuracy. By enabling quantitative analysis of retinal vasculature, these models contribute to the early detection and monitoring of various ocular pathologies, including diabetic retinopathy and hypertensive retinopathy.

The utilization of deep learning in inner ear segmentation has opened up novel pathways for comprehending the intricate anatomy of both the auditory and vestibular systems. Precise delineation of inner ear structures from medical imaging techniques such as MRI and CT scans has enhanced diagnostic precision in conditions impacting hearing and balance. This advancement allows for tailored treatments and surgical interventions. Despite these advancements, challenges remain, including the need for large annotated datasets, model interpretability, and robustness to diverse imaging conditions. Addressing these challenges will require multidisciplinary collaboration between computer scientists, clinicians, and imaging experts to refine existing algorithms and develop novel methodologies. Looking ahead, the integration of deep learning transformations into routine clinical practice holds immense potential for revolutionizing healthcare delivery. By streamlining image analysis workflows, improving diagnostic accuracy, and facilitating personalized treatment strategies, deep learning in medical imaging stands poised to enhance patient care and outcomes across diverse medical specialties. As we continue to push the boundaries of innovation, it is essential to prioritize ethical considerations, ensure algorithmic transparency, and promote equitable access to cutting-edge technologies for the benefit of patients worldwide.

References

Abbasi, M.M., Iqbal, S., Naveed, A. et al. (2023). LMBiS-Net: A lightweight multipath bidirectional skip connection based CNN for retinal blood vessel segmentation. *ArXiv (Cornell University) arXiv preprint arXiv:2309.04968*.

Akter, A., Nosheen, N., Ahmed, S. et al. (2024). Robust clinical applicable CNN and U-Net based algorithm for MRI classification and segmentation for brain tumor. *Expert Systems with Applications* 238 (122347): 122347. https://doi.org/10.1016/j.eswa.2023.122347.

Atli, I. and Gedik, O.S. (2021). Sine-Net: A fully convolutional deep learning architecture for retinal blood vessel segmentation. *Engineering Science and Technology, an International Journal* 24 (2): 271–283.

Bandyopadhyay, H. (2023). An introduction to image segmentation: Deep learning vs. Traditional [+examples].(Accessed on 24 April 2023) V7. https://www.v7labs.com/blog/image-segmentation-guide

Barbhuiya, R.K., Ahmad, N., and Akram, W. (2022). Application of convolutional neural networks in cancer diagnosis. In: *Computational Intelligence in Oncology: Applications in Diagnosis, Prognosis and Therapeutics of Cancers*, 95–109. Singapore, Springer Singapore.

Bhattacharya, S., Maddikunta, P.K.R., Pham, Q.V. et al. (2021). Deep learning and medical image processing for coronavirus (COVID-19) pandemic: A survey. *Sustainable Cities and Society* 65: 102589.

Biratu, E.S., Schwenker, F., Ayano, Y.M., and Debelee, T.G. (2021). A survey of brain tumor segmentation and classification algorithms. *Journal of Imaging* 7 (9): 179.

Chen, C., Chuah, J.H., Ali, R., and Wang, Y. (2021a). Retinal vessel segmentation using deep learning: a review. *IEEE Access* 9: 111985–112004.

Chen, J., Wan, Z., Zhang, J. et al. (2021b). Medical image segmentation and reconstruction of prostate tumor based on 3D AlexNet. *Computer Methods and Programs in Biomedicine* 200 (105878): 105878. https://doi.org/10.1016/j.cmpb.2020.105878.

Cheng, D., Gao, X., Mao, Y. et al. (2023). Brain tumor feature extraction and edge enhancement algorithm based on U-Net network. *Heliyon* 9 (11): e22536. https://doi.org/10.1016/j.heliyon.2023.e22536.

Dai, J., Li, Y., He, K., and Sun, J. (2016). R-fcn: Object detection via region-based fully convolutional networks. *Advances in neural information processing systems* 29.

Deepak, S. and Ameer, P.M. (2019). Brain tumor classification using deep CNN features via transfer learning. *Computers in Biology and Medicine* 111: 103345.

Gu, J., Wang, Z., Kuen, J. et al. (2018). Recent advances in convolutional neural networks. *Pattern Recognition* 77: 354–377. https://doi.org/10.1016/j.patcog.2017.10.013.

Gegundez-Arias, M.E., Marin-Santos, D., Perez-Borrero, I., and Vasallo-Vazquez, M.J. (2021). A new deep learning method for blood vessel segmentation in retinal images based on convolutional kernels and modified U-Net model. *Computer Methods and Programs in Biomedicine* 205: 106081.

Guo, X., Chen, C., Lu, Y. et al. (2020). Retinal vessel segmentation combined with generative adversarial networks and dense U-Net. *IEEE Access* 8: 194551–194560.

Ilesanmi, A.E., Ilesanmi, T., and Gbotoso, A.G. (2023). A systematic review of retinal fundus image segmentation and classification methods using convolutional neural networks. *Healthcare Analytics* 4: 100261.

Cheng, J., Huang, W., Cao, S. et al. (2015). Enhanced performance of brain tumor classification via tumor region augmentation and partition. *PloS one* 10 (10): e0140381.

Cheng, J., Yang, W., Huang, M. et al. (2016). Retrieval of brain tumors by adaptive spatial pooling and fisher vector representation. *PloS one* 11 (6): e0157112.

Jeevakala, S., Sreelakshmi, C., Ram, K. et al. (2020). Artificial intelligence in detection and segmentation of internal auditory canal and its nerves using deep learning techniques. *International Journal of Computer Assisted Radiology and Surgery* 15: 1859–1867.

Jiang, Z., Zhang, H., Wang, Y., and Ko, S.B. (2018). Retinal blood vessel segmentation using fully convolutional network with transfer learning. *Computerized Medical Imaging and Graphics* 68: 1–15.

Kayalibay, B., Jensen, G., and van der Smagt, P. (2017). CNN-based segmentation of medical imaging data. *ArXiv (Cornell University). arXiv preprint arXiv:1701.03056.*

Khan, A., Sohail, A., Zahoora, U., and Qureshi, A.S. (2020). A survey of the recent architectures of deep convolutional neural networks. *Artificial intelligence review* 53: 5455–5516.

Lei, T. and Nandi, A.K. (2022). *Image Segmentation: Principles, Techniques, and Applications*. John Wiley & Sons.

Liu, C., Gu, P., and Xiao, Z. (2022). Multiscale U-Net with spatial positional attention for retinal vessel segmentation. *Journal of Healthcare Engineering* .

Ma, J., He, Y., Li, F. et al. (2024). Segment anything in medical images. Nature. *Communications* 15 (1): https://doi.org/10.1038/s41467-024-44824-z.

Malhotra, P., Gupta, S., Koundal, D. et al. (2022). Deep neural networks for medical image segmentation. *Journal of Healthcare Engineering.*

Mall, P.K., Singh, P.K., Srivastav, S. et al. (2023). A comprehensive review of deep neural networks for medical image processing: Recent developments and future opportunities. *Healthcare Analytics* 4 (100216): 100216. https://doi.org/10.1016/j.health.2023.100216.

O'Shea, K. and Nash, R. (2015). An Introduction to Convolutional Neural Networks. *ArXiv (Cornell University).* https://doi.org/10.48550/ARXIV.1511.08458.

Pereira, S., Pinto, A., Alves, V., and Silva, C.A. (2016). Brain tumor segmentation using convolutional neural networks in MRI images. *IEEE Transactions on Medical Imaging* 35 (5): 1240–1251.

Priya, A. and Vasudevan, V. (2024). Brain tumor classification and detection via hybrid alexnet-gru based on deep learning. *Biomedical Signal Processing and Control* 89 (105716): 105716. https://doi.org/10.1016/j.bspc.2023.105716.

Ronneberger, O., Fischer, P., and Brox, T. (2015). U-Net: Convolutional Networks for Biomedical Image Segmentation. *ArXiv (Cornell University).* https://doi.org/10.48550/ARXIV.1505.04597.

Siddique, N., Paheding, S., Elkin, C.P., and Devabhaktuni, V. (2021). U-net and its variants for medical image segmentation: A review of theory and applications. *IEEE Access* 9: 82031–82057.

Szegedy, C., Liu, W., Jia, Y., Sermanet, P., Reed, S., Anguelov, D., and Rabinovich, A. (2015). Going deeper with convolutions. *Proceedings of the IEEE conference on computer vision and pattern recognition* (pp. 1–9).

Vaidyanathan, A., van der Lubbe, M.F., Leijenaar, R.T. et al. (2021). Deep learning for the fully automated segmentation of the inner ear on MRI. *Scientific Reports* 11 (1): 2885.

Wang, J., Noble, J.H., and Dawant, B.M. (2019). Metal artifact reduction for the segmentation of the intra cochlear anatomy in CT images of the ear with 3D-conditional GANs. *Medical Image Analysis* 58: 101553.

Zeng, X., Jiang, Z., Luo, W. et al. (2021). Efficient and accurate identification of ear diseases using an ensemble deep learning model. *Scientific Reports* 11 (1): 10839.

Zhao, H., Qiu, X., Lu, W. et al. (2020). High-quality retinal vessel segmentation using generative adversarial network with a large receptive field. *International Journal of Imaging Systems and Technology* 30 (3): 828–842.

6

Deep Learning-Based Image Segmentation for Early Detection of Diabetic Retinopathy and Other Retinal Disorders

Ankur Biswas[1] *and Rita Banik*[2]

[1] *Department of Computer Science & Engineering, Tripura Institute of Technology, Narsingarh, West Tripura, India*
[2] *Department of Electrical Engineering, ICFAI University Tripura, Kamalghat, West Tripura, India*

6.1 Introduction

Diabetic retinopathy (DR) and associated retinal illnesses pose important worldwide health issues, impacting millions of people and resulting in profound vision impairment if not treated (Aziz et al. 2021). The retina is a light-sensitive tissue located in the back of the eye that is essential for vision. However, over time, several medical disorders might harm the fragile retina, which could endanger vision. DR is a prevalent retinal condition that is particularly prevalent in the diabetic population. Elevated blood sugar levels linked to the condition may lead to gradual alterations in the retina by harming small blood vessels. DR can progress to the point of blindness if left untreated. (Aziz et al. 2021) In addition to diabetes, there are a number of additional retinal disorders that can arise and affect vision. Diabetes-related high blood sugar levels can lead to the blockage, enlargement, or leakage of fluid or blood from small blood vessels in the retina. An individual is more likely to acquire diabetes the longer they have the disease. Depending on the extent of retinal damage, DR can go through many phases. Microaneurysms, or tiny vascular bulges, appear in the early stages. As the disease advances, more severe retinal abnormalities such as hemorrhages, cotton-wool patches, and hard exudates appear. The most advanced form of retinopathy is proliferative retinopathy, in which new fragile blood vessels sprout on the retina or optic disc. These aberrant blood vessels can cause blindness by leaking blood or scarring the retina. Another vision-threatening consequence of proliferative retinopathy is retinal detachment, which occurs when the retina rips away from the back of the eye. Retinal detachment unrelated to diabetes, retinitis pigmentosa, age-related macular degeneration, and retinal artery occlusion are

Deep Learning Applications in Medical Image Segmentation: Overview, Approaches, and Challenges, First Edition. Edited by Sajid Yousuf Bhat, Aasia Rehman, and Muhammad Abulaish.

additional retinal illnesses. The macula, which is the center portion of the retina that provides clear, forward-looking vision, is harmed by age-related macular degeneration. It is the primary cause of blindness in the elderly. A retinal blood artery blockage, known as a retinal vascular occlusion, can result in loss or distortion of vision. A set of hereditary conditions, known as retinal pigmentosa, causes the retina's cells to gradually degrade and eventually disappear over time, resulting in tunnel vision and eventually blindness. The retina may peel away from the layer of support tissue behind it, a condition known as retinal detachment that frequently needs surgery to treat.

To identify retinal diseases early on and prevent irreversible vision loss, routine eye exams are essential. For those who have risk factors such as diabetes, high blood pressure, or a family history of eye illness, screenings are especially crucial. Many retinal problems can be treated early to help avoid additional vision loss and relieve discomfort (Wang et al. 2019). Therefore, early detection and precise diagnosis are crucial for the successful management and avoidance of irreversible visual impairment. Conventional approaches to diagnosing retinal problems are usually complicated, based on personal assessment, and susceptible to human fallibility. In order to overcome these constraints, there is a rising inclination toward investigating alternative sophisticated methods of image segmentation to enhance the early detection process. With the development of computer vision technology, scientists are investigating how to use fundus images and eye scans to identify different retinal illnesses using deep learning (DL). DL-based image segmentation has emerged as a viable approach to address these problems (Torre et al. 2020; Vij and Arora 2022). Artificial neural networks, which can be trained on enormous datasets, are used in DL to identify intricate patterns in images. Automating the segmentation procedure enables precise and efficient identification of retinal abnormalities (Mateen et al. 2020). This suggests that creating automated screening technologies might assist increase access to eye care. A common method involves training convolutional neural networks (CNNs) trained using extensive datasets of retinal images that have been manually rated and categorized by specialists. In order to differentiate scans that show no symptoms of diabetic retinopathy, age-related macular degeneration, glaucoma, or other disorders, the CNNs directly learn characteristics from pixel data (Alyoubi et al. 2020). Certain networks have proven to have accuracy levels similar to those of professional graders. DL has potential to identify individuals who require thorough eye exams by screening vast populations. It could assist in alleviating the global scarcity of resources for eye care by automating preliminary picture analysis (Sarki et al. 2020). Before the models can be used autonomously without human supervision, however, they still need to undergo thorough validation. To increase confidence in these algorithms' decisions, future research will also try to make them more explainable or easier to understand.

This chapter aims to explore the potential of DL-based image segmentation techniques in the early detection of DR and other retinal disorders. Through an extensive review of existing literature, (Li et al. 2019a; Yin et al. 2020) we will examine the current state of the field, and identify key challenges in this field. In this chapter, we also seek to contribute to the growing body of knowledge on this subject and provide insights that can guide future research and therapeutic practice. By utilizing the power of DL-based picture segmentation, we can improve the quality of care and outcomes for those affected by retinal illnesses (Playout et al. 2019). The initial section of this paper will furnish an overview of the frequency and consequences of DR and other retinal illnesses, emphasizing the significance of early detection and precisely diagnosing these conditions. We will explore the limitations of standard diagnostic techniques and the need for more efficient and accurate approaches. The second section will go into DL techniques for image segmentation, with a focus on CNNs. We will study the architecture and training procedures of CNNs, as well as the utilization of transfer learning and pretrained models in retinal image segmentation. Additionally, we will examine additional DL algorithms such as generative adversarial networks (GANs) (Jeong et al. 2022) and recurrent neural networks (RNNs) (Bonassi et al. 2022) and their potential applications in this sector. The third section will illustrate the uses and benefits of DL-based picture segmentation in the identification of DR and other retinal illnesses. We will describe how image segmentation can aid in recognizing early indicators of DR and how it can increase the accuracy and efficiency of diagnosis. Furthermore, we will study the potential for DL approaches to assist in the diagnosis and classification of various retinal abnormalities, as well as their function in quantitative analysis and disease progression monitoring. The fourth section will explore the issues and limits involved with DL-based image segmentation. These include the availability and quality of datasets, model interpretability and explainability, computational complexity and resource requirements, as well as ethical considerations (Shen et al. 2020). We will examine the need for standardized datasets, developments in model interpretability, optimization of computational resources, and the establishment of ethical frameworks for responsible application. Finally, the fifth section will recommend future possibilities for research, emphasizing the need for large-scale annotated datasets, breakthroughs in model interpretability, optimization of computational resources, and ethical considerations. We will close with a call to researchers and healthcare professionals for continuous collaboration and innovation in the field of DL-based picture segmentation for the early identification of DR and other retinal illnesses.

6.2 Deep Learning and Image Segmentation

DL methods, especially CNNs, have revolutionized image analysis in different disciplines. Image segmentation, a fundamental stage in medical image analysis, involves splitting a picture into different regions of interest. DL models trained on big datasets have exhibited outstanding performance in segmenting retinal pictures, enabling precise identification of aberrant characteristics associated with DR and other retinal disorders. While DL-based image segmentation shows considerable promise, numerous problems limit its wider use in clinical practice. Limited availability of labeled data, model interpretability, computational complexity, and potential ethical problems are among the primary barriers that need to be solved. Collaborative efforts between researchers, clinicians, and data scientists are important to overcome these issues and enable the responsible deployment of DL algorithms in healthcare settings. In medical image analysis, image segmentation is essential, especially when it comes to retinal problems. DL has completely changed the area of image segmentation by automatically learning and extracting complicated characteristics from images. CNNs, transfer learning, and other cutting-edge methods will be the main topics of discussion as we examine the numerous DL strategies used for image segmentation in this part.

6.2.1 Convolutional Neural Networks Architecture

Neural networks with convolutional architecture have been the mainstay of DL methods for image segmentation. CNNs are able to extract hierarchical characteristics from images because of their architecture, which is modeled after the visual cortex of the human brain. Convolutional, pooling, and fully linked layers are among the layers that make up these networks. In order to capture spatial relationships, CNNs use the power of convolutional layers to perform local calculations on image patches. Multiple convolutional layers with nonlinear activation functions are used to enable CNNs to extract ever-more-abstract and sophisticated features from the input pictures. The feature maps are then down-sampled using pooling layers, which keep the most noticeable characteristics while decreasing the spatial dimensions. Ultimately, the image is classified and segmented using fully linked layers in accordance with the learned characteristics. In a study, the authors presented an alternate solution using a hybrid technique for detecting DR based on retinal fundus pictures. (Hemanth et al. 2020) In particular, the hybrid technique is built on integrating both image processing and DL to improve the results.

6.2.2 Pretrained Models and Transfer Learning

Transfer learning is a method that uses models that are already trained to accomplish image segmentation tasks in another domain. CNNs that have been pretrained for broad image recognition tasks using extensive datasets, such as ImageNet, are known as pretrained models. Researchers may greatly minimize the training time and computer resources needed for certain segmentation tasks by beginning with these pretrained models. Through the use of a smaller labeled dataset unique to the retinal images, the weights of the network are adjusted via transfer learning to conform the pretrained model to the target segmentation task. By using this method, the model is able to learn properties unique to the retina and enhance its segmentation capabilities. Transfer learning lets researchers make use of the expertise and feature extraction skills of models trained on big datasets, which is especially helpful when labeled retinal datasets are hard to access. A study introduced CNN model for DR classification and compared it to different variations of pretrained DL models for initial DR recognition using binary and multi-class classification. (Biswas and Banik 2023) The achieved result of 97% accuracy demonstrates that the pretrained ResNet model is more effective in diagnosing DR.

6.2.3 Other Deep Learning Techniques

Other DL neural network architectures have also been the widely used techniques investigated for image segmentation in the context of retinal illnesses. A few CNN architecture employs a dilated convolutional filter to obtain a bigger receptive field, resulting in almost human-level accuracy in segmenting retinal blood vessels (Biswas et al. 2020). This also makes it take only a few iterations to train the network. U-Net architecture, which is intended especially for biomedical image segmentation, is another such method (Guo et al. 2021). The U-Net design is made up of an expanding route that allows for the exact localization of segmented areas and a contracting path that gathers context and geographical information. Because U-Net can handle little training data and generate reliable segmentations, it has been frequently employed in retinal image segmentation applications. Thus, U-shape-based techniques are among the most effective structures in the medical sector. However, the encoder's repeated downsampling processes result in the loss of spatial information, which is critical for medical picture segmentation. In research, the author proposed a unique lightweight end-to-end feature refinement network to overcome this issue. (Wang et al. 2021a) The network uses an encoder–decoder network as its backbone, with two extra routes, the spatial refinement path and the semantic refinement path, applied to the encoder and decoder, respectively, to increase the model's detailed representation and discriminative capacity. In addition, a feature adaptive fusion block (FAF block) is presented that successfully integrates features with varying depth. The proposed network can be taught end to end.

Additionally, RNNs and GANs have shown potential in retinal picture segmentation. A generator network and a discriminator network make up a GAN. The generator network learns to produce realistically segmented pictures, while the discriminator network learns to distinguish between created and actual images. The segmentation accuracy is increased using this adversarial training method, which also yields visually pleasing results. RNNs, on the other hand, work well with sequential data, such as volumetric pictures or image sequences. RNNs are able to provide more precise segmentation results by making use of the temporal dependencies present in the sequence. RNNs may be used in retinal imaging to segment pictures taken with multiple modalities or perspectives, or to follow the course of a disease over time. These cutting-edge DL methods provide viable paths for raising the precision and effectiveness of picture segmentation in retinal diseases. Researchers can reliably segment areas of interest and extract significant information from retinal pictures by using CNNs, transfer learning, U-Net architecture, GANs, and RNNs. Therefore, the area of image segmentation for retinal illnesses has undergone a revolution based on DL methods, especially CNNs. GANs, RNNs, U-Net architecture, transfer learning, and GANs all improve the efficiency and accuracy of segmentation. These methods show a lot of potential for enhancing the early identification and detection of retinal illnesses, increasing patient outcomes, and directing individualized therapy regimens. DL-based image segmentation is an area that will improve and lead to more effective healthcare treatments with further study and innovation.

6.3 Applications and Benefits of Deep Learning-Based Image Segmentation

Image segmentation using DL has many uses in many different fields. It helps in diagnosis and therapy planning in medical imaging by providing precise tumor delineation, organ, and anatomical structure identification. By segmenting objects of interest, it allows robots to see and interact with their surroundings in the field of robotics. DL-based picture segmentation is a significant tool in computer vision applications because of its advantages, which include increased accuracy, less subjectivity and human effort, and the potential for real-time analysis. In eye analysis, DL-based segmentation can be used for the following tasks.

6.3.1 Detection of Diabetic Retinopathy

As one of the primary causes of blindness in the world, DR must be detected early in order to effectively intervene. Techniques for segmenting images based on DL provide significant benefits in spotting early indicators of diabetic retinopathy. (Ting et al. 2019) DL algorithms are capable of precisely identifying anomalies linked to DR by segmenting retinal pictures into discrete areas, such as blood vessels, exudates, and microaneurysms. The publicly accessible Kaggle dataset of retina pictures is widely used to train the model. An ensemble of five deep CNN models (Resnet50, Inceptionv3, Xception, Dense121, and Dense169) are used to encode the rich information and enhance categorization for various phases of DR on Kaggle datasets. (Qummar et al. 2019) Through the isolation and analysis of certain areas of interest, image segmentation is essential in the identification of diabetic retinopathy. From a vast collection of retinal pictures, DL algorithms can pick up on minute patterns and characteristics that human viewers would overlook, allowing them to recognize tiny indicators of retinopathy. This increases diagnostic efficiency and accuracy, enabling prompt intervention and preventative steps to lower the risk of additional vision loss.

6.3.2 Determination of Additional Retinal Conditions

DL-based image segmentation methods have potential for diagnosing and categorizing a range of retinal conditions in addition to diabetic retinopathy. Utilizing the capabilities of CNNs and other cutting-edge methods, scientists are able to train models to precisely identify and categorize anomalies such as glaucoma, age-related macular degeneration, and retinal vascular occlusions. There are several advantages to being able to identify and categorize various retinal illnesses with DL-based picture segmentation. First of all, it makes early diagnosis possible, which permits quick treatment and may lead to better patient outcomes. Furthermore, it enables customized therapy strategies by offering comprehensive details on the unique traits and gravity of the retinal ailment. Better condition management and more focused therapies may result from this tailored strategy. However, the segmentation of retinal structures is critical for determining DR and other retinal diseases (Li et al. 2019b). The process of detecting and distinguishing distinct areas or structures within retinal pictures is known as segmentation. The following are the main structures for segmentation in the context of DR and other retinal conditions.

6.3.2.1 Optic Disc

The place on the retina where the optic nerve leaves the eye is called the optic disc, or optic nerve head. It is a region that resembles a circle or oval and is crucial for the transfer of visual data from the retina to the brain. Analyzing the optic disc's appearance is essential for detecting disorders such as glaucoma since abnormalities in it can be a sign of a number of other eye problems.

6.3.2.2 Microaneurysm

These are tiny, localized outpouchings or bulges in the walls of the retina's tiny blood vessels (Atli and Gedik 2021). They are frequently linked to the disease known as DR, which affects people who have diabetes. The early diagnosis and treatment of DR depend on the detection of microaneurysms in retinal imaging.

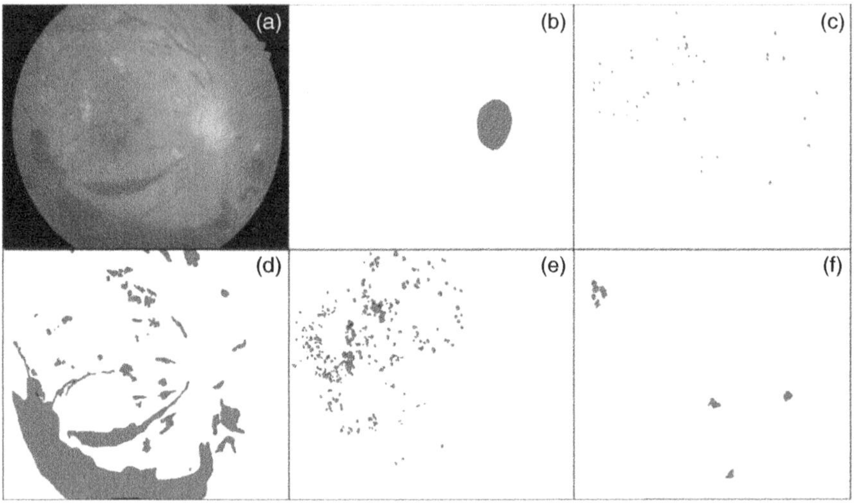

Figure 6.1 (a) Original image of eye, (b) optic disc, (c) microaneurysm, (d) hemorrhage, (e) hard exudates, and (f) soft exudates.

6.3.2.3 Hemorrhage

Blood leaking from blood vessels is referred to as hemorrhage. Hemorrhages may show up as abnormally red patches on retinal imaging because of blood. Conditions such as hypertensive retinopathy and DR are prone to hemorrhages. Hemorrhage patterns, sizes, and locations can all give important information for diagnosing and tracking these disorders.

6.3.2.4 Hard Exudates

Hard exudates are yellow or white deposits that form in the retina as a result of lipid leaking from injured blood vessels. They are frequently linked to disorders such as diabetic macular edema. Hard exudates in retinal imaging must be identified and monitored in order to determine the severity of retinopathy and guide treatment options (Wang et al. 2020).

6.3.2.5 Soft Exudates (Cotton-Wool Spots)

Soft exudates, commonly known as cotton-wool spots, are white or greyish lesions in the retina produced by inflammatory material buildup. They are frequently linked to disorders such as hypertensive retinopathy and diabetic retinopathy. Soft exudate detection is critical for determining the amount of retinal injury and directing suitable therapies. Figure 6.1 presents the segmentation of the main structures in the context of detecting DR and other retinal conditions.

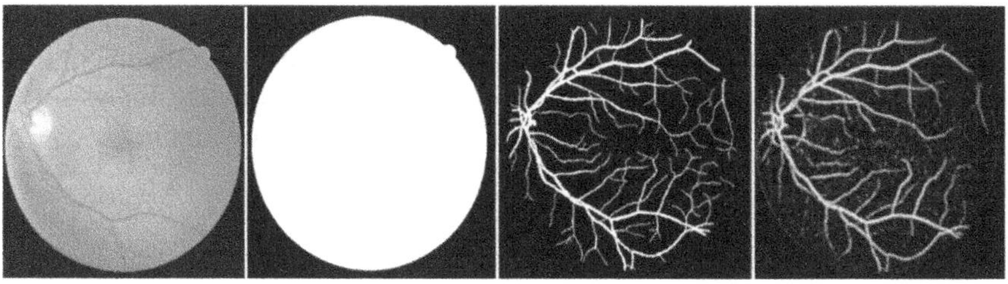

Figure 6.2 (a) Original image, (b) mask image, (c) ground truth, and (d) final segmentation result.

6.3.2.6 Retinal Vessel

Retinal vessel segmentation is a critical step in the processing of retinal pictures, and it is a valuable tool in ophthalmology for a variety of diagnostic and therapeutic applications (Ooi et al. 2021). This segmentation is crucial for the early diagnosis and monitoring of disorders such as diabetic retinopathy, glaucoma, and hypertensive retinopathy, in which changes in vascular shape give critical insights into disease development. Furthermore, retinal vessel segmentation assists in treatment planning, particularly for laser therapies, and provides a better knowledge of vascular anomalies associated with illnesses including age-related macular degeneration and retinopathy of prematurity. Its relevance extends to assisting research initiatives, clinical trials, and the creation of automated screening programs, therefore improving diagnostic efficiency and consistency. Furthermore, the incorporation of retinal vascular segmentation into telemedicine and artificial intelligence technologies has the potential to improve remote diagnostics and personalized healthcare methods, eventually enhancing patient outcomes in the field of ophthalmic care. Figure 6.2 presents the comparison of different images used for segmentation of retinal vessel.

6.3.3 Monitoring the Progression of the Disease and Quantitative Analysis

Techniques for segmenting images based on DL are also essential for quantitative analysis and tracking the course of illness. These methods allow automated measurements of retinal properties such as macular thickness, vascular caliber, and optic disc size by segmenting retinal pictures. These measures may provide insightful information about how a disease progresses and how it responds to therapy. There are several benefits of being able to use DL-based segmentation for quantitative analysis of retinal characteristics. First of all, it lessens the need for labor-intensive and prone to human mistakes' manual measurements. Second, it makes it possible to trace the course of an illness over time, giving medical practitioners the information, they need to assess the effectiveness of a treatment plan and choose the best course of action. In the end, this quantitative analysis may help provide patients with more individualized and focused treatment.

6.3.4 Healthcare Professionals' Assistive Tool

Healthcare practitioners may use DL-based image segmentation as a diagnostic aid for ocular problems. These strategies boost diagnostic efficiency and strengthen the skills of healthcare providers by offering dependable and precise retinal picture segmentation. In the past, ophthalmologists' skill and their subjective interpretation of retinal pictures were used to diagnose retinal abnormalities. By producing standardized and objective segmentation findings, DL-based picture segmentation reduces subjectivity. Afterward, medical experts may concentrate on examining the divided areas and using the quantitative data to guide their clinical judgments. Furthermore, by automating the segmentation process and saving time and resources, DL-based segmentation might improve the efficiency of healthcare professionals' workflow. This makes diagnosis more effective and frees up medical staff members to focus their knowledge and efforts on other vital aspects of patient care.

Thus, there are several uses and advantages for DL-based image segmentation methods in the area of retinal illnesses. These methods provide enhanced precision and efficacy in diagnosis, ranging from the early identification of DR to the detection of diverse retinal disorders. They also make it possible to do quantitative analysis, track the development of diseases, and provide healthcare providers with useful support tools. The capabilities of DL-based image segmentation will be improved, and further research and development in this field will help improve patient outcomes in the treatment of retinal illnesses. The commonly used datasets are IDRiD, DRIVE, STARE, HRF, FGADR, DDR, e-opthaEX, and e-opthaMA while performance metrics are accuracy, sensitivity, IoU, Dice coefficient, pixel-wise accuracy, precision, recall, etc. A comparison of DL-based image segmentation model for detection DR and other eye diseases (Deshmukh et al. 2023; Wang et al. 2021b; Suardika et al. 2022; Karmakar et al. 2022) is shown in Table 6.1.

6.4 Challenges and Limitations

There are a number of difficulties and restrictions with DL-based image segmentation. The requirement for vast quantities of labeled training data, which may

Table 6.1 Comparison of DL models.

Model	Architecture	Advantages	Limitations	Metrics	Metrics score
U-Net	Convolutional	High accuracy, handles complex structures	Requires large amounts of labeled data	Precision Accuracy	89.48 92.60 to 95.70
FCN	Fully convolutional	Efficient, real-time processing	Limited ability to handle object boundaries	Precision	84.30
FRNet	Convolutional	Lightweight end-to-end feature refinement network	Loss of spatial information, difficulty in handling blurred boundaries	Accuracy	0.968
DeepLab	Dilated convolutional	Captures fine details, handles large images	Computationally intensive.	Precision	95.79
Mask R-CNN	Regional convolutional	Combined object detection and segmentation	Higher computational complexity	Intersection over Union	0.843
RetinaMask	Feature pyramid network	High accuracy, handles class imbalance, real-time processing	Limited object boundary precision, sensitivity to parameter tuning	AUC	0.950 to 0.981
PSPNet	Pyramid pooling modules	Multi-scale contextual information, accurate object boundary delineation	Computationally intensive, sensitivity to hyperparameters	Precision	88.27

be expensive and time consuming to acquire, is one of the main obstacles. Furthermore, the implementation of DL models on devices with limited resources is restricted due to their high computing demands. The possibility of overfitting, in which the model performs well on training data but is unable to generalize to new, unseen pictures, is another drawback.

6.4.1 Dataset Quality and Availability

The scarcity of extensively annotated datasets for training poses a significant obstacle to the successful use of DL-based image segmentation methods. DL models are highly dependent on large quantities of high-quality labeled data, which are difficult to come by in the medical field, particularly in the case of uncommon retinal conditions (Gunduz et al. 2023). The lack of annotated datasets makes it more difficult to train reliable and accurate models as they could not fully reflect the complexity and diversity of real-world situations. Standardized datasets that may be used as benchmarks for comparing and assessing various segmentation techniques are required to overcome this difficulty. These datasets need to cover a broad spectrum of retinal conditions and include thorough annotations for reliable ground truth. The creation of these datasets will promote the development of DL methods for picture segmentation and allow for equitable comparisons between various strategies.

6.4.2 Explainability and Interpretability of the Model

CNNs in particular are DL models that are sometimes referred to as "black boxes" because of their sophisticated learning processes and complex topologies. In medical situations, where physicians must comprehend the logic behind the model's predictions in order to make confident decisions, this lack of interpretability presents difficulties. DL models must be transparent and easily interpreted for clinical practice to embrace and use them. The development of methods that may shed light on these models' decision-making process is underway. To improve interpretability and foster clinician trust, techniques such as saliency maps and attention mechanisms emphasize the areas of the picture that provide the most contributions to the model's predictions.

6.4.3 Complexity of Computation and Necessity for Resources

Techniques for segmenting images based on DL need a significant amount of computing resources, such as strong hardware and effective software. Deep neural network training may be computationally demanding, including lengthy processing times and significant memory use. Implementing this complexity may be difficult, especially in contexts with limited resources such as real-time apps or low-resource healthcare settings. In order to surmount these obstacles, scientists are investigating methods for enhancing the computational effectiveness of DL models. Included in this are model quantization and compression, which reduce the model's size and processing demands without appreciably compromising accuracy. Additionally, DL inference may be made more accessible and useful for real-world deployment by enhancing its efficiency via the use of distributed computing and specialized accelerators, two developments in hardware technology.

6.4.4 Ethical Issues

There are significant ethical issues with the use of DL-based image segmentation in the medical field (Fernandez-Quilez 2023). Ensuring privacy and data security are crucial when handling confidential medical data. Sustaining trust and safeguarding patient privacy requires making sure that patient data is anonymized, maintained securely, and used only for approved reasons. In addition, any biases in the data and algorithms used for picture segmentation must be addressed. Unbalanced datasets may introduce biases that cause variations in the segmentation accuracy for various demographic groups. In order to prevent the continuation of current healthcare inequities, it is imperative that we work toward justice. The correct use of DL models in clinical practice is also governed by ethical issues. Healthcare practitioners should use caution when interpreting and making decisions based on these models since they have limitations and may pose hazards. To guarantee patient safety and ethical treatment, openness and unambiguous communication on the models' capabilities and limits are crucial.

Therefore, there are a number of issues and restrictions that need to be resolved even if DL-based image segmentation approaches provide notable improvements in the field of retinal illnesses. These include the quality and accessibility of datasets, the interpretability and explainability of models, the computational complexity and resource needs, and ethical issues. Researchers and practitioners may improve the efficacy, dependability, and morality of DL-based picture segmentation in healthcare by addressing these issues.

6.5 Conclusions and Future Directions

DL-based image segmentation has a great deal of promise for the early diagnosis and treatment of retinal diseases including diabetic retinopathy. We can allow personalized treatment plans, increase the capacity of healthcare personnel, and improve diagnostic accuracy and efficiency by using DL methods. We must, however, address the difficulties and constraints covered in this paper, such as the quality and accessibility of datasets, the interpretability of models, computational complexity, and ethical issues. We can fully realize the promise of DL-based image segmentation and make great progress toward bettering patient outcomes in the field of retinal illnesses by working together and innovating in these areas. In order to achieve these objectives, researchers and medical professionals are encouraged to keep collaborating and making sure that patient-centered care, ethics, and openness serve as the cornerstones of our scientific progress.

More investigation is required to enhance the use of DL-based image segmentation in the early diagnosis of retinal illnesses. Important areas of research include the creation of large-scale annotated datasets, enhanced model interpretability, and computational resource optimization. In addition, to guarantee patient welfare and equality in the provision of healthcare, ethical issues pertaining to data privacy, patient consent, and algorithmic bias need to be properly addressed.

References

Alyoubi, W.L., Shalash, W.M., and Abulkhair, M.F. (2020). Diabetic retinopathy detection through deep learning techniques: a review. *Informatics in Medicine Unlocked* 20: 100377.

Atli, İ. and Gedik, O.S. (2021). Sine-Net: a fully convolutional deep learning architecture for retinal blood vessel segmentation. *Engineering Science and Technology, an International Journal* 24 (2): 271–283.

Aziz, T., Ilesanmi, A.E., and Charoenlarpnopparut, C. (2021). Efficient and accurate hemorrhages detection in retinal fundus images using smart window features. *Applied Sciences* 11 (14): 6391.

Biswas, A. and Banik, R. (2023). Deep learning system for assessing diabetic retinopathy prevalence and risk level estimation. *E3S Web of Conferences* 430: 01292.

Biswas, R., Vasan, A., and Roy, S.S. (2020). Dilated deep neural network for segmentation of retinal blood vessels in fundus images. *Iranian Journal of Science and Technology, Transactions of Electrical Engineering* 44 (1): 505–518.

Bonassi, F., Farina, M., Xie, J., Scattolini, R.2022. "On Recurrent Neural Networks for learning-based control: Recent results and ideas for future developments." *Journal of Process Control* 114: 92-104. doi:https://doi.org/10.1016/j.jprocont.2022.04.011.

Deshmukh, S. V., Roy, A., Agrawal, P.2023 "Retinal Image Segmentation for Diabetic Retinopathy Detection using U-Net Architecture", International Journal of Image, *Graphics and Signal Processing (IJIGSP)*, Vol.15, No.1, pp. 79-92. DOI:https://doi.org/10.5815/ijigsp.2023.01.0

Fernandez-Quilez, A. 2023. "Deep learning in radiology: ethics of data and on the value of algorithm transparency, interpretability and explainability." *AI Ethics* 3: 257–265. doi:https://doi.org/10.1007/s43681-022-00161-9.

Gündüz, H. A., Binder, M., To, X. Y., et al. 2023. "A self-supervised deep learning method for data-efficient training in genomics." *Communications Biology* 6: 928. doi:https://doi.org/10.1038/s42003-023-05310-2.

Guo, C., Szemenyei, M., Hu, Y., Wang, W., Zhou, W., Yi, Y.2021. "Channel attention residual U-net for retinal vessel segmentation. " In: *ICASSP 2021–2021 IEEE international conference on acoustics, speech and signal processing (ICASSP).* IEEE, pp 1185–1189.

Hemanth, D.J., Deperlioglu, O., and Kose, U. (2020). An enhanced diabetic retinopathy detection and classification approach using deep convolutional neural network. *Neural Computing and Applications* 32 (3): 707–721.

Jeong, J. J, Tariq, A., Adejumo, T. et al. 2022. "Systematic Review of Generative Adversarial Networks (GANs) for Medical Image Classification and Segmentation." *Journal of Digital Imaging* 35: 137–152. doi:https://doi.org/10.1007/s10278-021-00556-w.

Karmakar, R., Nooshabadi, S., and Eghrari, A. (2022). Mobile-RetinaNet : A Computationally Efficient DeepNet for Retinal Fundus Image Segmentation for Use in Low-resource Settings. *Investigative Ophthalmology & Visual Science* 63 (7): 2064–F0053.

Li, T., Gao, Y., Wang, K. et al. (2019a). Diagnostic assessment of deep learning algorithms for diabetic retinopathy screening. *Information Sciences* 501: 511–522.

Li, X., Hu, X., Yu, L. et al. (2019b). CANet: cross-disease attention network for joint diabetic retinopathy and diabetic macular edema grading. *IEEE Transactions on Medical Imaging* 39 (5): 1483–1493.

Mateen, M., Wen, J., Hassan, M. et al. (2020). Automatic detection of diabetic retinopathy: a review on datasets, methods and evaluation metrics. *IEEE Access* 8: 48784–48811.

Ooi, A.Z., Embong, Z., Abd Hamid, A.I. et al. (2021). Interactive blood vessel segmentation from retinal fundus image based on canny edge detector. *Sensors* 21 (19): 6380.

Playout, C., Duval, R., and Cheriet, F. (2019). A novel weakly supervised multitask architecture for retinal lesions segmentation on fundus images. *IEEE Transactions on Medical Imaging* 38: 2434–2444.

Qummar, S., Khan, F.G., Shah, S. et al. (2019). A deep learning ensemble approach for diabetic retinopathy detection. *IEEE Access* 7: 150530–150539.

Sarki, R., Ahmed, K., Wang, H., and Zhang, Y. (2020). Automatic detection of diabetic eye disease through deep learning using fundus images: a survey. *IEEE Access* 8: 151133–151149.

Shen, Y. et al. (2020). Domain-invariant interpretable fundus image quality assessment. *Medical Image Analysis.* 61: 101654.

Ting, D.S., Wu, W.C., and Toth, C. (2019). Deep learning for retinopathy of prematurity screening. *British Journal of Ophthalmology* 103 (5): 577–579.

Torre, J.d.L., Valls, A., and Puig, D. (2020). A deep learning interpretable classifier for diabetic retinopathy disease grading. *Neurocomputing* 396: 465–476.

Vij R, Arora S. 2022. "Computer vision with deep learning techniques for neurodegenerative diseases analysis using neuroimaging: a survey." In: *International conference on innovative computing and communications*, pp 179–189.

Wang, D., Hu, G., and Lyu, C. (2021a). Frnet: an end-to-end feature refinement neural network for medical image segmentation. *International journal of computer vision* 37: 1101–1112.

Wang, H., Yuan, G., Zhao, X. et al. (2020). Hard exudate detection based on deep model learned information and multi-feature joint representation for diabetic retinopathy screening. *Comput Methods Programs Biomed* 191: 105398.

Wang, X., Ju, L., Zhao, X, Ge, Z. 2019. "Retinal abnormalities recognition using regional multitask learning." *International conference on innovative computing and communications* (eds Shen, D. et al.): 30–38 (Springer).

Wang Z, Zhong Y, Yao M. et al. 2021b. "Automated segmentation of macular edema for the diagnosis of ocular disease using deep learning method". *Scientific reports* 11, 13392. doi:https://doi.org/10.1038/s41598-021-92458-8

Suardika IGPD, Maysanjaya IMD, Kesiman MWA. 2022 "Optic Disc Segmentation Based on Mask R-CNN in Retinal Fundus Images," *2022 4th International Conference on Biomedical Engineering (IBIOMED)*, Yogyakarta, Indonesia, pp. 71–74, doi: https://doi.org/10.1109/IBIOMED56408.2022.9987756.

Yin, P., Yuan, R., Cheng, Y., and Wu, Q. (2020). Deep guidance network for biomedical image segmentation. *IEEE Access* 16 (8): 116106–116116.

7

Analysis of Deep Learning Models for Lung Field Segmentation

Tairah Andrabi and Sajid Yousuf Bhat

Department of Computer Science, University of Kashmir, Srinagar, Jammu & Kashmir, India

7.1 Introduction

Lung diseases cover a broad spectrum of health issues impacting breathing and overall well-being. Ranging from infectious diseases such as pneumonia to persistent disorders such as emphysema, "chronic obstructive pulmonary disease (COPD)," and even potentially life-threatening conditions such as lung cancer and COVID-19, these pose significant challenges to healthcare globally. To diagnose diseases related to the lungs, healthcare professionals utilize an array of advanced medical imaging modalities, including magnetic resonance imaging (MRI), chest X-rays (CXR), computed tomography (CT) scans, and positron emission tomography (PET). Among these, Chest X-rays stand out as a pivotal diagnostic tool. Chest X-rays (CXR), also known as chest radiographs, are a fundamental imaging modality in the field of medical diagnostics. Chest X-rays (CXRs) provide crucial insights about the heart, lungs, ribs, and surrounding tissue. They are known for their cost-effectiveness, widespread availability, low radiation dose, and ability to provide valuable insights that other imaging techniques may not offer as easily. Due to these advantages, a substantial volume of X-rays is generated daily, making them a cornerstone of medical diagnostics. Despite its affordability, interpreting CXRs demands considerable expertise and poses challenges due to their complexity. Manual examination of X-rays is both time-consuming and labor-demanding, emphasizing the requirement for an automated diagnostic system.

Computer-aided diagnosis (CAD) tools are a category of software applications designed to assist healthcare professionals, particularly radiologists, in interpreting medical images and making accurate diagnoses. CAD has seen rapid

Deep Learning Applications in Medical Image Segmentation: Overview, Approaches, and Challenges, First Edition. Edited by Sajid Yousuf Bhat, Aasia Rehman, and Muhammad Abulaish.

advancements, and its incorporation into clinical practice not only enhances diagnostic accuracy but also accelerates the decision-making process, leading to more prompt interventions and improved patient outcomes.

In recent years, medical image analysis has seen remarkable progress, with image segmentation, an integral aspect, extracting crucial and meaningful information from medical images. Lung field segmentation (LFS), a prerequisite step, precisely delineates the region of interest. However, this task comes with its own set of challenges such as (i) variations in patient positioning, (ii) the presence of superimposed anatomical structures such as the heart, diaphragm, clavicles, and rib cage influenced by factors due to age and gender (Agrawal and Choudhary 2023), (iii) potential distortions in lung appearance due to underlying pathologies, and (iv) variations in image quality, contrast, and brightness settings across different imaging devices. Furthermore, achieving precise segmentation of the lung apex is complicated by the diverse intensity levels present in the upper clavicle bone region. Addressing these obstacles is crucial for ensuring the accuracy and reliability of segmentation algorithms.

Over the past 40 years, LFS has attracted significant attention, witnessing advancements from basic rule-based approaches to sophisticated deep-learning methods, as reflected in various high-quality publications. Van Ginneken et al. provided a foundational classification of LFS techniques, organizing them into four primary categories(Van Ginneken et al. 2001): "(i) rule-based, (ii) pixel-classification (PC)-based, (iii) deformable model-based, and (iv) hybrid methods." Initially, lung segmentation methods in CAD systems relied on specific rules that defined the relationships between the lungs and neighboring structures. Later, in the 1990s, pixel-level classification emerged, categorizing individual pixels as either lung or non-lung based on manually derived features (considered shallow learning). In the 2000s, deformable model-based methods utilized models capable of adapting under internal and external influences to outline lung shapes. Despite the existence of several LFS methods, ongoing research strives to elevate their efficacy. Presently, researchers focus on automatic feature extraction through deep learning, emphasizing a promising area for advancement within this domain.

LFS using deep learning employs a diverse range of sophisticated models such as "convolutional neural networks (CNNs), recurrent neural networks (RNNs), generative adversarial networks (GANs), encoder decoder architectures," and other advanced architectures. Among these, U-Net based on encoder–decoder architecture has emerged as a popular choice for semantic segmentation, particularly in the context of lung segmentation. Its effectiveness in capturing contextual information makes it well suited for the intricate structures present in medical images obtained from chest X-rays or CT scans. DeepLab, a state-of-the-art architecture utilizing atrous convolutions, has also been adapted for lung segmentation tasks. Notably, DeepLab excels in handling diverse image resolutions, showcasing success in precisely segmenting lung fields. Additionally, "Mask R-CNN," a refinement of "Faster R-CNN" designed for instance segmentation, has found application in lung segmentation, providing accurate pixel-wise delineation of lung structures. Attention mechanisms, such as self-attention or channel attention, have further enhanced the capability of deep learning models to focus on relevant regions, discarding irrelevant information and thereby improving the precision of lung segmentation. The integration of these diverse models with their respective strengths contributes to the development of robust and efficient lung segmentation methods, addressing the various image resolutions and achieving high levels of accuracy in delineating lung boundaries.

The following sections of this chapter are structured as follows: Section 7.2 provides a brief overview of medical imaging modalities. Section 7.3 provides an overview of the classical approaches for lung segmentation in chest X-rays. Section 7.4 offers a summary of deep learning models for lung segmentation in both chest X-rays and CT scans. Section 7.5 enumerates several publicly accessible chest X-rays and CT scans. Different evaluation metrics used for assessing model performance are covered in Section 7.6. Last, Section 7.7 encapsulates the conclusive findings and prospective future directions derived from the systematic review.

7.2 Medical Imaging Modalities

In clinical settings, diverse medical imaging modalities play crucial roles by offering distinct information tailored to specific diagnostic needs. Among the prevalent modalities are "CT, MRI, PET, ultrasound imaging, and optical coherence tomography (OCT)," as depicted in Figure 7.1. However, in the context of lung segmentation, the focus is on utilizing two modalities – CT scans and X-rays. The selection of CT scans and X-rays is driven by their distinctive attributes and appropriateness for capturing pertinent details in lung imaging.

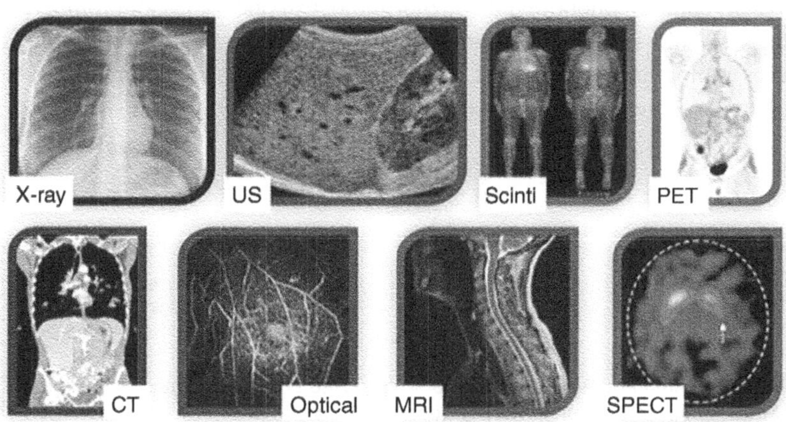

Figure 7.1 Overview of diverse medical imaging techniques. Source: Beyer et al. (2020) /Springer Nature/CC BY 4.0.

7.3 Overview of Classical Approaches for Lung Segmentation in Chest X-rays

Traditional methods for LFS typically cover various techniques and approaches, which are discussed as follows.

7.3.1 Rule-Based Methods

Rule-based methods include techniques that rely on predefined rules or criteria to delineate and describe the borders and areas corresponding to the lungs. These rules are like step-by-step instructions applied in a specific order to accurately outline the lungs. The rules consider factors such as where the lungs are located, how bright or dark they appear, their texture, and shape, and how they relate to other body structures. These methods provide flexibility by allowing the application of rules in various sequences allowing adaptation to various situations. (Gados and Horvath n.d.) (Figure 7.2).

Intensity thresholding, edge detection, and knowledge-based rules are techniques utilized in rule-based segmentation.

Intensity thresholding categorizes each pixel into either non-lung or lung regions based on a predefined grayscale threshold. The key challenge lies in determining an optimal threshold value because a low setting may lead to unclear lung contour while a high value might merge or blur the boundary between the lung and non-lung regions. Cheng and Goldberg introduced one of the earliest methods in this category, (Cheng and Goldberg 1988) employing a distinct gray-level threshold value to individually segment the left and right lungs. In contrast, Armato et al. presented a method that combines iterative gray-level thresholding, (S. G. Armato et al. 1998) incorporating both global and local aspects, with contour smoothing using morphological operations and rolling-ball techniques. While iterative thresholding improves segmentation precision, it introduces computational overhead. Conversely, static threshold values may lead to suboptimal segmentation, especially in images with varying contrast.

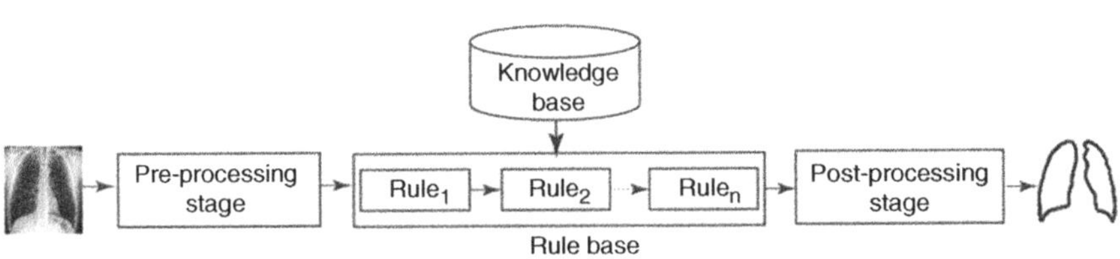

Figure 7.2 Diagrammatic Representation of Rule-Based Lung Segmentation Workflow. Source: Mittal et al. (2017) /John Wiley & Sons.

Edge detection-based lung segmentation is used to highlight the edges or contours of the lungs, allowing for accurate segmentation. It depends on variations in pixel intensity between non-lung lung areas, capitalizing on sharp intensity changes near lung edges. Powell et al. originally used derivatives to identify rib cage boundaries, (Powell et al. 1988) a method subsequently enhanced by Xu et al. who applied the "second-order derivative" for contour identification to capture intricate details, (Xu and Doi 1995) albeit with a susceptibility to noise. Duryea et al. adopted a "heuristic technique" for edge tracing, (Duryea and Boone 1995) independently segmenting both lungs with an average processing duration of 0.84 seconds per image across 802 images. Li et al. further addressed challenges such as rib structure hindrance and false contours, (Li et al. 2001) achieving lung contours in 0.775 seconds per image by utilizing the first derivative. In the domain of intensity and edge-based segmentation, the challenges associated with deformed anatomical structures are addressed by methods incorporating prior understanding of texture, lung spatial, and shape characteristics. Luo et al. proposed a comprehensive approach that employs knowledge-based characteristics, (Luo et al. 2000) utilizing an object-oriented anatomical model, with robust initial contour construction and boundary detection using a snake model. Brown et al. also presented a similar method utilizing an anatomical model for both normal lung shapes and deformities. (Brown et al. 1998) While these approaches contribute to enhancing robustness in lung segmentation, they also face challenges in threshold determination, computational efficiency, and noise susceptibility in edge-based approaches. The choice of a rule-based technique depends on specific requirements and image characteristics.

7.3.2 Deformable Methods

These are the techniques that can adapt their shape and boundaries to accurately follow the complex and potentially irregular contours of the lungs. Unlike fixed models that rely on rigid templates or predefined shapes, deformable methods offer greater flexibility and can handle challenges like variability in lung shape and the presence of overlapped structures. Deformable models fall into two categories: "parametric and geometric." (Figure 7.3).

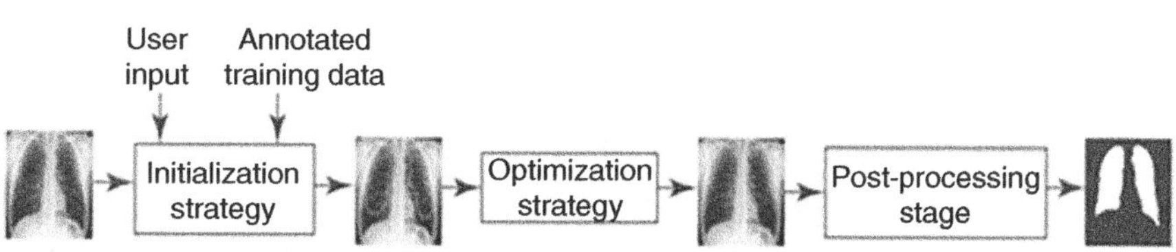

Figure 7.3 Deformable-based lung segmentation process. Source: Mittal et al. (2017) /John Wiley & Sons.

7.3.3 Parametric Methods

"Active Shape Model (ASM)" and "Active Appearance Model (AAM)", both belonging to parametric, use a limited set of parameters for lung segmentation in CXRs. These incorporate shape and appearance information to adapt to the variations in lung structures and textures.

In 1995, Cootes et al. introduced the "ASM" (Cootes et al. 1995), which was subsequently refined by other researchers. Wu et al. enhanced the performance of the ASM (Wu et al. 2015) by introducing weighted components and incorporating additional constraints. This modification yielded better accuracy compared to the standard ASM technique. The deformable model proposed by Shi et al. integrates shape statistics at both "patient-specific and population-based" (Shi et al. 2008) levels through hierarchical Principle component Analysis (PCA). The aim was to employ statistical shape modeling for reliable lung segmentation across various anatomies, with the inclusion of scale-invariant feature transform (SIFT) to enhance accuracy. Iakovidis and Savelonas automated landmark extraction for lung segmentation, (Iakovidis and Savelonas 2009) offering an advantage in initial boundary detection but facing challenges in low-contrast images. Dawoud integrated shape information with intensity-based thresholding, (Dawoud 2011) demonstrating improved results compared to ASM. However, it necessitated the use of images with identical resolution for optimal performance. Zhang et al. (Zhang et al. 2014) suggested a comparable approach that combines intensity information and shape priors for lung segmentation. Both studies employed the JSRT dataset for the training and evaluation of their models. The limitation of ASM lies in its exclusive focus on the object's shape, neglecting factors such as texture and color variations. To resolve this, AAM was introduced, extending ASM to consider both shape and appearance. While AAM is more powerful, it also requires more computational effort. Li et al. (Li et al. 2016) introduced an innovative approach that integrates both shape and appearance models to enhance the segmentation of lung fields. Their approach incorporated a multi-scale and multi-step-size strategy, contributing to improved accuracy. Additionally, Shao et al. proposed the AAM method using learning-based landmark detection and a hierarchical framework, (Shao et al. 2014) ensuring a thorough and strong segmentation process.

7.3.4 Geometric Deformable Models

Deformable models based on geometry, such as the theory of curve evolution and the level set approach, were proposed by Caselles et al. to ensure smooth evolution and effective handling of topology changes, (Caselles et al. 1993) providing advantages in capturing complex lung shapes, while being independent of parameters. Employing the prior shape information, Annangi et al. used an active contour technique for the segmentation task, (Annangi et al. 2010) combining level set minimal energy and Otsu thresholding with extracted edge characteristics, corners, and region-specific data. This method proficiently addressed challenges related to local minima and accomplished the segmentation of lung structures within seven seconds per image for both lungs.

By incorporating graph-cut techniques, Candemir et al. aimed to address challenges related to variable lung shapes and high computation time. This method initially calculated the average lung shape and determined the boundary using graph-cut techniques. Despite encountering challenges in static shape modeling and facing high computation time, they proposed a method that employed a multi-class classifier approach, (Candemir et al. 2013) achieving segmentation in 8 seconds at a resolution of 1024×1024. The approach was further enhanced by incorporating anatomical atlases and non-registration, (Candemir et al. 2014) resulting in a faster execution time of 20–25 seconds at a resolution of 256×256.

Overall, deformable methods, including AAMs, active shape models, and geometric deformable models, exhibit the potential for precise segmentation of lung structures in chest radiography.

7.3.5 Pixel Classifier-Based Segmentation

From the early 1990s onward, various "Machine learning techniques such as k-nearest neighbors (kNNs) and Support vector machines (SVMs)" have been extensively employed for LFS. This pixel classifier (PC)-based approaches use grayscale values to assign pixels to anatomical structures, ensuring stable performance even in situations involving absent or significantly deformed anatomical structures, assuming the classifier is adequately trained. Training these classifiers is, however, challenging due to difficulties in obtaining diverse and high-quality annotated medical training data. PC-based methods are categorized into two groups: one based on shallow learning and the other based on deep learning, depending on the process of extracting features, which can be either manual or automatic (Figure 7.4).

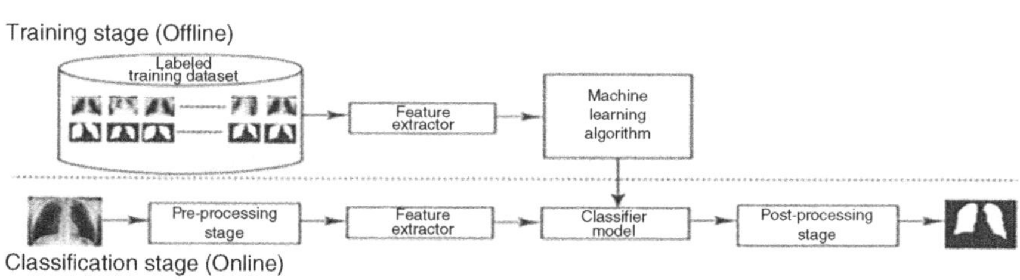

Figure 7.4 Pixel-based lung segmentation process. Source: Mittal et al. (2017) /John Wiley & Sons.

7.3.6 Shallow Learning

In shallow learning, machine learning methods are employed to extract important information. The challenge lies in identifying a fitting class for the extracted features. With growing trends in research, (McNitt-Gray et al. 1993) aimed to build a segmentation technique using the "pattern classification approach." Numerous classifiers include "linear discriminant, k-nearest neighbor, and feed-forward back-propagation neural network (FFBPNN)" to categorize pixels based on local texture and gray-level features. Each classifier was trained on a dataset comprising 17 CXR images and trained classifiers were evaluated on a distinct set of 16 images. Although the neural network outperformed KNN and LDA, accurately predicting over 76% of pixels, limitations existed. Vittitoe et al. addressed these limitations by introducing Markov random field modeling (MRFM) to identify lung regions and non-lung regions, achieving 94.8%-pixel classification accuracy on a test set of 115 CXRs, (Vittitoe et al. 1998) outperforming some previous methods. However, the computational expense of MRFM was acknowledged as a drawback. Finally, Shi et al. and Jangam et al. in their respective works individually modified the fuzzy c-means clustering algorithm for the segmentation of lungs. Shi et al. implemented an unsupervised approach using a "Gaussian kernel-based fuzzy C-means," (Shi et al. 2009) achieving 97.8% accuracy on 52 CXRs from the JSRT dataset. On the other hand, Jangam et al. proposed an "optimized fuzzy c-means clustering" method, (Jangam and Rao 2019) incorporating a level set algorithm and spatial fuzzy clustering for segmentation. However, Jangam et al.'s method had a longer computation time of 25–30 seconds. Both studies differ in computational efficiency.

7.4 Deep Learning Approaches

7.4.1 Lung Field Segmentation in Chest X-rays

Accurate lung segmentation is crucial in medical imaging because losing even a small part of the lung during the process can have serious consequences. Shallow learning methods for segmentation rely on manually defined features, which can be tedious and error-prone. In contrast, deep learning automatically extracts features from the data, rendering it a robust and efficient approach for lung segmentation.

Deep learning approaches for lung segmentation use advanced neural network architectures to automatically discern lung structures in CXR images. These models comprise several layers of nonlinear processing, which include the input layer, intermediate layers, and output layer. Deep learning offers various computationally efficient approaches for the computer vision task of lung segmentation, including convolutional neural networks such as "Fully Convolutional Networks (FCNs), dilated convolutions like DeepLab v3 and encoder–decoder-based models like UNet" and its variants. These architectures significantly contribute to improving segmentation accuracy. Additionally, innovative methods, such as "GANs," "attention-based mechanisms," and "multistage or hybrid frameworks," further enhance the segmentation process. The networks learn to distinguish between lung and non-lung regions, addressing challenges such as variations in anatomy and image quality. Training is typically performed on large datasets, allowing the model to generalize to diverse cases.

7.4.1.1 CNN-Based Approaches

In the past few years, with the rise of deep learning techniques, especially "CNNs," the field of artificial intelligence has undergone a remarkable evolution. This study emphasizes the effectiveness of CNNs in automating segmentation processes, thereby reducing the manual effort and time required. Certainly, CNNs can be employed for various applications, including but not limited to image recognition, computer vision, natural language processing, and speech recognition. In medical image analysis, CNNs prove effective for different organ segmentation, automatically extracting features and identifying intricate patterns challenging for human detection. Crucially, this capability enhances accurate and efficient lung segmentation, vital for diagnosing, treating, and monitoring deadly lung diseases. To address challenges such as model overfitting, reducing parameters, and handling imbalanced data, Novikov et al. (2018) developed a robust "fully convolutional network (FCN)" architecture. The three variants – All-Dropout, incorporating Gaussian dropout layers to prevent overfitting; All-Convolutional, which replaced pooling layers with convolutional layers for denser feature extraction; and "InvertedNet", (Novikov et al. 2018) utilizing inverted residual blocks and Exponential Linear Units (ELUs) for accelerated training – were thoroughly evaluated. The study used the JSRT dataset, which comprises 247 chest X-rays. The training time for InvertedNet was 33 hours, involving 3,140,771 parameters. The study's findings revealed that InvertedNet performed better than others, showing good results in terms of the Jaccard score, as proven by the study's results.

Furthermore, Adel Sulaiman and colleagues introduced a lung segmentation model using deep CNNs. The model incorporates convolutional and concatenate blocks, (Sulaiman et al. 2023) with convolutional layers capturing essential features and a transpose layer enhancing spatial resolution of feature maps. Performance metrics such as accuracy, Intersection over Union (IoU), and Dice coefficient were used to evaluate the model's effectiveness, yielding impressive results. Trained with k-fold validation ($k = 5$), the model achieved 97% accuracy with minimal loss.

The neural network architecture known as encoder–decoder, widely used for image segmentation, consists of two essential parts: the encoder and the decoder. The encoder, often referred to as the contracting path, utilizes convolutional layers to downsample the input image, extracting crucial features and reducing spatial dimensions. Conversely, the decoder, known as the expansion path, employs upsampling layers to enhance spatial resolution and generate a segmentation mask. U-Net, a specialized encoder–decoder network initially created for biomedical image segmentation by "Olaf Ronnenberger," (Ronneberger et al. 2015) incorporates skip connections and additional convolutional layers to refine segmentation accuracy.

7.4.1.2 U-Net-Based Approaches

The "U-Net architecture" has significantly influenced medical image segmentation, marking a pivotal advancement. Researchers have made remarkable contributions to U-Net studies. Here are some contributions made to the U-Net-based model by numerous researchers (Figure 7.5).

In this context, Islam et al. put forward a "U-Net-based deep CNN" for lung segmentation, incorporating enhancements such as advanced data augmentation techniques, refined skip connections, and modifications to the contracting-expanding pathway. These improvements aim to better capture the complexities

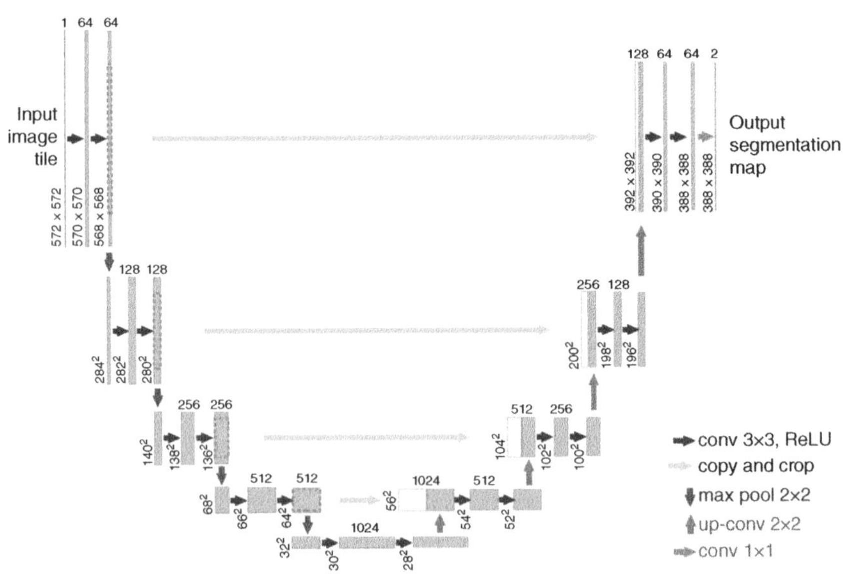

Figure 7.5 Basic U-Net architecture for medical image segmentation. Source: Ronneberger et al. 2015/Springer Nature.

and variations present in chest X-rays. The model achieves a Dice score of 98.6% and undergoes evaluation on two benchmark chest X-ray datasets: "Shenzhen Hospital (SH) dataset and Montgomery County (MC)" dataset demonstrating the performance of U-Net enhancements in advancing medical image segmentation. Deep learning models exhibit impressive performance in anatomical structure segmentation, but a high number of training parameters is a potential issue. This leads to increased memory usage and reduced model generalization, connecting with our earlier U-Net architecture discussion. To address this, Yahyatabar et al. introduced "Dense-Unet," (Yahyatabar and Jouvet 2020) an extension of U-Net with dense connectivity. Enhancing information flow between layers. The model offers "compact and normal" versions, incorporating squeeze-and-excitation (SE) blocks. The study used JSRT and Montgomery datasets, achieving Dice and Jaccard scores of 97.6/95.3 and 97.9/95.59, respectively, illustrating improved segmentation. Similarly, as in previous studies for automatically segmenting lung regions in chest radiographs, Liu et al. proposed an "Improved U-Net" (Liu et al. 2022) network that incorporates a pretraining EfficientNet-b4 backbone in the encoder, LeakyReLU activation function, and residual block in the decoder to efficiently extract lung field features and prevent gradient instability. The suggested approach was tested on public CXR datasets, JSRT and MC, as well as a private Haut lung segmentation dataset, and it outperformed the traditional U-Net model in terms of "Jaccard Index and Dice sensitivity coefficient (DSC)." Both studies use data augmentation techniques to overcome the training set's limited size, enhancing generalization to diverse datasets. (Liu et al. 2022; Yahyatabar and Jouvet (2020).

The U-Net architecture has been extensively preferred in recent medical studies; however, it exhibited shortcomings, the most prominent being the presence of a single dropout function at the final convolution layer, which leads to overfitting and poor model generalization. To address these concerns, Arvind et al. proposed a refined and relatively lightweight variant of the U-Net model, (Arvind et al. 2023) incorporating multiple dropouts in both convolution and deconvolution layers for improved semantic segmentation of lung images in chest X-rays. Their improvements in the architectural components of U-Net, such as batch normalization and fewer convolutions, resulted in fewer model parameters and lower model complexity while maintaining performance metrics. The study offered improved performance on multiple datasets with a generalization accuracy of 93.87%.

Continuing the discussion on encoder–decoder approaches, the researchers introduced the "DED-CNN (dual encoder–decoder CNN)" (Ullah et al. 2023) for precise segmentation of multiorgan anatomical structures in chest X-ray images. The model utilizes a pretrained VGG19 as an encoder, incorporates a SE block for better representation, and employs "Attention Gating Modules (AGMs)" to improve the segmentation of smaller regions in the second encoder–decoder.

Evaluation of benchmark datasets (JSRT, MCCXR, and SCXR) demonstrated DED-CNN's superior performance in anatomical structure segmentation compared to existing CNN architectures.

Chest X-rays are vital for diagnosing lung conditions, including cancer and other chest infections. In response, the authors proposed "CSR-Net" (Kumar et al. 2023), a fully CNN, integrating "Transfer Learning (TL) with ResNet-101 as a feature extractor," along with "U-Net serving as a Backbone." TL proves valuable for overcoming data limitations, enhancing generalization, and reducing training time. CSR-Net's performance is evaluated on the JSRT database, with metrics such as Dice score, precision, recall, accuracy, and Jaccard similarity coefficient (JSC) quantitatively measured.

7.4.1.3 Dilated Convolution-Based Approaches

Deeplabv3+ stands as a pivotal architecture, (Chen et al. 2018) offering a robust encoder–decoder framework for accurate image analysis. While its predecessor, deeplabv3, excelled at capturing multi-scale contextual information but faced challenges in accurately delineating object boundaries deeplabv3+ addressed this limitation by integrating a decoder module to improve segmentation results, especially along object borders and object edges. Building upon this foundation, researchers have explored various advancements to further enhance its performance and handle specific challenges.

Singh et al. developed Deep LF-Net, (Singh et al. 2021) an encoder–decoder network building upon deeplabv3+, designed to robustly segment lungs in Indian patients with diverse abnormalities. The encoder incorporates atrous convolutions and spatial pyramid pooling for capturing multi-scale contextual information, while the decoder refines segmentation, addressing challenges such as opacities and pleural effusions. Post-processing, including area filtering, effectively eliminates false positives. Evaluated on an in-house Indian dataset and public datasets (Shenzhen, JSRT, and MC), Deep LF-Net demonstrated outstanding performance, achieving 99.37% on JSRT, 99.09% on MC, and 98.31% accuracy on Shenzhen, outperforming existing methods. In a recent study by Boudoukhani et al., (Boudoukhani et al. 2023) a unique methodology was adopted to address common challenges in lung segmentation such as shape/scale variations, device artifacts, false positives, and poor generalizability across devices. Attention gates in the encoder filter out noise, focus on relevant lung features, and minimize false positives, while residual convolutions in the decoder preserve crucial details, leading to sharp, accurate lung boundaries across diverse X-ray datasets, boosting the generalizability of this model. Based on EfficientNet-b4 and ResNet-50 architectures, it outperforms prior models, achieving "Dice coefficient of 98.03% and Jaccard index 96.14%" without pre-/post-processing (Figure 7.6).

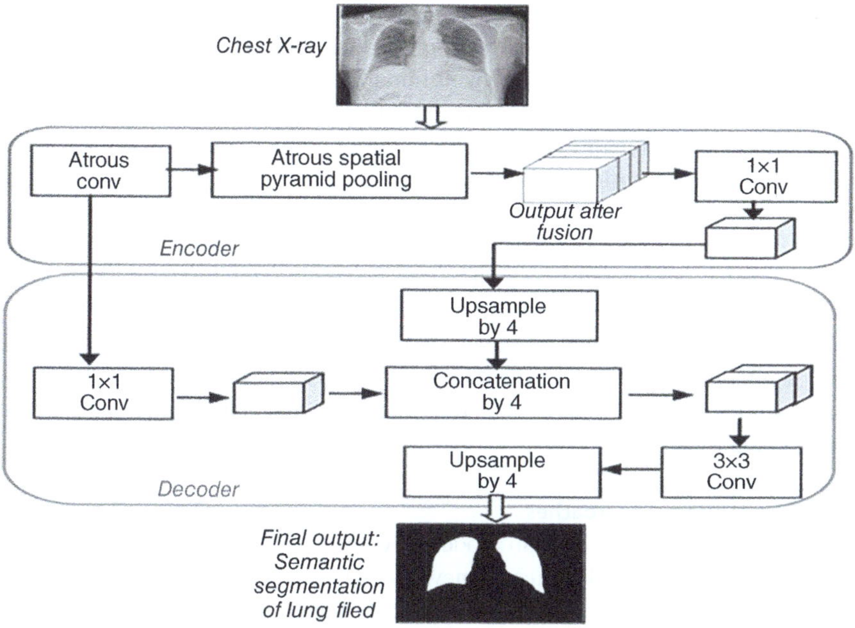

Figure 7.6 Architectural overview of Deeplabv3+ for semantic lung segmentation. Source: Singh et al. 2021/with permission of ELSEVIER.

7.4.1.4 Attention-Based Approaches

Numerous studies adopted the attention mechanism in their segmentation framework attention-based models have emerged as powerful tools. Unlike the conventional U-Net architecture, these models strategically integrate attention modules within both contracting and expanding paths, resulting in capturing essential features relevant to the lung region and overall segmentation accuracy. Kim et al. presented a self-attention-based deep learning model consisting of "X-attention and Y-attention modules" (Kim and Lee 2021). The X-attention module concentrates on local features, while the Y-attention module incorporates global context from deeper layers to effectively utilize global features. Both attention modules employ channel and spatial attention, enhancing the feature extraction process. The attention maps derived from these modules are multiplied and utilized in subsequent layers through residual learning. The proposed attention modules contribute to accurate pixel-level attention information, resulting in smooth segmentation masks with reduced noise. To overcome issues faced by previous models in properly segmenting lung areas, particularly in the presence of rib cage edges, irregularities, and changes in size and shape, researchers have introduced a novel segmentation model named "Attention RegSeg (ARSeg)" (Ghali and Akhloufi 2022). This method utilizes an attention mechanism to eliminate irrelevant features. The ARSeg architecture employs RegNety-32GF as a backbone for detecting and extracting lung features. The decoder consists of three Deconv blocks and a 1×1 convolutional layer that generates a lung mask. The primary aim is to overcome these limitations and improve the lung segmentation tasks. In the meantime, authors proposed a novel attention UW-Net that addresses U-Net limitations and directly segments both large and small regions of interest in chest X-rays, (Pal et al. 2022) without pre-/post-processing steps. The model incorporates an intermediate layer with fully connected convolutions and attention gates, specifically designed to improve segmentation accuracy for small lesions. This method shows promising results even, when trained on a subset (200 images) of the NIH X-ray dataset, suggesting potential for efficient and accurate lung segmentation. The generalizability of the model across diverse chest X-ray datasets remains uncertain, as the study did not investigate its performance on different datasets.

7.4.1.5 GAN-Based Approaches

The "GAN," introduced by "Ian Goodfellow et al." in 2014, (Goodfellow et al. 2020) is an artificial intelligence framework that employs a competitive training approach involving dual neural networks: "a generator and a discriminator." The generator's goal is to produce synthetic data, such as images, that are virtually identical to real data, while the discriminator distinguishes between the training data and the generated data, to determine the originality of the input. Using both neural networks, researchers extended the applications of GANs to propose an innovative model. Their model, (Munawar et al. 2020) equipped with a generator structured like a U-net, was trained to produce segmented masks, while four discriminators ("D1, D2, D3, and D4"), acting as binary classifiers, were used to differentiate between ground truth masks and generated one. The "Montgomery County, JSRT, and Shenzhen" datasets were used for evaluation, where the model achieved an "IOU score of 0.943 and a Dice similarity coefficient (DSC) of 0.9740." In a related study, (El Mansouri et al. 2022) authors explored more about GAN-based lung segmentation, utilizing a similar GAN architecture with a U-Net design. Their focus was on chest X-ray segmentation, specifically employing the JSRT dataset consisting of 240 images (40 for validation, 40 for testing, and 160 for training). The proposed model achieved a notable Dice score of 0.9778. Despite this success, the study acknowledged the computational intensity associated with GANs, highlighting the need for future research to explore diverse datasets and assess performance across varying image sizes.

In response to the challenges of instability and diversity in GANs, Lyu et al. introduced the "Multiple Tasking Wasserstein Generative Adversarial U-Shape Network (MWG-UNet)" (Lyu and Tian 2023). This architecture includes a generator to match the distribution of generated samples with real data and a

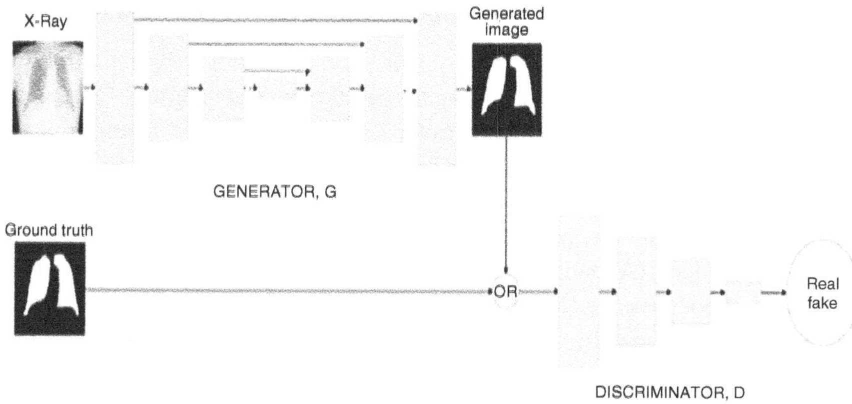

Figure 7.7 GAN architecture overview. Source: Munawar et al. 2020/IEEE/CC-BY-4.0.

discriminator to differentiate between authentic and synthetic data. The generator employs an enhanced U-Net, termed ARU-Net. The primary purpose of multitask learning in MWG-UNet is to enhance performance and generalization (Figure 7.7).

7.4.1.6 Multistage and Ensemble Approaches

The use of multistage and ensemble learning frameworks has significantly improved segmentation outcomes in various studies. Ciano et al. proposed a multi-organ segmentation approach, (Ciano et al. 2021) employing a GAN with a multistage algorithm for X-ray images. Using PGGANs, Pix2PixHD, and SMANet, the study highlights the importance of accurate segmentation in CAD, particularly in scenarios with limited training data, showcasing advanced segmentation techniques. Similarly, researchers introduced a sophisticated lung segmentation approach, (Souza et al. 2019) presenting a cascaded two-stage model. The method employs a reconstruction technique for segmenting lungs, initially using AlexNet on lung patches. In cases with opacities or consolidations, a secondary CNN, ResNet-18, is trained for lung reconstruction. The results from the initial segmentation and subsequent reconstruction stages are combined, resulting in enhanced accuracy in the final segmentation results. Expanding the study of ensemble frameworks for lung segmentation, Rahman et al. conducted studies (Rahman et al. 2021; Rahman et al. 2022) that introduced ensemble deep learning frameworks for lung segmentation using a two-stage approach. While later method employed a conventional CNN for patch classification in the first stage. Both studies incorporated post-processing techniques and a modified U-Net architecture to enhance final segmentation accuracy, providing an alternative for the cases where we have small datasets available for training CNNs.

7.4.2 Overview of Deep Learning Approaches for Lung Segmentation in CT Scans

Deep learning techniques have recently emerged as powerful tools for LFS in medical images, particularly in the context of CT scans. This review focuses on the advancements and applications of deep learning-based methods for LFS, emphasizing their significance in medical diagnosis.

Early attempts at lung segmentation relied on conventional techniques such as numerical methods, (Abdani et al. 2022) gray-level thresholding, (Zulkifley et al. 2022), and shape-based techniques. However, these methods faced limitations in handling the complexity of medical images. The emergence of deep learning, with CNNs leading the charge, has brought about a transformative impact on the domain of medical image segmentation.

Recent studies have suggested several CNN-based approaches for segmenting lung fields, (Stofa et al. 2021) leveraging the capabilities of 2D CNNs, 2.5D CNNs, and 3D CNNs. These techniques have shown significant improvements over traditional methods, enabling more accurate and efficient segmentation.

The study presented by Xu et al. proposed a straightforward CNN model for lung segmentation, (Xu et al. 2019) using a training dataset generated through a "clustering algorithm-based" approach. The k-means clustering algorithm utilized the mean and minimum intensities of image patches, effectively dividing CT slices into two groups. To ensure accuracy and completeness, the final dataset was generated through a multi-step process involving cross-shaped verification for shape consistency, volume intersection for overlap removal, connected component analysis for region identification, and patch expansion for data augmentation. The network architecture consisted of a single convolutional layer with six kernels for extracting features, a maximum pooling layer for downsampling, and two fully connected layers used for final classification. The model's performance was rigorously evaluated using an eightfold cross-validation approach on the generated datasets.

A complementary approach introduced by Lyu et al. developed algorithms for the automatic segmentation of lung fields aimed at filtering noise from CT images of lungs while preserving lung boundaries. This was achieved by employing a filtering approach based on image decomposition, followed by the application of wavelet transformation and diverse morphological operations to delineate the lung boundaries accurately. The resulting lung outlines underwent correction and smoothing as part of a segmentation refinement process, (Liu and Pang 2020) incorporating a method for adjusting contours. This comprehensive set of methodologies illustrates the diverse strategies employed in the domain of lung segmentation, showcasing the efficacy of clustering algorithms, CNN architectures, and image-processing techniques. (Liu and Pang 2020; Xu et al. 2019).

An effective approach involves employing a "U-Net architecture with a false-positive" (Khanna et al. 2020) strategy illustrating the efficacy of a more advanced network for lung segmentation. In another study, (Comelli et al. 2020) the performance of "U-Net and E-Net models" was compared, highlighting their effectiveness in segmenting parenchyma among patients with pulmonary fibrosis.

A U-Net architecture featuring separate paths for recovering global context and extracting fine details (Ait Skourt et al. 2018) has shown high performance with a Dice coefficient of 0.9502. Additionally, (Hu et al. 2020) an integrated approach combining supervised and unsupervised machine learning techniques within a Mask R-CNN methodology demonstrated quick and accurate segmentation with 97.68% accuracy and an average processing time of 11.2 seconds.

Multi-view convolutional networks have been employed to identify lung nodules, (Setio et al. 2016) targeting different nodule types. Combining multiple streams of 2D ConvNets with a robust classification approach yielded promising results, with an average of 4 False-Positives/Scan and a "detection sensitivity" of 85.4% achieved.

Moving beyond 2D approaches, some researchers focused on training "3D CNNs" for the autonomous detection of lung nodules. These networks were trained on volumes of interest (VOIs) extracted from datasets such as LIDC, which is a valuable resource for detecting "lung nodules." Researchers also analyzed the performance of 3D FCNN to generate score maps for the whole volume in a single iteration, thereby showcasing the effectiveness of 3D CNNs, (Negahdar et al. 2018) showcasing the efficiency of 3D CNNs. With ongoing advancements, Roy et al. proposed an innovative model for the segmentation of lung nodules, (Roy et al. 2019) incorporating a complementary fusion of "deep learning and shape-driven level sets." The method utilized "coarse segmentation maps" generated by deep FCNs, facilitating the segmentation process with an initial, broad delineation to refine accurate boundary detection. Initially, shape-driven evolution of level sets was employed for fine segmentation. Moreover, these level sets played a vital role in automatically initializing the model, (Thanoon et al. 2023) utilizing seed points derived from the coarse segmentation of the deep network. Segmenting lung nodules is a complex task due to variations in their shapes, contours, textures, and locations. Some nodules may be connected to surrounding tissues, further complicating the determination of their contours. The main objective of lung nodule segmentation is to precisely identify the nodule's contour and separate it from the lung region. Despite various approaches employed for lung nodule segmentation, challenges persist, particularly in accurately segmenting different types of lung nodules. Zhang et al. (Zhang et al. 2021) proposed a robust lung nodule segmentation method using an enhanced U-Net convolutional network. This approach demonstrates precise segmentation for various types of lung nodules. The methodology involves lung parenchyma segmentation with contour correction using the α-hull algorithm. CT slices containing lung nodules undergo preprocessing steps, and an "improved U-Net with Batch Normalization" is employed for accurate segmentation. The training utilizes patches with corresponding ground truth from the "Lung Image Database Consortium and Image Database Resource Initiative (LIDC/IDRI)." The model surpasses state-of-the-art algorithms and achieves a Dice score of 0.8623. Meanwhile, the authors developed the "Hierarchical Segmentation Network (CHS-Net)" (Punn and Agarwal 2022) to identify lung regions affected by COVID-19-infected CT scans. The model was evaluated on combined datasets that are publicly available. CHS-Net addresses the scarcity of COVID-19 data. The model, inspired by advanced architectures such as U-Net, Google's Inception, and residual networks, employs a multistage approach for the segmentation and extraction of features. CHS-Net achieves a 95% accuracy in segmenting the lung mask and the infected region. Recently, the authors introduced a novel approach named "Wavelet U-Net++", (Akila Agnes et al. 2024) merging the "U-Net++ architecture with wavelet pooling." This approach uses Haar wavelet transform to downsample the feature maps in the encoder, capturing both high- and low-frequency details to improve segmentation accuracy, especially for small and irregular nodules. Evaluation conducted on the LIDC-IDRI dataset, consisting of 1018 CT images, yielded promising findings, with a mean Dice coefficient of 0.936 and a mean IoU of 0.878.

Furthermore, these advancements underscore the ongoing challenges in lung segmentation, necessitating innovative solutions for improved diagnostic accuracy (Table 7.1).

7.5 Data Sources and Datasets

Data plays a vital role in advancing computerized methods, particularly in the domain of "CAD" systems. Developing these systems requires substantial sets of images as they provide a foundation for training algorithms, testing their effectiveness, and comparing the performance of different techniques. However, assembling a sizable medical dataset presents challenges due to legal and privacy concerns. Despite this, specific research organizations have prepared datasets for both "chest X-rays and CT scans," making them publicly accessible for research purposes. Numerous researchers depend on the datasets listed below for their studies, which are fundamental for training and evaluating deep learning models.

Table 7.1 Comparative analysis of the lung segmentation models.

S. no.	References	Model	Modality	Dataset	Accuracy	DSC	JC	F1-score
01	Yahyatabar and Jouvet (2020)	Dense U-Net	X-rays	JSRT MC		97.6 97.9	95.3 95.59	
02	Arvind et al. (2023)	Enhanced U-Net	X-rays	JSRT MC Shenzhen	93.87%.			
03	Boudoukhani et al. (2023)	Attention-gated Residual DeepLabV3+		JSRT MC Shenzhen		98.03%	96.14%	
04	Ghali and Akhloufi (2022)	Vision transformers	X-rays	JSRT MC Shenzhen	97.47%			
05	Zhang et al. (2021)	Improved U-Net	CT	LIDC/IDRI		0.8623		
06	Punn and Agarwal (2022)	Hierarchical segmentation network	CT	"COVID-19 CT dataset, COVID-19 CT Lung and Infection Segmentation Dataset"	95%	81%	89%	
07	Novikov et al. (2018)	Fully convolutional network (FCN)	X-rays	JSRT			95 %	
08	Sulaiman et al. (2023)	Deep convolutional neural networks	X-rays	MC Shenzhen	0.97	0.93	0.96	
09	Liu et al. (2022)	Improved U-Net	X -rays	JSRT MC Haut	98.55 98.94 99.41	97.92 97.82 98.84	95.73 95.55 97.43	
10	Islam et al. (2018)	U-Net based	X-rays	MC Shenzhen		98.6%		
11	Ait Skourt et al. (2018)	U-Net based	CT	LIDC/IDRI		0.9502		
12	Hu et al. (2020)	Mask R-CNN	CT		97.68			

(continued)

Table 7.1 (Continued)

S. no.	References	Model	Modality	Dataset	Accuracy	DSC	JC	F1-score
13	Singh et al. (2021)	Deep LF-Net	X-rays	JSRT MC Shenzhen	99.37% 99.37% 98.31%			
14	Ullah et al. (2023)	DED-CNN	X-rays	JSRT MC Shenzhen		97.60% 97.67% 95.68%	95.50% 95.48% 91.84%	
15	Ghali and Akhloufi (2022)	Attention RegSeg	X-rays	JSRT MC Shenzhen	95.69%			95.63%
16	Munawar et al. (2020)	GAN	X-rays	JSRT MC Shenzhen		0.9740	0.943	
17	Khanna et al. (2020)	Residual U-Net	CT	LUNA16, VESSEL12, HUG-ILD		98.63 99.62 98.68		
18	El Mansouri et al. (2022)	GAN	X-rays	JSRT		0.9778		
19	Kim and Lee (2021)	Self-attention DNN	X-rays	MC JSRT Shenzhen		0.982 0.968 0.954		
20	Liu et al. (2022)	Wavelet transformation	CT	Multimedia database of interstitial lung diseases (ilds)		98.04%	94.91%	
21	Lyu and Tian (2023)	MWG-UNet:	X-rays	JSRT Shenzhen	95.28%	92.31%		95.79 %
22	Agnes et al. (2024)	Wavelet U- Net++	CT	LIDC-IDRI		0.936	0.878.	
23	Pal et al. (2022)	Attention UW-Net	X-rays	NIH				95.7%

7.5.1 Chest X-Ray Datasets

7.5.1.1 JSRT ("Japanese Society of Radiological Technology")

The "Standard Digital Image Database of chest radiographs" with and without lung nodules was created by the "Academic Committee of the Japanese Society of Radiological Technology" in 1998, (Shiraishi et al. 2000) supported by the Japan Radiological Society (JRS) and collaborated with healthcare facilities in the United States and Japan. JSRT stands as the most frequently used dataset with renowned usage in "nodule detection and lung segmentation research," comprising "247 posteroanterior (PA) chest X-rays" with a "resolution of 2048×2048" pixels. Among these 154 CXR images are "with lung nodules" (54 benign and 100 malignant nodules) and "93 without nodules." These CXRs are stored as PNG files with a 12-bit grayscale depth. In addition, the database includes patients' details such as age, gender, diagnosis (benign or malignant), X and Y coordinates of nodules, and a basic diagram showing nodule location. Regarded as a valuable repository, this dataset has found widespread usage in various research studies focusing on the identification of lung nodules from chest X-rays. (Kaggle (2020)).

7.5.1.2 Montgomery County (MC) Dataset

The "Montgomery County (MC)" dataset is a collaborative effort between the "Department of Health and Human Services in Montgomery County, Maryland and US National Library of Medicine (USNLM)." The Montgomery dataset comprises labeled X-ray images captured in a frontal view. This data repository contains "138 posteroanterior (PA) chest X-rays" obtained through the tuberculosis (TB) screening program. Among these CXRs, 80 CXRs depict normal chest conditions without TB manifestations, while 58 exhibit indications of TB. The dataset is accompanied by ground truth masks corresponding to each X-ray image in the dataset. These masks are binary images that provide delineation of lung areas and aid in the identification of specific pulmonary regions within the X-ray images. Each CXR in the dataset is accompanied by clinical readings stored in text files (.txt), and individual ground truth masks are provided for both right and left lungs in the form of .png files. These X-ray images maintain high image quality, with a "resolution of 12 bits per pixel and a pixel size of 0.0875 mm". (Kaggle (2018)).

7.5.1.3 Shenzhen Dataset

The Shenzhen dataset, created collaboratively by "USNLM and Shenzhen No. 3 People's Hospital, Guangdong Medical College, China," comprises 662 PA chest X-rays. Out of these, 326 CXRs depict normal cases, while 336 X-rays show manifestations of TB, including some pediatric anteroposterior (AP) X-rays. The dataset contains images of different sizes, with widths ranging from 1130 to 3001 pixels and heights from 948 to 3001 pixels. Most images are approximately 3K × 3K pixels in size. The CXR images are saved with the file extension ".jpeg" and were captured using a "Philips DR Digital Diagnostic System." Only 566 ground masks are provided for these images. These images are notably high-resolution, boasting dimensions of 4020 × 4892 or 4892 × 4020 pixels. Each X-ray image within this dataset exhibits a grayscale depth of 12 bits, allowing for a comprehensive range of 4096 gray-scale levels for enhanced imaging. This repository serves as a precious asset for detailed chest imaging research and analysis due to its high-resolution images and the availability of corresponding masks for further analysis and identification of anatomical features.

7.5.1.4 Indian Dataset

The Indian dataset includes a total of 7470 medical images, corresponding to these images, 3955 detailed radiology reports are utilized for various medical applications or studies. The dataset is sourced from various hospitals affiliated with Indiana University. These hospitals likely contribute their medical images and associated reports to form this comprehensive dataset. These images and reports contribute to a comprehensive repository supporting diverse medical applications. Utilizing text-mining techniques, the dataset incorporates eight disease labels per image, enabling the association of multiple labels with individual images. This diverse labeling system facilitates image classification based on pathology, encompassing a wide range of medical conditions. The radiographs vary in dimensions from 1024 to 4248 pixels, both in width and height, initially existing in "Digital Imaging and Communications in Medicine (DICOM) format." Later, these were converted to PNG format for enhanced accessibility and standardized usage. Researchers at the US National Library of Medicine have used this dataset for distinct studies, such as CXR view classification, (Xue et al. 2015) identification of image rotations, (Santosh et al. 2015) and detection of foreign objects in these images.

7.5.1.5 National Institutes of Health Chest X-Ray Dataset (NIH)

The NIH dataset, also referred to as "chest X-ray 14", (Wang et al. 2017) is a significant repository comprising "112,120" CXR images annotated with "disease labels from 30,805 unique patients." These labels were derived using "Natural Language Processing (NLP) techniques," extracting disease classifications from the related radiological findings. This dataset encompasses 14 different thorax disease categories, along with an additional category indicating "no findings." However, the absence of definitive ground truth masks posed a significant challenge. This dataset presents a broad spectrum of pathological conditions. By providing access to this dataset, this publication aims to equip scientists with resources to enhance algorithmic training for disease identification and diagnosis, ultimately aiding physicians in making more informed and accurate diagnostic decisions.

7.5.1.6 COVID-19 Radiography Database

The "COVID-19 Chest X-ray Database" is a vast repository of medical images assembled by scholars from the "The University of Dhaka, Qatar University, Doha, and Bangladesh," in collaboration with partners from "Pakistan and Malaysia," along with medical professionals. This dataset has been progressively released in stages, with subsequent updates increasing the volume of images across different categories. All the CXR images are in PNG format and have a resolution of 299×299 pixels. The dataset is continuously evolving, with updates provided in stages. As of the latest information, it includes "3616 COVID-19 positive cases," "10,192 normal images," "6012 lung opacity images," and "1345 viral pneumonia images." The commitment is to regularly update the database with new radiographs for COVID-19 pneumonia patients. This database serves as a great resource for scientists to generate significant scholarly contributions toward addressing the COVID-19 pandemic. (Kaggle (2022)).

Type of CXR	Image Count	Source
Normal	10,192	RSNA: 8,851, Kaggle: 1,341
Lung opacity	6,012	RSNA CXR dataset
COVID-19	3,616	PadChest dataset: 2,473, German medical school: 183, Various sources: 559, Github source: 400
Viral pneumonia	1,345	"Chest X-Ray Images (pneumonia) database"

PadChest: The PadChest dataset comprises 160,868 chest X-rays derived from 109,931 studies and involves 67,000 at "San Juan Hospital" (Bustos et al. 2020) in Spain over a period from 2009 to 2017. The images are stored as 16-bit grayscale images, preserving detailed information. Among the reports associated with the X-rays, 27,593 were manually annotated by physicians. An innovative approach involved training a RNN on these labeled reports. The trained RNN was then employed to automatically label the remaining dataset based on the information extracted from the reports. The labels adhere to a hierarchical taxonomy that aligns with the standards of the Unified Medical Language System (UMLS). (Bodenreider 2004).

RSNA-Pneumonia: The RSNA-Pneumonia (RP) dataset, derived from chest X-ray 14, includes 30,000 chest X-rays (CXR) images with meticulous annotations for pneumonia. The dataset consists of 16,248 posteroanterior views, 13,752 AP views, and 4,527 test images. These digital radiographs were converted from PNG to DICOM format, containing patient details. The resolution of each radiograph is 1024 × 1024, and they are presented in 8-bit grayscale format and labeled with bounding boxes for lung opacities. The categories are normal, lung opacity, and not normal. Widely used in the "RSNA Pneumonia Detection Challenge (2018)" on Kaggle, this dataset is crucial for training and assessing machine learning models for automated pneumonia detection in Chest X-rays. (Kaggle n.d.).

7.5.2 CT Scan Datasets

With the advancement of medical imaging technology, CT scan datasets have emerged as vital tools for examining lung diseases, offering researchers access to a rich repository of medical images and associated clinical data. Some of the commonly used CT datasets for lung diseases are the following.

LIDC-IDRI: Armato et al. introduced the LIDC-IDRI dataset in "The Lung Image Database Consortium (LIDC) and Image Database Resource Initiative (IDRI): a completed reference database of lung nodules on CT scans." This dataset is a collaborative effort by the Lung Tissue Research Consortium, consisting of 1,018 low-dose lung CT scans from 1,200 patients. Enriched with lesion annotations meticulously provided by experienced thoracic radiologists, the dataset includes associated characteristics such as calcification and malignancy. This resource plays a crucial role in advancing research in lung tissue analysis and serves as a valuable reference for studying various lung conditions. The CT images in this dataset are in the DICOM format, with a total size of 125 GB and a resolution of [65,764] × 512 × 512 voxels for each scan, along with its associated metadata file. An average scan has 240 slices, with an average slice thickness of 1.73 mm. (Armato et al. 2010).

LUNA 16: The LUNA16 dataset, specialized in lung nodule detection, contains 888 sets of 3D CT images. Focused on pulmonary nodule segmentation, LUNA16 provides a rich resource for the creation and assessment of algorithms targeting the detection and characterization of pulmonary nodules.

LOLA11, an acronym for Lobe and Lung Analysis Challenge, (Lola11 n.d.) is a dataset specifically designed for challenges related to the analysis of lung lobes. Comprising 55 volumetric chest CT scans from various sources, this dataset offers a diverse range of scans that include significant pathologies and abnormalities.

SPIE-AAPM: Initiated by the "SPIE Medical Imaging Conference in collaboration with the National Cancer Institute (NCI) and the American Association of Physicists in Medicine (AAPM)," enables researchers to evaluate and contrast their methods in employing quantitative image analysis to categorize nodules as either benign or malignant. This dataset was last updated in 2014 and includes

22,489 CT scans totaling 12.1 GB in size, together with 70 patient records and supporting data that provide ground-truth information in addition to the picture. Scientists and healthcare professionals use these datasets to develop and assess deep learning algorithms, machine learning models, and various computational methods aimed at comprehending, diagnosing, and prognosticating various lung diseases. (National Lung Screening Trial (NLST) n.d.)

Lung CT-Diagnosis Dataset: This dataset was updated in 2014 and is accessible to the public through TCIA. Consisting of 61 patient's data, the dataset is kept up to date by Moffitt Cancer Center. The dataset comprises 4682 images, with a cumulative size of 2.5 GB. These images represent the CT medical imaging modality saved in DICOM format, with the "slice width ranging from 3–6 mm." Each file contains metadata containing patient details and the instance number of tumor slices. (Cancer imaging archive n.d.).

NLST dataset: The NLST dataset, updated in 2013, is a restricted-access repository, a crucial clinical study that evaluates the effectiveness of low radiation CT screening in decreasing mortality rates associated with lung cancer. In addition to pathological images, the dataset encompasses radiological images paired with pertinent clinical data. The collaborative efforts of the "National Cancer Institute's Division of Cancer Prevention and Division of Cancer Treatment and Diagnosis" underpin this project. This dataset comprises nearly 21,082,502 CT scans amounting to 11.3 TB, involving 26,254 individuals (NLST 2013). (National Cancer Institute - Cancer Data Access System n.d.).

7.6 Evaluation Metrics

Evaluation metrics are the quantitative measures used to measure the performance of a model or an algorithm. These metrics help in determining how well a model performs on a specific task. Their significance lies in facilitating comparisons between various algorithms and plays a vital role in ensuring the precision of a model in a practical context. The metrics assess the performance of the model by comparing the predicted results of the model with those of the ground truth. Ground truth means the actual lung segmentation results obtained manually by medical experts. Here's a summary of the commonly used metrics for lung segmentation in medical images.

True Positive (TP): When the model predicts something as positive which is positive. In the case of lung segmentation, the model correctly identifies the image pixels as lung pixels when they are lung pixels.

True Negative (TN): When the model predicts something as negative which is negative. In the case of lung segmentation when the system correctly classifies image pixels as non-lung pixels that do not belong to the lung region.

False Positive (FP): When the model predicts something as positive which is negative. In the case of lung segmentation when the model classifies image pixels as the lung pixels that belong to the non-lung region.

False Negative (FN): When the model classifies something as negative which is positive. In the case of lung segmentation when the model classifies image pixels as background pixels that belong to the lung region.

Here's a summary of the commonly used metrics for lung segmentation in medical images.

Accuracy: Accuracy serves as a pivotal metric for evaluating deep learning models, providing insight into their prediction capabilities. It measures the ratio of accurate predictions to the total predictions made by the model, determining the percentage of image pixels correctly classified as lung or non-lung. This computation is achieved through the following formula:

$$Accuracy = \frac{TP + TN}{TP + TN + FP + FN}$$

Jaccard Index: Also known as an overlap measure, it is the measure of similarity between ground truth mask and segmented image. It is also called IoU. It is calculated using the below formula:

$$Jaccard\ Index = \frac{TP}{TP + FP + FN}$$

Its value ranges between 0 and 1, where 0 indicates no overlap or similarity between both the predicted image and ground truth image, and 1 signifies perfect overlap, that is, both segmented image and ground truth are identical. The higher value of the Jaccard Index indicates better similarity and accuracy in the segmentation results. The Jaccard Index is considered balanced because it takes both false positives and false negatives into account. It penalizes the model for either missing or including regions that are not present in the ground truth.

Dice coefficient: The DSC measures the similarity between two sets, typically used in tasks such as image segmentation and natural language processing. This metric quantifies the overlap between the predicted segmentation and the ground truth. Again, higher DSC indicates better segmentation accuracy. It is also known as "Sorensen Dice coefficient" calculated as follows:

$$DC = \frac{2 \times TP}{2 \times TP + FP + FN}$$

Precision: Precision is a metric that measures the accuracy of positive predictions made by a model. It is calculated as the ratio of TP predictions to the total number of instances classified as positive by the model, regardless of whether those predictions are correct or incorrect. In the case of lung segmentation, it is the number of correctly classified pixels divided by the total number of pixels classified as lung pixels. Precision is an important evaluation metric when false positive predictions are costly. For example, if a model incorrectly classifies healthy tissues as cancerous. High precision means that the errors of incorrectly identifying positive values are minimized. Precision gives us the measure of the accuracy of positive predictions made by the model. It is calculated as follows:

$$Preciaion = \frac{TP}{TP + FP}$$

Recall: Also known as sensitivity, it is a measure of the ability of the model to correctly capture and identify the TPs. In case of lung segmentation, it is the probability of correctly classifying the lung pixels from an image. It is a useful metric when false negatives are more critical than false positives. It is calculated using the below formula:

$$Recall = \frac{TP}{TP + FN}$$

Specificity: In contrast to sensitivity or recall, specificity is the measure of the ability of the model to correctly identify the TNs. In the case of lung segmentation, it is the probability of correctly classifying a background (or a non-lung) pixel. It becomes a useful metric when the cost of false positives is high or when there is a focus on the accuracy of negative predictions. It offers insight into the model's capacity to filter out irrelevant data. This metric is derived using the following formula:

$$Specificity = \frac{TN}{TN + FN}$$

Specificity tells us how accurately a model can make correct negative predictions. A higher value of specificity means the model is effective at correctly identifying TNs, minimizing the occurrence of false positives. A lower value means that the model is incorrectly predicting negative instances as positive, leading to false positives.

F1-score: The F1-score is a crucial evaluation metric, offering a balanced assessment of a model's performance by considering both precision and recall. By computing the harmonic mean of precision and recall, the F1-score provides a symmetric representation of both metrics in a single value. With a maximum value of 1 representing perfect precision and recall, and a minimum value of 0 indicating either precision or recall being zero, the F1-score serves as a reliable indicator of a model's accuracy and is calculated as follows:

$$F1\ Score = \frac{2 \times Precsion \times Recall}{Precsion + Recall}$$

Hausdorff distance: Measures the maximum distance between any two points on the predicted and ground truth segmentation boundaries. Lower Hausdorff distance indicates better alignment between the segmentations.

The choice of evaluation metrics for lung segmentation or any medical image segmentation task depends on several factors, including specific goals of the segmentation, dataset characteristics, and the specific qualities desired in the evaluation metric.

7.7 Conclusion

This research study gives a broader picture of the transformative role of deep learning-based techniques, particularly in LFS, representing a significant move from traditional computer vision algorithms. Emphasis is placed on prioritizing robustness and generalizability in evaluations to mitigate the risks of overfitting to low-variability or inadequately annotated data. The review underscores the critical need for standardized datasets to effectively evaluate diverse models designed for segmentation and disease classification. Proposing future research directions, the study suggests exploring multi-modal imaging and integrating clinical data to enhance the precision of lung segmentation. Amid continuous advancements in deep learning models for medical image analysis, particularly in the context of CXR images, the study recognizes the persistent challenges in lung segmentation due to organ overlap and the presence of various anatomical structures. The ongoing research efforts, reflected in the proposed architectures, aim at improving the accuracy and robustness of segmentation. Importantly, the discussed segmentation framework holds promise for adaptation to other medical imaging modalities such as CT, thereby extending its applicability beyond CXR images. This versatility positions deep learning as a pivotal technology for diverse diagnostic and monitoring tasks in the realm of medical imaging.

References

Abdani, S.R., Zulkifley, M.A., Shahrimin, M.I., and Zulkifley, N.H. (2022). Computer-Assisted Pterygium Screening System: A Review. *Diagnostics (Basel, Switzerland)* 12 (3): 639. https://doi.org/10.3390/diagnostics12030639.

Agrawal, T. and Choudhary, P. (2023). Segmentation and classification on chest radiography: a systematic survey. *The Visual Computer* 39 (3): 875–913. https://doi.org/10.1007/s00371-021-02352-7.

Ait Skourt, B., El Hassani, A., and Majda, A. (2018). Lung CT Image Segmentation Using Deep Neural Networks. *Procedia Computer Science* 127: 109–113. https://doi.org/10.1016/j.procs.2018.01.104.

Akila Agnes, S., Arun Solomon, A., and Karthick, K. (2024). Wavelet U-Net++ for accurate lung nodule segmentation in CT scans: Improving early detection and diagnosis of lung cancer. *Biomedical Signal Processing and Control* 105: 105509. https://doi.org/10.1016/j.bspc.2023.105509.

Annangi, P., Thiruvenkadam, S., Raja, A., Xu, H., Sun, X., and Mao, L. (2010). A region based active contour method for x-ray lung segmentation using prior shape and low level features. *2010 IEEE International Symposium on Biomedical Imaging: From Nano to Macro*. https://doi.org/10.1109/isbi.2010.5490130.

Armato, S., McLennan, G., McNitt-Gray, M. et al. (2010). WE-B-201B-02: The Lung Image Database Consortium (LIDC) and Image Database Resource Initiative (IDRI): A Completed Public Database of CT scans for Lung Nodule Analysis. *Medical Physics* 37 (6Part6): 3416–3417. https://doi.org/10.1118/1.3469350.

Armato, S.G., Giger, M.L., and Mac Mahon, H. (1998). Automated lung segmentation in digitized posteroanterior chest radiographs. *Academic Radiology* 5 (4): 245–255. https://doi.org/10.1016/s1076-6332(98)80223-7.

Arvind, S., Tembhurne, J.V., Diwan, T., and Sahare, P. (2023). Improvised light weight deep CNN based U-Net for the semantic segmentation of lungs from chest X-rays. *Results in Engineering* 17: 100929. https://doi.org/10.1016/j.rineng.2023.100929.

Beyer, T., Bidaut, L., Dickson, J. et al. (2020). What scans we will read: imaging instrumentation trends in clinical oncology. *Cancer Imaging* 20 (1): https://doi.org/10.1186/s40644-020-00312-3.

Bodenreider, O. (2004). The Unified Medical Language System (UMLS): integrating biomedical terminology. *Nucleic Acids Research* 32 (Database issue): D267–D270. https://doi.org/10.1093/nar/gkh061.

Boudoukhani, N., Elberrichi, Z., Oulladji, L., and Dif, N. (2023). New attention-gated residual deep convolutional network for accurate lung segmentation in chest x-rays. *Evolving Systems.* https://doi.org/10.1007/s12530-023-09516-x.

Brown, M.S., Wilson, L.S., Doust, B.D. et al. (1998). Knowledge-based method for segmentation and analysis of lung boundaries in chest X-ray images. *Computerized Medical Imaging and Graphics* 22 (6): 463–477. https://doi.org/10.1016/s0895-6111(98)00051-2.

Bustos, A., Pertusa, A., Salinas, J.-M., and de la Iglesia-Vayá, M. (2020). PadChest: A large chest x-ray image dataset with multi-label annotated reports. *Medical Image Analysis* 66: 101797. https://doi.org/10.1016/j.media.2020.101797.

Cancer imaging archive A large-scale CT and PET/CT dataset for lung cancer diagnosis (lung-pet-ct-DX). *(*n.d.*)*. Retrieved from Https://Wiki .Cancerimagingarchive.Net/Pages/Viewpage.Action?PageId=70224216.

Candemir, S., Jaeger, S., Palaniappan, K. et al. (2014). Lung Segmentation in Chest Radiographs Using Anatomical Atlases With Nonrigid Registration. *IEEE Transactions on Medical Imaging* 33 (2): 577–590. https://doi.org/10.1109/tmi.2013.2290491.

Candemir, S., Palaniappan, K., and Akgul, Y. S. (2013, April). Multi-class regularization parameter learning for graph cut image segmentation. *2013 IEEE*

10th International Symposium on Biomedical Imaging. https://doi.org/10.1109/isbi.2013.6556813

Caselles, V., Catte, F., Coll, T., and Dibos, F. (1993). A geometric model for active contours in image processing. *Numerische Mathematik* 66 (1): 1–31. https://doi.org/10.1007/bf01385685.

Chen, L.-C., Zhu, Y., Papandreou, G. et al. (2018). Encoder-Decoder with Atrous Separable Convolution for Semantic Image Segmentation. In: *Lecture Notes in Computer Science*, 833–851. Springer International Publishing https://doi.org/10.1007/978-3-030-01234-2_49.

Cheng, D. and Goldberg, M. (1988). An Algorithm For Segmenting Chest Radiographs. In: *Visual Communications and Image Processing '88: Third in a Series* (ed. T.R. Hsing). Washington, USA: SPIE https://doi.org/10.1117/12.968961.

Ciano, G., Andreini, P., Mazzierli, T. et al. (2021). A Multi-Stage GAN for Multi-Organ Chest X-ray Image Generation and Segmentation. *Mathematics* 9 (22): 2896. https://doi.org/10.3390/math9222896.

Comelli, A., Coronnello, C., Dahiya, N. et al. (2020). Lung Segmentation on High-Resolution Computerized Tomography Images Using Deep Learning: A Preliminary Step for Radiomics Studies. *Journal of Imaging* 6 (11): 125. https://doi.org/10.3390/jimaging6110125.

Cootes, T.F., Taylor, C.J., Cooper, D.H., and Graham, J. (1995). Active Shape Models-Their Training and Application. *Computer Vision and Image Understanding* 61 (1): 38–59. https://doi.org/10.1006/cviu.1995.1004.

Dawoud, A. (2011). Lung segmentation in chest radiographs by fusing shape information in iterative thresholding. *IET Computer Vision* 5 (3): 185. https://doi.org/10.1049/iet-cvi.2009.0141.

Duryea, J. and Boone, J.M. (1995). A fully automated algorithm for the segmentation of lung fields on digital chest radiographic images. *Medical Physics* 22 (2): 183–191. https://doi.org/10.1118/1.597539.

El Mansouri, O., El Mourabit, Y., and El Habouz, Y. (2022). System segmentation of Lungs in images chest x-ray using the generative adversarial network. *ITM Web of Conferences* 43: 01020. https://doi.org/10.1051/itmconf/20224301020.

Gados, D. and Horvath, G. (n.d.). Using Heuristics for the Lung Fields Segmentation in Chest Radiographs. In: *IFMBE Proceedings*, 802–805. Berlin Heidelberg: Springer https://doi.org/10.1007/978-3-540-73044-6_208.

Ghali, R., and Akhloufi, M. A. (2022, August). ARSeg: An attention RegSeg architecture for CXR lung segmentation. *2022 IEEE 23rd International Conference on Information Reuse and Integration for Data Science (IRI)*. https://doi.org/10.1109/iri54793.2022.00068

Goodfellow, I., Pouget-Abadie, J., Mirza, M. et al. (2020). Generative adversarial networks. *Communications of the ACM* 63 (11): 139–144. https://doi.org/10.1145/3422622.

Hu, Q., Souza, L.F.D.F., Holanda, G.B. et al. (2020). An effective approach for CT lung segmentation using mask region-based convolutional neural networks. *Artificial Intelligence in Medicine* 103: 101792. https://doi.org/10.1016/j.artmed.2020.101792.

Iakovidis, D. K., and Savelonas, M. (2009, November). Active shape model aided by selective thresholding for lung field segmentation in chest radiographs. *2009 9th International Conference on Information Technology and Applications in Biomedicine*. https://doi.org/10.1109/itab. 2009.5394326

Islam, J., and Zhang, Y. (2018). Towards robust lung segmentation in chest radiographs with deep learning. arXiv. https://arxiv.org/abs/1811.12638.

Jangam, E. and Rao, A.C.S. (2019). Segmentation of Lungs from Chest X Rays Using Firefly Optimized Fuzzy C-Means and Level Set Algorithm. In: *Recent Trends in Image Processing and Pattern Recognition*, 303–311. Springer Singapore https://doi.org/10.1007/978-981-13-9184-2_27.

Kaggle. (2018) Pulmonary Chest X-Ray Abnormalities. Https://Www.Kaggle.Com/Datasets/Kmader/Pulmonary-Chest-Xray-Abnormalities?Select=Montgomery.

Kaggle. (2020) *Nodules in Chest X-rays (JSRT)*. https://Www.Kaggle.Com/Datasets/Raddar/Nodules-in-Chest-Xrays-Jsrt.

Kaggle (2022). COVID-19 Radiography Database. Kaggle. Https://Www.Kaggle.Com/Datasets/Tawsifurrahman/Covid19-Radiography-Database.

Kaggle. (n.d.). *RSNA Pneumonia Detection Challenge* | . https://Www.Kaggle.Com/c/Rsna-Pneumonia-Detection-Challenge/Data.

Khanna, A., Londhe, N.D., Gupta, S., and Semwal, A. (2020). A deep Residual U-Net convolutional neural network for automated lung segmentation in computed tomography images. *Biocybernetics and Biomedical Engineering* 40 (3): 1314–1327. https://doi.org/10.1016/j.bbe.2020.07.007.

Kim, M. and Lee, B.-D. (2021). Automatic lung segmentation on chest X-rays using self-attention deep neural network. *Sensors (Basel, Switzerland)* 21 (2): 369. https://doi.org/10.3390/s21020369.

Kumar, P., Raja, L., and Soni, P.K. (2023). CSR-NeT: lung segmentation from chest radiographs using transfer learning technique. *Proceedings of the Indian National Science Academy*. https://doi.org/10.1007/s43538-023-00223-4.

Li, L., Zheng, Y., Kallergi, M., and Clark, R.A. (2001). Improved method for automatic identification of lung regions on chest radiographs. *Academic Radiology* 8 (7): 629–638. https://doi.org/10.1016/s1076-6332(03)80688-8.

Li, X., Luo, S., Hu, Q. et al. (2016). Automatic lung field segmentation in X-ray radiographs using statistical shape and appearance models. *Journal of Medical Imaging and Health Informatics* 6 (2): 338–348. https://doi.org/10.1166/jmihi.2016.1714.

Liu, C. and Pang, M. (2020). Automatic lung segmentation based on image decomposition and wavelet transform. *Biomedical Signal Processing and Control* 61: 102032. https://doi.org/10.1016/j.bspc.2020.102032.

Liu, W., Luo, J., Yang, Y. et al. (2022). Automatic lung segmentation in chest X-ray images using improved U-Net. *Scientific Reports* 12 (1): 8649. https://doi.org/10.1038/s41598-022-12743-y.

Lola11- *Grand Challenge*. (n.d.). Retrieved from https://Lola11.Grand-Challenge.Org/.

Luo, H., Gaborski, R., and Acharya, R. (2000). Automatic segmentation of lung regions in chest radiographs: a model guided approach. *Proceedings 2000 International Conference on Image Processing (Cat. No.00CH37101)*. https://doi.org/10.1109/icip.2000.899459

Lyu, Y. and Tian, X. (2023). MWG-UNet: hybrid deep learning framework for lung fields and heart segmentation in chest X-ray images. *Bioengineering (Basel, Switzerland)* 10 (9): 1091. https://doi.org/10.3390/bioengineering10091091.

McNitt-Gray, M. F., Sayre, J. W., Huang, H. K., and Razavi, M. (1993). Pattern classification approach to segmentation of chest radiographs ; In M. H. Loew (Ed.), *Proceedings Medical Imaging 1993: Image Processing. SPIE*. https://doi.org/10.1117/12.154500

Mittal, A., Hooda, R., and Sofat, S. (2017). Lung field segmentation in chest radiographs: a historical review, current status, and expectations from deep learning. *IET Image Processing* 11 (11): 937–952. https://doi.org/10.1049/iet-ipr.2016.0526.

Munawar, F., Azmat, S., Iqbal, T. et al. (2020). Segmentation of Lungs in Chest X-Ray Image Using Generative Adversarial Networks. *IEEE Access* 8: 153535–153545. https://doi.org/10.1109/access.2020.3017915.

National Cancer Institute - Cancer Data Access System. (n.d.). NLST - the Cancer Data Access System. https://Cdas.Cancer.Gov/Nlst/.

National Lung Screening Trial (NLST) (National Lung Screening Trial (NLST) - National Lung Screening Trial (NLST) Public Access - Cancer Imaging Archive Wiki. (n.d.). *Available at:* Https://Wiki.Cancerimagingarchive.Net/Display/NLST.

Negahdar, M., Beymer, D., and Syeda-Mahmood, T. F. (2018). Automated volumetric lung segmentation of thoracic CT images using fully convolutional neural network. In K. Mori and N. Petrick (Eds.), *Proceedings Medical Imaging 2018: Computer-Aided Diagnosis*. SPIE. https://doi.org/10.1117/12.2293723

Novikov, A.A., Lenis, D., Major, D. et al. (2018). Fully Convolutional Architectures for Multiclass Segmentation in Chest Radiographs. *IEEE Transactions on Medical Imaging* 37 (8): 1865–1876. https://doi.org/10.1109/tmi.2018.2806086.

Pal, D., Reddy, P.B., and Roy, S. (2022). Attention UW-Net: A fully connected model for automatic segmentation and annotation of chest X-ray. *Computers in Biology and Medicine* 150: 106083. https://doi.org/10.1016/j.compbiomed.2022.106083.

Powell, G.F., Doi, K., and Katsuragawa, S. (1988). Localization of inter-rib spaces for lung texture analysis and computer-aided diagnosis in digital chest images. *Medical Physics* 15 (4): 581–587. https://doi.org/10.1118/1.596209.

Punn, N.S. and Agarwal, S. (2022). CHS-Net: A Deep Learning Approach for Hierarchical Segmentation of COVID-19 via CT Images. *Neural Processing Letters* 54 (5): 3771–3792. https://doi.org/10.1007/s11063-022-10785-x.

Rahman, M. F., Tseng, T.-L. B., Pokojovy, M., Qian, W., Totada, B., and Xu, H. (2021). An automatic approach to lung region segmentation in chest x-ray images using adapted U-Net architecture. In H. Bosmans, W. Zhao, and L. Yu (Eds.), *Proceedings Medical Imaging 2021: Physics of Medical Imaging. SPIE*. https://doi.org/10.1117/12.2581882

Rahman, M.F., Zhuang, Y., Tseng, T.-L. et al. (2022). Improving lung region segmentation accuracy in chest X-ray images using a two-model deep learning ensemble approach. *Journal of Visual Communication and Image Representation* 85: 103521. https://doi.org/10.1016/j.jvcir.2022.103521.

Ronneberger, O., Fischer, P., and Brox, T. (2015). U-Net: Convolutional Networks for Biomedical Image Segmentation. In: *Medical Image Computing and Computer-Assisted Intervention– MICCAI 2015*, 234–241. Springer International Publishing https://doi.org/10.1007/978-3-319-24574-4_28.

Roy, R., Chakraborti, T., and Chowdhury, A.S. (2019). A deep learning-shape driven level set synergism for pulmonary nodule segmentation. *Pattern Recognition Letters* 123: 31–38. https://doi.org/10.1016/j.patrec.2019.03.004.

Santosh, K.C., Candemir, S., Jaeger, S. et al. (2015). Automatically Detecting Rotation in Chest Radiographs Using Principal Rib-Orientation Measure for Quality Control. *International Journal of Pattern Recognition and Artificial Intelligence* 29 (02): 1557001. https://doi.org/10.1142/s0218001415570013.

Setio, A.A.A., Ciompi, F., Litjens, G. et al. (2016). Pulmonary Nodule Detection in CT Images: False Positive Reduction Using Multi-View Convolutional Networks. *IEEE Transactions on Medical Imaging* 35 (5): 1160–1169. https://doi.org/10.1109/tmi.2016.2536809.

Shao, Y., Gao, Y., Guo, Y. et al. (2014). Hierarchical Lung Field Segmentation With Joint Shape and Appearance Sparse Learning. *IEEE Transactions on Medical Imaging* 33 (9): 1761–1780. https://doi.org/10.1109/tmi.2014.2305691.

Shi, Y., Qi, F., Xue, Z. et al. (2008). Segmenting Lung Fields in Serial Chest Radiographs Using Both Population-Based and Patient-Specific Shape Statistics. *IEEE Transactions on Medical Imaging* 27 (4): 481–494. https://doi.org/10.1109/tmi.2007.908130.

Shi, Z., Zhou, P., He, L., Nakamura, T., Yao, Q., and Itoh, H. (2009). Lung segmentation in chest radiographs by means of gaussian kernel-based FCM with spatial constraints. *2009 Sixth International Conference on Fuzzy Systems and Knowledge Discovery*. https://doi.org/10.1109/fskd.2009.811

Shiraishi, J., Katsuragawa, S., Ikezoe, J. et al. (2000). Development of a Digital Image Database for Chest Radiographs With and Without a Lung Nodule. *American Journal of Roentgenology* 174 (1): 71–74. https://doi.org/10.2214/ajr.174.1.1740071.

Singh, A., Lall, B., Panigrahi, B.K. et al. (2021). Deep LF-Net: Semantic lung segmentation from Indian chest radiographs including severely unhealthy images. *Biomedical Signal Processing and Control* 68: 102666. https://doi.org/10.1016/j.bspc.2021.102666.

Souza, J.C., Bandeira Diniz, J.O., Ferreira, J.L. et al. (2019). An automatic method for lung segmentation and reconstruction in chest X-ray using deep neural networks. *Computer Methods and Programs in Biomedicine* 177: 285–296. https://doi.org/10.1016/j.cmpb.2019.06.005.

Stofa, M.M., Zulkifley, M.A., and Zainuri, M.A.A.M. (2021). Skin Lesions Classification and Segmentation: A Review. *International Journal of Advanced Computer Science and Applications* 12 (10): https://doi.org/10.14569/ijacsa.2021.0121060.

Sulaiman, A., Anand, V., Gupta, S. et al. (2023). A Convolutional Neural Network Architecture for Segmentation of Lung Diseases Using Chest X-ray Images. *Diagnostics (Basel, Switzerland)* 13 (9): 1651. https://doi.org/10.3390/diagnostics13091651.

Thanoon, M.A., Zulkifley, M.A., Mohd Zainuri, M.A.A., and Abdani, S.R. (2023). A Review of Deep Learning Techniques for Lung Cancer Screening and Diagnosis Based on CT Images. *Diagnostics (Basel, Switzerland)* 13 (16): 2617. https://doi.org/10.3390/diagnostics13162617.

Ullah, I., Ali, F., Shah, B. et al. (2023). A deep learning based dual encoder-decoder framework for anatomical structure segmentation in chest X-ray images. *Scientific Reports* 13 (1): 791. https://doi.org/10.1038/s41598-023-27815-w.

Van Ginneken, B., Ter Haar Romeny, B.M., and Viergever, M.A. (2001). Computer-aided diagnosis in chest radiography: a survey. *IEEE Transactions on Medical Imaging* 20 (12): 1228–1241. https://doi.org/10.1109/42.974918.

Vittitoe, N.F., Vargas-Voracek, R., and Floyd, C.E. (1998). Identification of lung regions in chest radiographs using Markov random field modeling. *Medical Physics* 25 (6): 976–985. https://doi.org/10.1118/1.598405.

Wang, X., Peng, Y., Lu, L., Lu, Z., Bagheri, M., and Summers, R. M. (2017, July). ChestX-Ray8: Hospital-Scale chest X-ray database and benchmarks on weakly-supervised classification and localization of common thorax diseases. *2017 IEEE Conference on Computer Vision and Pattern Recognition (CVPR)*. https://doi.org/10.1109/cvpr.2017.369

Wu, G., Zhang, X., Luo, S., and Hu, Q. (2015). Lung segmentation based on customized active shape model from digital radiography chest images. *Journal of Medical Imaging and Health Informatics* 5 (2): 184–191. https://doi.org/10.1166/jmihi.2015.1382.

Xu, M., Qi, S., Yue, Y. et al. (2019). Segmentation of lung parenchyma in CT images using CNN trained with the clustering algorithm generated dataset. *Biomedical Engineering Online* 18 (1): 2. https://doi.org/10.1186/s12938-018-0619-9.

Xu, X. and Doi, K. (1995). Image feature analysis for computer-aided diagnosis: Accurate determination of ribcage boundary in chest radiographs. *Medical Physics* 22 (5): 617–626. https://doi.org/10.1118/1.597549.

Xue, Z., You, D., Candemir, S., Jaeger, S., Antani, S., Long, L. R., and Thoma, G. R. (2015, June). Chest X-ray image view classification. *2015 IEEE 28th International Symposium on Computer-Based Medical Systems*. https://doi.org/10.1109/cbms.2015.49

Yahyatabar, M., Jouvet, P., and Cheriet, F. (2020, July). Dense-Unet: a light model for lung fields segmentation in Chest X-Ray images. *2020 42nd Annual International Conference of the IEEE Engineering in Medicine andamp; Biology Society (EMBC)*. https://doi.org/10.1109/embc44109.2020.9176033

Zhang, G., Cong, L., Wang, L., and Guo, W. (2014). Lung Fields Segmentation Algorithm in Chest Radiography. In: *Advances in Image and Graphics Technologies*, 137–144. Berlin Heidelberg: Springer https://doi.org/10.1007/978-3-662-45498-5_16.

Zhang, X., Li, S., Zhang, B. et al. (2021). Automatic detection and segmentation of lung nodules in different locations from CT images based on adaptive α-hull algorithm and DenseNetconvolutional network. *International Journal of Imaging Systems and Technology* 31 (4): 1882–1893. https://doi.org/10.1002/ima.22580.

Zhang, X., Liu, X., Zhang, B., Dong, J., Zhang, B., Zhao, S., and Li, S. (2021). Accurate segmentation for different types of lung nodules on CT images using improved U-Net convolutional network. Medicine, 100 (40)): e27491. https://doi.org/10.1097/MD.0000000000027491.

Zulkifley, M.A., Moubark, A.M., Saputro, A.H., and Abdani, S.R. (2022). Automated apple recognition system using semantic segmentation networks with group and shuffle operators. *Agriculture* 12 (6): 756. https://doi.org/10.3390/agriculture12060756.

8

Generative Adversarial Networks in the Field of Medical Image Segmentation

Bisma Sultan, Aasia Rehman, and Lubna Riyaz

Department of Computer Science, University of Kashmir, Srinagar, Jammu and Kashmir, India

8.1 Introduction

Recently, a lot of people in the medical imaging field have become interested in using deep learning (DL) to separate out normal or abnormal structures. It has been found to work amazingly well in a wide range of imaging methods and clinical settings to help doctors with computer-assisted diagnosis, therapy, or planning surgeries. The growing amount of medical data that doctors need to look at for diagnosis, treatment, or surgical planning has led to the creation of computer-aided image analysis tools that can use the accurate, quick, repeatable, and objective measurements that computers can make. Medical image segmentation, which aims to identify the boundaries of anatomical or pathological entities from medical images, is still one of the most important analysis jobs now in use. Image segmentation, a fundamental component of many computer-aided detection and diagnosis techniques, is used to analyze various imaging modalities, such as computed tomography (CT), magnetic resonance imaging (MRI), positron emission tomography (PET), or ultrasound (US).

Traditionally, medical images are manually delineated for anatomical or pathological structures. To obtain clinically useful outlines, this task is time-consuming and requires appropriate clinical knowledge. This does not apply to significant amounts of data usually generated in clinical or research projects. Manual segmentation is vulnerable to significant intra- and inter-expert variability because of the possible weariness of human specialists and the large variances in expertise. Prior to the development of learning approaches, segmentation was achieved by the widespread use of mathematical models and low-level image

Deep Learning Applications in Medical Image Segmentation: Overview, Approaches, and Challenges, First Edition. Edited by Sajid Yousuf Bhat, Aasia Rehman, and Muhammad Abulaish.

processing. In clinical settings, model-based segmentation using statistical shape models has been used (Heimann and Meinzer 2009). Internal shape fitting and auto-correction have improved these models by guiding delineation with shape information (Kim et al. 2017). Additionally, certain hybrid techniques that use statistical shape models restricted by probabilistic atlases have been studied. Bayesian methods utilizing expectation–maximization (Van Leemput et al. 1999), possibility clustering (Barra and Boire 2002), histogram-based thresholding, followed by region growth (Purushwalkam et al. 2013), active contours (Zhou et al. 2016), and, more recently, machine learning (ML) (Conze et al. 2017) techniques have all been used to segment images. High levels of intersubject shape variability, weak borders, and noticeable variations in tissue appearance make the aforementioned techniques less than ideal. Typically, their resilience falls short when confronted with the intrinsic challenges of medical imaging, including noise, nonuniform contrasts, and motion aberrations. In addition, there are significant computational costs involved with these methods because many of them are semi-automatic and, as a result, require prior information. Because of this, DL methods have been developed to take advantage of image features (such as variations in contrast, orientation, form, and texture patterns) more effectively using data-driven means.

Recently, Artificial Intelligence (AI) and DL models have excelled in medical image segmentation, becoming the current state-of-the-art. There is now a shift occurring between systems that rely on manually created features (ML) and systems that derive features directly from data (DL). Convolutional neural networks (CNNs) are the foundation of the most popular models in use today. The U-Net convolutional architecture (Ronneberger et al. 2015) in particular has been widely accepted due to its capacity to output comprehensive delineations with a relatively small quantity of training data. However, new attention-based paradigms have emerged alongside the growing interest in models based on pure and hybrid Transformers (Shamshad et al. 2023).

Since its inception in 2014, generative adversarial networks (GANs), a DL model, has garnered substantial attention in both academic and industrial circles, experiencing rapid growth in popularity. Currently, numerous high-caliber papers have been published and discussed extensively, while various AI-focused companies dedicate considerable efforts to advancing and advocating GAN models. Our analysis reveals that GAN's utilization in medical image segmentation emerged around 2016. In recent years, owing to GAN's distinct advantages like reduced training data requirements, impressive generation capabilities, and seamless integration with other neural networks, GAN-based segmentation methods have seen a notable rise in their application within medical image research. The utilization of GANs has demonstrated significant enhancements in the outcomes of medical image segmentation, showcasing their efficacy and impact in this specific domain. This indicates a positive trend toward the integration of advanced DL techniques, particularly GANs, in the field of medical imaging, contributing to improved accuracy and reliability in segmentation processes. A review of the GAN-based image segmentation techniques is presented in this paper. For completeness, the recent non-DL image segmentation techniques are also discussed briefly. GAN principles and its representatives are described. Various image segmentation methods, utilizing these GAN models, are reviewed. The segmentation techniques are classified here into three main categories: the segmentation regions, imaging modality, and classification methods. The main ideas of the important GAN-based segmentation techniques are described. In our quest for relevant research papers, we engaged in thorough exploration across academic platforms such as Google Scholar and PubMed. Our search strategy involved employing specific keywords such as "segmentation," "medical image," and "GAN." Furthermore, we expanded our inquiry by conducting additional searches on Semantic Scholar, Springer, and arXiv, as well as exploring leading conferences in computer science. The primary focus during these searches was on keywords associated with GAN, ensuring a comprehensive and exhaustive approach to identifying pertinent literature.

The rest of the paper is organized as follows: Section 2 discusses methods for accessing the effectiveness of image segmentation methods. Section 3 gives a preview of image segmentation techniques. Section 4 presents the GAN model and its key variants. Section 5 gives the classification of GAN-based image segmentation methods. Results and discussions are presented in Section 6. The conclusion is finally presented in Section 7.

8.2 Overview of Image Segmentation Techniques

The recent medical image segmentation approaches are reviewed in this section.

8.2.1 Traditional Methods for Segmentation of Images

Traditional approaches for medical image segmentation encompass a range of established techniques rooted in classical computer vision and image processing. These methods, such as thresholding, edge-based models, region-growing models, and graph-cut models, rely on mathematical and algorithmic principles to partition medical images into distinct regions or structures.

Thresholding involves dividing an input image into regions based on a chosen threshold, and multiple thresholds can be employed in multi-threshold segmentation (Senthilkumaran and Vaithegi 2016). Selecting an appropriate threshold is challenging, as higher values may lead to fragmented boundaries and overlook subtle segments. Thresholding is sensitive to noise and lacks spatial linkage awareness between different image characteristics. Thresholding has been applied in a number of applications, like brain tumor detection from MRI images and its combination with other techniques. Wittke et al. (Wittke et al. 2007) employed classification-based thresholding to produce a binary image from histological slide sections of prostate carcinoma. While thresholding is easy and fast, finding the optimal threshold automatically can be complex, and iterative thresholding may be necessary for noisy images like CT scans or ultrasound images. Overall, thresholding is a widely used method but requires careful consideration for effective application.

Edge-based methods rely on edge detection to identify boundaries and object contours. Various edge detection operators rely on gradient (derivative) functions, including but not limited to Roberts, Prewitt, Sobel, Marr–Hildreth, Laplacian, and Canny edge detectors (Song et al. 2017). The Canny edge detector, in particular, is highlighted for its optimization involving edge enhancement and tracing. Edge-based segmentation addresses challenges like under-segmentation, over-segmentation, and false edges. Kattire et al. (Shah (n.d.)) presented a two-stage method wherein they initially acquire edge information by considering the magnitude and direction of the image gradient, and subsequently generate the edge map based on the texture. While edge-based methods are simple, they may perform poorly in the presence of noise, and some edge detectors are suitable for X-ray pre-processing.

In the Region Growing Method, pixels are grouped into homogeneous regions by iteratively expanding from seed points. The growth of each region is guided by a similarity criterion, often defined as the difference between a pixel's intensity value and the mean intensity of the region. However, region-growing methods often need manual seed setting, making them sensitive to noise and resulting in regions with holes. Challenges include finding appropriate thresholding values, especially in noisy images. Despite their simplicity and ease of implementation, region-growing approaches have drawbacks, including the need for manual interaction, sensitivity to initialization, high processing time, and the potential for non-connected regions. Tan et al. (Tan et al. 2017) suggested an approach for detecting tumors in PET images by employing adaptive region growth with a maximum curvature strategy (ARG-MC).

Graph-cut-based segmentation methods have proven effective for optimal global segmentation. These methods transform segmentation into a maximum flow problem with polynomial time complexity, treating the image as a graph where nodes represent pixels/voxels, including special nodes for the source (S) and sink (t) connected by t-edges and other nodes connected by n-edges. Object (O) and background (B) seeds are denoted, and the goal is to achieve an optimal cut distinguishing objects from the background. Popular algorithms include normalized cuts and minimum cuts. The methods, suitable for various image modalities, are not considered complex, generally moderate in speed, and yield excellent results when prior shape information is available. Multiple graph-based contributions in the literature share similarities but differ in defining hard constraints and designing energy functions for optimization. Chen et al. (Chen et al. 2012) employed a blend of graph cuts and graph search for the segmentation of symptomatic exudate-associated derangement (SEAD). In their method, they skillfully integrated a classifier based on probability constraints into the approach utilizing graph search/graph cuts. The method demonstrated excellent accuracy.

8.2.2 Deep Learning Methods for Segmentation of Images

Medical images enable detailed examination of organ structures and facilitate quantitative analysis to assess clinical features related to shape and volume, particularly in studies of organs like the brain and heart. This analysis is achieved through the segmentation of organs and anatomical features. Various DL methodologies have been developed for segmenting organs in medical image analysis.

Several studies have proposed using DL for brain segmentation. For instance, H. Chen et al. (2018b) introduced a voxel-wise residual network (VoxResNet), which incorporates residual units to address the degradation issue that can occur when training very deep neural networks. This approach ensures performance improvements with increased network depth are fully realized. Authors (Borne et al. (n.d.)) proposed a cascaded V-Net approach for brain tumor segmentation, breaking the task into two steps: segmenting the entire tumor and delineating its distinct regions.

In the domain of retinal imaging, segmentation of blood vessels is crucial for diagnosing various eye conditions. The pioneering work of Liskowski and Krawiec (Liskowski and Krawiec 2016) employed a deep CNN for retinal blood vessel segmentation. Following this, CNNs have been extensively used for this task. Authors in Guo et al. (2019) presented a method involving pre-processing techniques to enhance low-contrast retinal images using a multi-scale, multilevel CNN with short connections to extract retinal vessels. Authors in Yan, Yang and Cheng (2019) developed a three-stage DL model to segment both thick and thin retinal vessels.

Lung image segmentation is essential for the accurate analysis of lung CT images in lung cancer detection. Authors in Ait Skourt, El Hassani, and Majda (2018) used the U-Net architecture for lung segmentation in CT images. Authors in Yahyatabar, Jouvet, and Cheriet (2020) tackled lung segmentation in chest X-rays, introducing Dense-U-Net based on U-Net to enhance information flow, facilitating faster model convergence and reducing parameters while maintaining high performance. Authors in Guo et al. (2019) introduced CE-Net, which uses dense atrous convolution and residual multi-kernel pooling for feature extraction, applied to various 2D medical image segmentation tasks, including lung and retinal optical coherence tomography (OCT) layer segmentation.

In abdominal imaging from CT and MRI scans, segmentation identifies structures such as the liver, pancreas, and kidneys. Authors in Christ et al. (2017) developed cascaded fully convolutional neural networks (CFCNs) for automatic segmentation of the liver and lesions in abdominal images. This network uses two cascaded fully convolutional networks (FCNs), where the first segments the liver's region of interest (ROI), and the second identifies lesions within this ROI. Authors in Zhao et al. (2020) introduced a multi-scale supervised 3D U-Net (MSS) for segmenting kidneys and kidney tumors in CT images. Authors in Man et al. (2019) proposed a method inspired by a deep Q-network (DQN) with a deformable U-Net for pancreas segmentation, using 3D volume split into 2D slices along three axes.

For cardiac imaging, achieving automated heart region segmentation is crucial due to the significant threat posed by cardiac diseases. Authors in Xu, Wu, and Feng (2018) combined Faster R-CNN for rapid detection with 3D U-Net for powerful segmentation, introducing Conditional Function (CFUN) for comprehensive heart segmentation. Authors in Yan, Yang, and Cheng (2019) developed a deep-supervised 3D U-Net to enhance contextual information extraction at various network depths. Authors in Xia et al. (2019) introduced a two-stage framework for automated segmentation of atrial catheters, using a 3D U-Net for initial atrial center identification and another 3D U-Net for precise segmentation.

In breast ultrasound imaging, authors in Xia et al. (2019) divided images into four primary tissues – skin, fibro glandular tissue, mass, and fatty tissue – using three orthogonal image planes. A CNN was used to identify the tissue class of the central pixel within image blocks.

8.3 Generative Adversarial Networks

This section presents the core principles of GANs and elucidates various notable variations. These variants encompass a spectrum of advancements within the GAN framework, incorporating conditional generative adversarial networks (CGANs), deep convolutional generative adversarial networks (DCGANs), information generative adversarial networks (InfoGANs), auxiliary classifier generative adversarial networks (AC-GANs), Wasserstein generative adversarial networks (Wasserstein-GANs), cycle generative adversarial networks (Cycle-GANs), and progressively growing generative adversarial networks (ProGANs), among others.

8.3.1 Vanilla GAN

One of the most highly contested subjects within the field of ML is the concept of GANs, a generative technique introduced by Goodfellow and his colleagues in 2014 (Goodfellow et al. 2020). The remarkable success of GANs in a range of applications such as image processing (Ledig et al. 2017; Kazeminia et al. 2020), artistic style transfer (Knyaz et al. 2019; Zhang et al. 2019), classification (Israel et al. 2017), medical imaging, and image generation (Li et al. 2018; Lin et al. 2017) underscores the substantial progress GANs have made in various computer vision tasks. GAN models have been proposed in numerous variations across different domains over time. In recent years, GANs have emerged as one of the most actively researched algorithms in the realm of DL.

Within GANs, there are two crucial components: the generator and the discriminator. These two components can be implemented using any differentiable system that transforms data from one space to another, although neural networks are commonly employed for this purpose. MLPs were utilized in the generator G and discriminator D of the initial GANs. The role of the generator is to create new data samples while attempting to mimic the distribution of real-world examples. On the other hand, the discriminator typically functions as a binary classifier, aiming to distinguish between generated instances and real instances.

GANs are optimized through a Minimax optimization problem. This optimization process converges at a saddle point, which represents the maximum for the discriminator and the minimum for the generator. In essence, the goal of GAN optimization is to reach Nash equilibrium, at which point the generator accurately captures the distribution of real-world examples.

8.3.1.1 GAN Framework

The GAN framework (as illustrated in Figure 8.1) proves to be quite straightforward when both models are neural networks. To grasp the generator distribution, p_g, regarding the data, x, a prior is established for input noise variables known as $p_z(z)$ (Goodfellow et al. 2020), with z representing the noise variable. The generator then functions as a mapping from the noise space to the data space, denoted as $G(z, \theta_g)$. This mapping is executed using a neural network with parameters θ_g. On the other hand, another neural network, $D(x, \theta_d)$, is defined, also equipped with parameters θ_d. The output of $D(x)$ provides a singular scalar, representing the likelihood that x originates from the real training data rather than being a product of the GAN model G. The aim of training the discriminator, D, is to enhance its

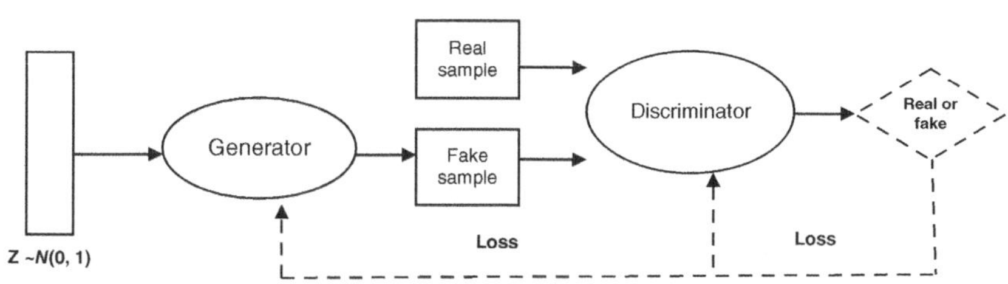

Figure 8.1 GAN framework.

ability to correctly classify both genuine training data and synthetic instances produced by the generator G. Simultaneously, G is trained to minimize the term log $(1-D(G(z)))$.

In the realm of GANs, various objective functions can be applied. The initial objective function in GANs involves a minimax game between G and D, which can be expressed as follows (Equation 8.1):

$$\underset{G}{Min}\,\underset{D}{Max}\,V(D,G) = E_{x\sim p_{data}(x)}[\log D(x)] + E_{z\sim p_z(z)}[\log(1-D(G(z)))] \tag{8.1}$$

$\log D(x)$ denotes the cross-entropy between $[1\ 0]^T$ and $[D(x)\ 1-D(x)]^T$

$\log(1-D(G(z)))$ denotes the cross-entropy between $[1\ 0]^T$ and $[D(G(z))\ 1-D(G(z))]^T$

The ideal solution for a fixed G is given in Equation 8.2:

$$D^*{}_G(x) = \frac{p_{data}(x)}{p_{data}(x) + p_g(x)} \tag{8.2}$$

In certain situations, the gradient produced by Equation 8.1 may prove insufficient for effective learning by G. Early in the training process, G may generate examples that significantly deviate from the training data, leading to D's confident rejection of these initially generated instances. This often results in $\log(1-D(G(z)))$ becoming saturated. As an alternative, instead of minimizing $\log(1-D(G(z)))$, G can be trained to maximize $\log(D(G(z)))$. Consequently, the generator's cost can be expressed in Equation 8.3:

$$J(G) = E_{z\sim p_z(z)}[-\log(D(G(z)))] = E_{x\sim p_g}[-\log D(x)] \tag{8.3}$$

8.3.2 GAN Variants

In the following subsection, we will provide an introduction to a noteworthy GAN variant.

8.3.2.1 InfoGAN

The InfoGAN (Chen et al. 2016) introduced a different approach to noise vectors. Instead of using a single unstructured noise vector, it proposed decomposing the input noise into two distinct components: z, which represents incompressible noise, and c, known as the latent code. This latent code is designed to capture the essential structured semantic features found in the real data distribution. InfoGAN (Chen et al. 2016) seeks to minimize the objective function given in Equation 8.4:

$$\underset{G}{min}\,\underset{D}{max}\,V_{info}(D,G) = V(D,G) - \lambda\, I(c; G(z,c)) \tag{8.4}$$

- $V(D, G)$ stands for the original GANs' objective function
- $G(z, c)$ represents the generated example

- I denotes mutual information
- λ serves as a customizable regularization parameter.

The objective is to maximize $I(c; G(z, c))$, which enhances the mutual information between c and $G(z, c)$, ensuring that c contains as many critical and meaningful features from real examples as possible. However, in practice, optimizing $I(c; G(z,c))$ directly is challenging since it necessitates access to the posterior distribution $P(c|x)$.

A viable solution is to establish a lower bound for $I(c; G(z, c))$ by introducing an auxiliary distribution, $Q(c|x)$, to approximate $P(c|x)$. The final objective function for InfoGAN (Chen et al. 2016) is then defined as in Equation 8.5:

$$\frac{min}{G}\frac{max}{D}V_{info}(D,G) = V(D,G) - \lambda\, L_{info}(c;Q) \tag{8.5}$$

- $l_{info}\ (c; Q)$ represents the lower bound for $I\ (c; G(z, c))$.

InfoGAN also features various variants, including causal InfoGAN (Kurutach et al. 2018) and semi-supervised InfoGAN (ss-InfoGAN) (Spurr et al. 2017).

8.3.2.2 DCGAN

DCGAN (Radford et al. 2016) unites GANs with CNNs, a powerful approach to computer vision. DCGAN introduces specific constraints on the network architecture of CNN to ensure stable training and to leverage learned feature representations for image classification. DCGAN enhances the quality of generated images through the following three key improvements.

- DCGAN employs strided convolutions for the discriminator and fractional strided convolutions for the generator, replacing conventional pooling layers. While CNNs are typically used for feature extraction, the CNN structure in DCGAN is tasked with generating samples, marking a departure from its usual role in feature extraction. Strided and fractional-strided convolutions efficiently transmit the majority of information to the subsequent layer, ensuring the completeness and clarity of the generated samples.
- DCGAN incorporates the batch normalization algorithm to tackle the problem of vanishing gradients. This algorithm resolves issues stemming from poor initializations, facilitates the propagation of gradients through each layer, and prevents the generator from converging all samples to a single point.
- DCGAN embraces various activation functions, including the Adam optimization method, the ReLU activation function, and the leakyReLU activation function. Empirical results affirm the strong performance of DCGAN in practical applications, underscoring the GAN structure's ability to generate samples. DCGAN is widely acknowledged as the gold standard when compared to other GAN models.

8.3.2.3 cGAN

GAN, as an unsupervised learning technique, derives the probability distribution patterns from unannotated datasets and expresses them in a gradual and unconstrained manner. Yet, when dealing with intricate or extensive datasets, GAN faces challenges in managing the outcomes it generates. To address this issue, a straightforward approach is to introduce constraints and establish specific objectives for the generator. GANs can be expanded into a conditional model when both the discriminator and the generator take extra information y into account. The objective function for conditional GANs (Mirza and Osindero 2014) can be compared to that of InfoGAN, as seen in Equations (8.5) and (8.6). However, in InfoGAN, the latent code c is not known in advance; it is actually discovered during training. Additionally, InfoGAN incorporates an extra network, Q, which outputs the conditional variables Q(c|x).

$$\frac{min}{G}\frac{max}{D} = E_{x\sim p_{data}(x)}[\log(x/y)] + E_{z\sim p_z(z)}[\log(1 - D(G(z/y)))] \tag{8.6}$$

Building upon the foundation of CGANs, it becomes possible to generate examples conditioned on various factors such as class labels, text bounding boxes, and key points.

8.3.2.4 ACGAN

Auxiliary Classifier Generative Adversarial Network (ACGAN) (Odena et al. 2017) is an advanced CGAN specialized in image synthesis. By simply providing a class label, it can generate an image from scratch. Notably, ACGAN produces images with higher resolution compared to earlier methods. The ACGAN's loss function is divided into two parts as given in Equations 8.7 and 8.8:

$$L_G = E[\log P(S = real\ |X_{real})] + E[\log P(S = Fake\ |X_{fake})] \tag{8.7}$$

$$L_C = E[\log P(C = c\ |X_{real})] + E[\log P(C = c\ |X_{fake})] \tag{8.8}$$

In this context, L_G represents the log-likelihood for evaluating the source's authenticity, while L_C corresponds to the log-likelihood for classifying the category or class. The training process involves the generator aiming to maximize the difference between L_C and L_G, while the discriminator is trained to maximize their sum, $L_C + L_G$.

AC-GAN achieved a significant milestone as the first GAN variant capable of generating recognizable samples for all classes in the ImageNet dataset (Fei-Fei et al. 2010).

8.3.2.5 WGAN

In reference (Arjovsky et al. 2017), the authors introduced the Wasserstein distance, also known as the Earth-Mover (EM) distance, in the context of GANs for quantifying the dissimilarity between real and generated samples, as opposed to using the JavaScript (JS) divergence. The Wasserstein distance is defined in Equation 8.9:

$$W(p_r, p_g) = \frac{inf}{\gamma \sim \prod(p_r, p_g)} E_{(x,y)\sim\gamma}[||x - y||] \tag{8.9}$$

where $\Pi(p_r, p_g)$ represents the set of all possible joint distributions combining p_r and p_g, and γ encompasses all conceivable distributions.

The Wasserstein distance offers several advantages. It can calculate distances between distributions even when they do not overlap, possesses excellent smoothing characteristics, and mitigates the issue of gradient vanishing to some extent. Furthermore, the Wasserstein GAN (WGAN) addresses training instability problems and enhances the diversity of generated samples, eliminating the need for intricate balancing in the training of the generator (G) and discriminator (D).

8.4 Classification of GAN-Based Image Segmentation Techniques

The categorization of medical image segmentation techniques utilizing GANs is delineated into three overarching classifications as shown in Figure 8.2, each contingent on the employed segmentation strategy. These categories encompass segmentation area, modality, and the specific GAN model employed in the process. This systematic classification provides a structured framework for understanding and organizing the diverse approaches within the realm of medical image segmentation based on GANs. This three-tiered classification system not only facilitates a comprehensive understanding of the diverse approaches within GAN-based medical image segmentation but also serves as a valuable framework for researchers and practitioners in navigating the evolving landscape of this specialized field.

8.4.1 Classification on the Basis of Segmentation Area

This section categorizes different medical image segmentation methods that utilize GAN, focusing on the specific anatomical regions targeted for segmentation. The study comprehensively examines several segmentation areas, encompassing the brain, eyes, chest and breast, heart, abdomen, pelvis, and bones. In essence, it systematically analyzes and classifies GAN-based techniques with a specific emphasis on the anatomical structures they are designed to segment.

8.4.1.1 Brain Segmentation Using GAN

Identifying and distinguishing between healthy and abnormal brain tissues is a widely studied area within medical image processing. This field aims to differentiate diseased parts from normal ones, enabling precise brain analysis for accurate

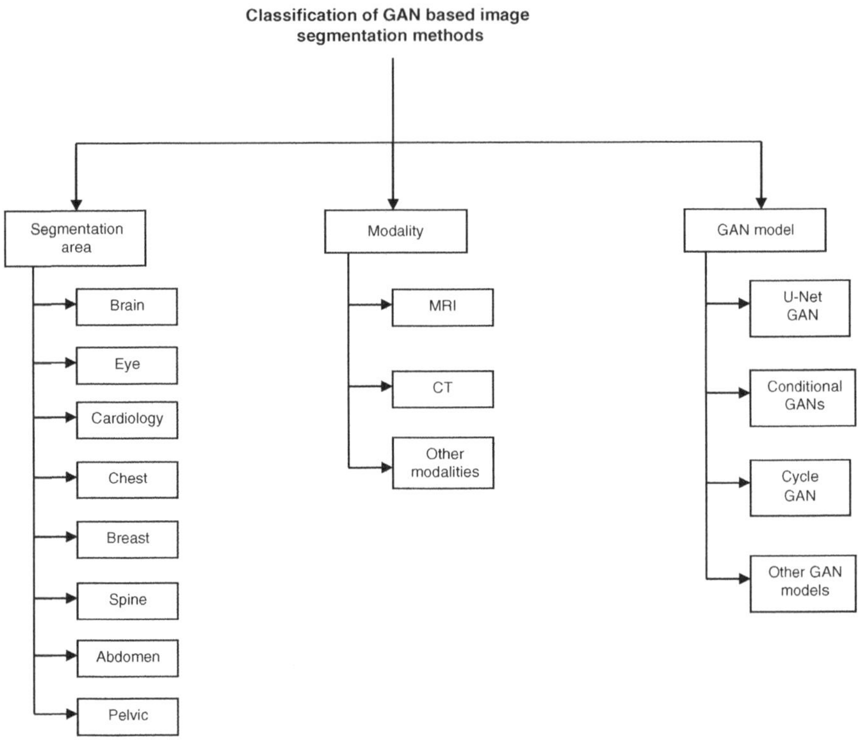

Figure 8.2 Classification of GAN-based medical image segmentation methods.

disease diagnosis and the identification and categorization of abnormalities. The most prevalent malignant tumor affecting the central nervous system is a brain tumor. Li and colleagues employed a GAN-based approach in their studies (Li et al. 2018; Xue et al. 2018; Yuan et al. 2019; Li et al. 2020; Nema et al. 2020; Cheng et al. 2021; Conte et al. 2021) to successfully segment these tumors. Xue et al. (2018) utilized U-Net as the generator for the GAN and introduced a multi-scale L1 loss method, enabling direct and efficient brain tumor segmentation. Additionally, Cheng et al. (2021) employed GAN to reweight and correct labels on samples, resulting in enhanced image quality for manually segmented labels and subsequently improving the accuracy of brain tumor segmentation. Moeskops et al. utilized GAN techniques for segmenting various brain tissues like gray matter and white matter (Moeskops et al. 2017; Mondal et al. 2018; Oh et al. 2020; Delisle et al. 2021). In their work, Mondal et al. (2018) were the first to employ GAN for semi-supervised segmentation of 3D multimodal brain images, showing considerable enhancement in segmentation performance compared to fully supervised methods. Delannoy et al.

Table 8.1 GAN-based segmentation method for brain.

Reference	Modality	Method	Data		Performance		
					Whole	Core	Enhanced
Cheng et al. (2021)	MRI	GAN	BraTS 2017	DSC	0.87	0.86	0.87
				Sen	0.87	0.72	0.68
((Borne et al. (n.d.))	MRI	U-Net GAN	BraTS 2013	DSC	0.84	0.70	0.65
				Sen	0.83	0.74	0.72
Conze et al. (2017)	MRI	U-Net GAN	BraTS 2017	DSC	0.901	0.781	0.682
Conze et al. (2021)	MRI	VGG GAN	BraTS 2017	DSC	0.82	0.71	0.92

(2020) and Li et al. (2021a) applied GAN methodologies to segment neonatal brain images, offering valuable assistance in diagnosing neonatal diseases.

Furthermore, GAN-based approaches have proven effective in segmenting various other brain lesions and abnormalities (Alex et al. 2017; Kamnitsas et al. 2017; Finck et al. 2020; Kuang et al. 2020; La Rosa et al. 2021).

Authors in Altun Güven and Talu (2023) introduce SSimDCL, a novel GAN for brain MRI segmentation, showcasing its superior performance compared to established architectures, its efficiency in various dataset analyses, and its promising potential for automated brain MRI segmentation. Authors in Khaled et al. (2022) introduced a multistage GAN model for brain segmentation, enhancing accuracy with a coarse-to-fine approach and achieving improved Dice Coefficient accuracy compared to one-stage models (Table 8.1).

8.4.1.2 Eye Segmentation Using GAN

The challenges stemming from fundus image acquisition limitations, such as prevalent image noise and the intricate, variable nature of the retina, pose significant hurdles for segmentation. Surprisingly, numerous GAN-based approaches outperform human experts in segmenting fundus images. Automatically segmenting fundus images presents significant challenges due to the intricate branching patterns of vessels and the prevalent background noise. Lahiri et al. achieved precise retinal blood vessel segmentation in their works (Lahiri et al. 2017; Mahapatra et al. 2017; Iqbal and Ali 2018; Javanmardi and Tasdizen 2018; Son et al. 2019; Yang et al. 2020). In their 2017 study (Lahiri et al. 2017), Lahiri et al. pioneered the use of GAN semi-supervised learning, marking an effective approach to segmenting retinal blood vessels. Iqbal and Ali (2018) (Iqbal and Ali 2018) redefined a set of loss functions to generate more realistic retinal images, aiding in the segmentation process. Yang et al. (2020) enhanced both the generator and discriminator network structures to accurately capture vessel edge details

Table 8.2 GAN-based segmentation method for eye.

Reference	Modality	Method	Dataset	Performance	
				Acc.	Sen
Guo et al. (2020)	Funduscopy	SRGAN	DRIVE	0.96	0.77
			STARE	0.96	0.87
			CHASE	0.95	0.82
Huang et al. (2021)	Funduscopy	SUD-GAN	DRIVE	0.9560	0.9663
			STARE	0.8340	0.8334
Huo et al. (2018b)	ICGA	CGAN	Private	0.9892	0.7763
Iqbal and Ali (2018)	OCT	WGAN	Private	–	0.8091

during segmentation. Schlegl et al. conducted the segmentation of abnormal lesions within fundus images (Schlegl et al. 2017, 2019; Jiang et al. 2019; Wang et al. 2021a), contributing to the diagnosis of ocular diseases. Glaucoma stands as one of the prevalent eye diseases, where accurate segmentation of the optic cup and optic disc, determining the cup-to-disc ratio (CDR), holds crucial significance. Shankaranarayana et al. employed various adversarial learning methods to address this challenge (Shankaranarayana et al. 2017; Wang et al. 2019; Kadambi et al. 2020; Luo et al. 2021). In contrast to the previously mentioned studies, (Liu et al. 2019c) and Tennakoon et al. (2018) employed GAN techniques to segment layer and fluid regions within OCT images. Furthermore, Ouyang et al. (2019) and Yildiz et al. (2021) utilized distinct GAN-based methods to segment the cornea. MedRegNet (Santarossa et al. 2022), an unsupervised GAN-based descriptor module, enhances multimodal retinal image registration without requiring expert annotation, demonstrating improved performance over classical algorithms, even in cases of substantial visual disparity between modalities, offering adaptability and potential application beyond retinal imaging (Table 8.2).

8.4.1.3 Cardiology Segmentation Using GAN

Cardiology is the medical specialty primarily focused on the study, diagnosis, and treatment of the heart and its associated circulatory system. Another term that can be used as a synonym for cardiology is "cardiovascular medicine" or "vascular medicine." These terms encompass a broader scope, including the heart and blood vessels, highlighting the comprehensive nature of the field beyond just the heart itself.

Segmenting the heart in medical images poses greater complexity compared to other anatomical regions due to its dynamic nature as a continuously functioning organ, whose shape varies during physical activity. Consequently, precise computation, modeling, and analysis of the complete heart structure hold immense significance for medical research and practical applications. Because each region within the heart exhibits distinct shapes and operational characteristics, the segmentation methods and challenges also vary across these regions.

Building on this understanding, Dou et al. conducted segmentation of various regions of interest across references (Chartsias et al. 2018; Zhang et al. 2018b; Dong et al. 2018; Joyce et al. 2018; Rezaei et al. 2018b; Upendra et al. 2019; Liu et al. 2019a; Xu et al. 2020; Decourt and Duong 2020; Shi et al. 2020; Wu et al. 2021; Yang et al. 2021; Cui et al. 2021; Gilbert et al. 2021; Chen et al. 2022). At the same time, Xu et al. (2020) introduced a deep spatiotemporal adversarial network, enabling simultaneous segmentation and measurement of the myocardial infarction area. Decourt and Duong (2020) proposed a novel loss function to enhance the accuracy of segmenting boundary pixels, notably improving segmentation precision for the myocardium, endocardium, and epicardium, particularly when dealing with limited annotation data. The implementation of GAN-based methodologies for automatic cardiac region segmentation addresses practical challenges in the field of cardiac medicine to a considerable extent (Table 8.3).

8.4.1.4 Chest Segmentation Using GAN

Chest and breast X-rays stand among the prevalent medical diagnostic methods, utilizing minimal radiation doses to generate quick, cost-effective images of these areas. These images aid in diagnosing and monitoring the treatment of a variety of

Table 8.3 GAN-based segmentation method for cardiology.

Reference	Modality	Method	Dataset	Performance (DSC)	
Li et al. (2021b)	CT	ConvNets GAN	MICCAI-2017	Ascending artery (AA)	0.748
				Left atrial blood (LA blood)	0.552
				Left ventricular blood (LV blood)	0.572
				Left ventricular myocardium (LVmyo)	0.478
Li et al. (2018)	CT, MRI	U-NET GAN	MICCAI-2017	CT	0.5
				MRI	0.66
Luo et al. (2021)	CT, MRI	Cycle GAN	MICCAI-2017	CT	0.815
				MRI	0.592
Mahapatra et al. (2017)	CMRI	U-Net GAN	ACDC	Left ventricular (LV)	0.88
				Right ventricular (RV)	0.90
				Myocardium (Myo)	0.89
Man et al. (2019)	CMRI	GAN	Private	Left atrium (LA)	0.946
				Atrial scars	0.821

Table 8.4 GAN-based segmentation method for chest.

Reference	Modality	Method	Dataset	Performance (DSC)	
Knyaz et al. (2019)	X-ray	SeUDA (semantic-aware GAN for unsupervised domain adaptation)	Montgomery	Right lung	0.9559
				Left lung	0.9342
Kuang et al. (2020)	CT	CGAN Pix2Pix	Private	0.814	
Lahiri et al. (2017)	CT	GAN	LIDC-IDRI	0.7986	
Ledig et al. (2017)	X-ray	SCAN (structure correcting adversarial network)	JSRT	0.973	
Li et al. (2021a)	Mammography	U-Net GAN	Private	0.9703	

cardiopulmonary conditions. Accurate pulmonary segmentation holds significant importance in diagnosing various pulmonary conditions. Chen et al. (2018a), Tan et al. (2021), and Stiehl et al. (2021) conducted lung segmentation across diverse medical images. Within the spectrum of lung diseases, lung cancer stands as a leading cause of mortality. Jin et al. (2018) introduced a novel multi-mask reconstruction loss within GAN to generate more realistic pulmonary nodule images. For accurate lung cancer detection, Jain et al. (2021) enhanced the GAN model by integrating the salp shuffled shepherd optimization algorithm for lung nodule segmentation. Moreover, Dai et al. employed various GAN models for automating the segmentation of multiple critical thoracic organs (Dai et al. 2018; Dong et al. 2019; Trullo et al. 2019), significantly streamlining the creation of radiotherapy plans (Table 8.4).

8.4.1.5 Breast Segmentation Using GANs

Breast cancer ranks among the most prevalent cancers, particularly affecting females. Zhu et al. achieved precise segmentation of breast masses (Zhu and Xie 2016; Shen et al. 2019; Han et al. 2020; Ma et al. 2020; Xing et al. 2021; Li et al. 2021c), a crucial step for computer-assisted breast cancer diagnosis. Shen et al. (2019) pioneered the use of CGAN to produce X-ray breast mass images, incorporating U-Net to enhance segmentation precision. Additionally, merged CycleGAN with FCN for breast lesion segmentation, alleviating the burden on radiologists for annotation tasks (Table 8.5).

8.4.1.6 Spine Segmentation Using GANs

Segmenting bone images encounters several hurdles, including low signal-to-noise ratio, imaging artifacts, and bone surfaces often just a few millimeters thick. To

Table 8.5 GAN-based segmentation method for breast.

Reference	Modality	Method	Dataset	Performance (DSC)
Kamnitsas et al. (2017)	Mammography	FCN-CRF GAN	INBreast	0.9097
Kan et al. (2021)	X-ray	CGAN	INBreast	0.8881
Kazeminia et al. (2020)	Breast Ultrasound	BUS-GAN (Breast Ultrasound with GAN)	Private	0.8712
Kessler et al. (2020)	Breast Ultrasound	SPCGAN (semi-pixel-wise cycle GAN)	Private	0.92
Kim et al. (2017)	Mammography	CGAN	INBreast	0.9154

address these challenges, several methods for bone segmentation and registration have been introduced.

Han et al. (2018) and Sekuboyina et al. (2018) employed GAN for spine segmentation. Han et al. focused on synchronously segmenting semantics of over 160 spinal structures, whereas Sekuboyina et al. concentrated on local spine segmentation. Meanwhile, Liu et al. integrated GAN with various neural networks for knee joint segmentation in MRI images across references (Liu 2019; Gaj et al. 2020; Kessler et al. 2020). Gong et al. (2021) utilized GAN for simultaneous segmentation and disease diagnosis of discs, neural foramens, thecal sacs, and posterior arches on axial MRI images (Table 8.6).

Table 8.6 GAN-based segmentation method for spine.

Reference	Modality	Model	Dataset	Performance (DSC)	
Sekuboyina et al. (2018)	MRI	Spine-GAN (recurrent GAN)	Private	0.87	
Shah (no date)	MRI	CycleGAN	T2FSE	**Femur bone**	0.97
				Tibia bone	0.95
				Femoral cartilage	0.66
				Tibial cartilage	0.65
Shen et al. (2019)	X-ray	DCGAN	Private	**Femur**	0.9762
				Femoral head	0.9786
Shi et al. (2020)	Ultrasound	CGAN	Private	0.9603	
Shi et al. (2019)	MRI	GAN	Private	0.949	

8.4.1.7 Abdomen Segmentation Using GANs

Deep neural networks have found extensive application in automating the segmentation of organs in abdominal CT scans. In abdominal scan images, distinguishing the spatial boundaries between adjacent organs poses a challenge, compounded by the substantial variations in size among different target organs. Traditional DL approaches struggle to accurately segment each organ due to these complexities.

Yang et al. (2017) and Kim and Ye (2018) applied GAN techniques specifically for liver segmentation, significantly enhancing both segmentation accuracy and processing speed. Using GAN, Liu et al. (2019a) (Liu et al. (2019b)) performed label assignments and generated probabilistic maps, enabling accurate segmentation of colorectal tumors. Ruan et al. (2020) integrated a multi-scale feature extractor and an area-of-interest locator into GAN for swift and accurate kidney tumor segmentation. For stomach and pancreas segmentation, Huang et al. (2021) and Li et al. (2021b) employed diverse adversarial networks (Table 8.7).

8.4.1.8 Pelvic Segmentation Using GANs

The intricate pelvic structure in the human body exhibits significant variability, leading to diverse clinical challenges, including shape variations, signal similarities among different structures, and a scarcity of annotated data. Automatic segmentation and modeling of the pelvic structure hold immense importance in supporting doctors' clinical practices. Accurately segmenting the prostate and surrounding critical structures is crucial for prostate radiation planning. Kohl

Table 8.7 GAN-based Segmentation Methods for Abdomen.

Reference	Modality	Model	Dataset	Performance (DSC)
Moeskops et al. (2017)	CT (3D)	DI2IN GAN	MICCAI (SLiver07)	0.95
Odena et al. (2017)	CT	LAGAN	Private	0.9154
Oh et al. (2020)	Colonoscopy image	Pix2Pix CGAN	CVC-Clinic	0.8848
Oh et al. (2020)	CT	MB-FSGAN (multi-branch feature sharing GAN)	Private	0.690, 0.722
Ouyang et al. (2019)	MRI	CycleGAN 3D Res-U-Net PatchGAN	NIH pancreas dataset	0.8393

et al. (2017), Jia et al. (2020), and Wang et al. (2021b) utilized GAN techniques for segmenting the prostate, a male reproductive organ situated within the pelvic cavity. Sultana et al. conducted simultaneous segmentation of multiple organs within the pelvic cavity across references (Sultana et al. 2020; Brion et al. 2021; Lei et al. 2021; Zhang et al. 2021) (Table 8.8).

8.4.2 Classification on the Basis of Image Modality

In this section, GAN-based medical segmentation methods are organized and categorized according to the specific image modalities they utilize. The section thoroughly examines several image modalities, including MRI, CT, and OCT.

8.4.2.1 Segmentation of Magnetic Resonance Imaging (MRI) Using GAN

MRI is a medical imaging method employing powerful magnetic fields and radio waves to produce detailed visuals of the body's internal structures. This technology produces high-resolution three-dimensional images, facilitating the visualization of soft tissues, organs, and various structures such as the brain, muscles, joints, and blood vessels. Notably, MRI stands out as a safer alternative for certain diagnostic needs compared to X-rays or CT scans, as it does not involve the use of ionizing radiation.

Authors in Conte et al. (2021) utilized GAN to generate missing MRI sequences, demonstrating the effectiveness of GAN-generated images in assisting other DL models in segmentation tasks. Authors in Chen et al. (2020) achieved precise segmentation of craniomaxillofacial (CMF) bony structures in MRI images. Authors in Yang et al. (2021) introduced a dilated block adversarial network for segmenting the left ventricle, right ventricle, and myocardium in short-axis cardiac MRI images. Authors in Conze et al. (2021) harnessed GAN for automatic multi-organ segmentation in abdominal MR images, effectively achieving simultaneous segmentation of multiple organs. Authors in Gadermayr et al. (2019) employed GAN for segmenting muscle tissue in MRI images (Table 8.9).

8.4.2.2 Segmentation of Computed Tomography (CT) Images Using GAN

CT is a medical imaging method that employs X-rays to produce detailed cross-sectional images of the body, offering comprehensive views of internal structures. This enables the detailed visualization of bones, organs, and tissues. CT scans play a crucial role in diagnosing a range of medical conditions, including injuries, infections, and tumors. The process involves the use of a rotating X-ray machine and a computer to generate detailed two-dimensional images or three-dimensional reconstructions. Due to its rapidity and capacity to capture precise anatomical details, CT imaging is widely utilized in medical diagnostics across various specialties.

Table 8.8 GAN-based segmentation method for pelvic.

Reference	Modality	Model	Dataset	Performance (DSC)				
Rezaei et al. (2018a)	MRI	FCN-GAN	Private	0.41				
Rezaei et al. (2018b)	MRI	3D APA-Net (3D adversarial pyramid anisotropic convolutional deep neural network)	PROMISE12	Whole	Base		Apex	
				0.906	0.891		0.869	
Ronneberger et al. (2015)	MRI	U-Net GAN	PROMISE12	0.8624				
La Rosa et al. (2021)	CT	U-Net CGAN Pix2Pix	Private	Prostrate		Uterus		
				0.929		0.724		
Ruan et al. (2020)	CT	FCN GAN U-Net	Private	Prostrate	Bladder		Rectum	
				0.868	0.762		0.719	
Schlegl et al. (2019)	CT, MRI	CycleGAN	Private	Bladder	Prostrate	Rectum	Left femoral head	Right femoral head
				0.93	0.88	0.88	0.94	0.94

Table 8.9 GAN-based segmentation method using MRI as modality.

Reference	Region of Interest	Model	Dataset	Performance
Conze et al. (2021)	Whole lesion, the FLAIR hyperintensities, and the contrast-enhanced areas	GAN	BraTS 2017	DSC = 0.82
Dong et al. (2018)	Craniomaxillofacial bone structure	U-Net CycleGAN	ADNI	DSC = 0.8856
Mahapatra et al. (2017)	Left ventricle (LV), right ventricle (RV), and myocardium (MYO)	U-Net GAN	ACDC	DSC = 0.96, 0.92, 0.87
Radford et al. (2016)	Liver, right kidney, left kidney, spleen, multi-organ	U-Net CGAN	CHAOS	(Liver, right kidney, left kidney, spleen, multi-organ) F-score = 85.53, 70.17, 70.39, 64.77, 69.92, 68.78

Table 8.10 Segmentation of CT images using GAN based Methods.

Reference	Region of Interest	Model	Dataset	Performance
Decourt and Duong (2020)	White matter	CGAN pix2pix	ADNI	DSC = 0.817
Kohl et al. (2017)	Brain tissue	GAN	MICCAI 2012	DSC = 0.92
			MRBrainS13	DSC = 0.85
Radford et al. (2016)	Liver, right kidney, left kidney, spleen, multi-organ	U-Net CGAN	CHAOS	(Liver, right kidney, left kidney, spleen, multi-organ) F-score = 85.53, 70.17, 70.39, 64.77, 69.92, 68.78

Authors in Oh et al. (2020) segment white matter in CT images, achieving precise delineation of brain tissues. Authors in Tan et al. (2021) integrated an EM distance-based loss function with GAN to precisely segment lungs in input CT scans. Authors in Conze et al. (2021) harnessed GAN for automatic multi-organ segmentation in abdominal CT images, effectively achieving simultaneous segmentation of multiple organs (Table 8.10).

8.4.2.3 Segmentation of Other Modalities Using GAN

X-ray imaging is a widely used medical diagnostic technique that utilizes ionizing radiation to create detailed pictures of the inside of the body. X-rays are particularly effective in visualizing bones and can help diagnose fractures, infections, and certain diseases. The procedure involves exposing a part of the body to a small amount of ionizing radiation, and the resulting X-ray images provide valuable

Table 8.11 Segmentation of other modalities using GAN based Methods.

Reference	Region of Interest	Modality	Model	Dataset	Performance
Israel et al. (2017)	Retinal anomaly	OCT	CycleGAN	K's dataset	DSC = 0.8239
Kan et al. (2021)	Breast lumps	X-ray	CGAN	INbreast	DSC = 88.81
Kurutach et al. (2018)	Pulmonary nodules	CT	3D CGAN	LIDC	DSC = 0.989
Lahiri et al. (2017)	Lung nodule	CT	GAN	LIDC-IDRI	DSC = 0.7986
Son et al. (2019)	Lungs	CT(3D)	TD-GAN	Private	DSC = 0.894
	heart				DSC = 0.870
	liver				DSC = 0.817
	bones				DSC = 0.835

information for healthcare professionals in various medical specialties, such as orthopedics and dentistry. OCT is a noninvasive imaging technology that uses light waves to capture high-resolution, cross-sectional images of biological tissues. It is commonly employed in ophthalmology to visualize the layers of the retina, allowing for early detection and monitoring of eye conditions such as macular degeneration and glaucoma. Additionally, OCT has applications in other medical fields, including cardiology and dermatology, where it provides detailed insights into tissue structures without the need for ionizing radiation (Table 8.11).

Authors in Wang et al. (2021b) proposed a weakly supervised learning network for segmenting lesions in OCT images. Authors in Shen et al. (2019) produced X-ray breast mass images using CycleGAN. Authors in Jin et al. (2018) presented an innovative multi-mask reconstruction loss incorporated into a GAN to produce pulmonary nodule images with heightened realism. Authors in Jain et al. (2021) improved the GAN model for precise lung cancer detection by integrating the salp shuffled shepherd optimization algorithm specifically for lung nodule segmentation. In their 2020 study (Sultana et al. 2020), Sultana et al. employed a multi-class 3D U-Net for coarse segmentation of pelvic structures, followed by an improved GAN for finer organ segmentation. In their study, Zhang et al. (Zhang et al. 2018a) used unsupervised segmentation of multiple organs on X-ray images.

8.4.3 Classification on the Basis of GAN Model Employed

Within this section, segmentation techniques for medical images using GANs are organized according to the specific GAN variants implemented. The assortment of models considered encompasses U-Net-based GAN, CycleGAN, DCGAN (deep convolutional GAN), CGAN (conditional GAN), and Pix-2-Pix GAN. This classification serves to distinguish and categorize the diverse GAN architectures utilized in the context of medical image segmentation. Each model represents a distinct approach, reflecting the nuanced strategies and methodologies employed in various studies within this domain.

8.4.3.1 Segmentation Using U-Net Based GAN

Authors in Xue et al. (2018) utilized U-Net as the generator for the GAN and introduced a multi-scale L1 loss method, enabling direct and efficient brain tumor segmentation. Authors in Shi et al. (2019) introduced the UG-net (a modified U-Net within a GAN) specifically designed for segmenting hippocampal subfields. Authors in Guo et al. (2020) utilized U-Net to recognize boundaries and GAN for shape prediction, specifically targeting the segmentation of pectoral muscle regions. Authors in Guo et al. (2020) utilized U-Net and a pyramid structure as the generator and discriminator, respectively, to extract intricate features from coronary arteries. Authors in Sultana et al. (2020) utilized a 3D U-Net with multi-class capabilities for the preliminary segmentation of pelvic structures, followed by the implementation of an enhanced GAN for more precise organ segmentation. Authors in Wang et al. (2020) incorporated the structural elements of U-Net into a GAN to improve the segmentation of the esophagus in OCT images (Table 8.12).

8.4.3.2 Segmentation Using Conditional GANs (CGAN, pix2pix GAN, and ACGAN)

Authors in Oh et al. (2020) utilized a CGAN implemented within a pix2pix framework to accurately segment white matter in 18F-FDG PET/CT images. This approach led to the precise delineation of brain tissues. Authors in Jiang et al. (2018) introduced CGAN along with the Dice loss function, pioneering lacquer crack segmentation. Authors in Shen et al. (2019) were the first to employ CGAN

Table 8.12 Segmentation using U-Net based GAN models.

Reference	Region of Interest	Modality	Dataset	Performance	
(Borne et al. (n.d.))	The entire tumor	MRI	BraTS 2013	Whole	DSC = 0.84
	The tumor core			Core	DSC = 0.70
	The GD-enhanced tumor core			Enhanced	DSC = 0.65
Dong et al. (2019)	Hippocampus (CA1, CA2, DG, CA3, head, tail, SUB, ERC and PHG)	MRI	CIND Center	DSC = 0.919	
Li et al. (2021a)	Chest muscle	Mammogram	Private	DSC = 0.9703	
Ruan et al. (2020)	Prostate	CT	Private	DSC = 0.90,	
	bladder			DSC = 0.96	
	rectum			DSC = 0.91	

Table 8.13 Segmentation Using Conditional GAN based Models.

Reference	Region of Interest	Modality	Dataset	Performance
Decourt and Duong (2020)	White matter	PET/ CTMRI	ADNI	DSC = 0.817
Kan et al. (2021)	Breast lumps	X-ray	INbreast	DSC = 88.81
Oh et al. (2020)	Colon polyps	Colonoscope image	CVC-Clinic	DSC = 0.8848
Shi et al. (2020)	Bone shadow	Ultrasound	Private	DSC = 0.9603
Wittke et al. (2007)	Eyes diseases	Cell (2D)	Private	DSC = 0.89

for the generation of X-ray breast mass images. They integrated U-Net to improve the precision of segmentation in the process. Authors in Huo et al. (2018a), Huo et al. (2018b) introduced a splenomegaly segmentation network based on CGAN, followed by an end-to-end synthesis and segmentation network, achieving precise spleen segmentation. In Poomeshwaran et al. (2019), authors presented an improved pix2pix framework for segmenting colon polyp regions. Authors in Kan et al. (2021) integrated a built-in auxiliary classifier into GAN to segment both the prostate and the female reproductive organ, the uterus. Authors in Alsinan et al. (2020) enhanced CGAN, enabling real-time segmentation of bone shadows in ultrasound images. Authors in Liu et al. (2021) merged a statistical model with CGAN to efficiently produce high-quality annotated images, facilitating cell segmentation. Authors in Nishiyama et al. (2021) utilized CGAN for accurate evaluation of gluteus medius volume (Table 8.13).

8.4.3.3 Segmentation Using CycleGAN

In 2021, Wang and colleagues (Wang et al. 2021b) introduced a weakly supervised learning network that relies on CycleGAN for the segmentation of lesions in OCT images. Authors in Xing et al. (2021) combined CycleGAN with FCN for the segmentation of breast lesions. This integration aimed to reduce the workload on radiologists by easing annotation tasks. Authors in Lei et al. (2021) utilized dual pyramid networks for feature extraction and CycleGAN to generate synthetic MRI images, supplementing information for simultaneous segmentation of multiple organs. Authors in de Bel et al. (2021) enhanced the standard CycleGAN by integrating residual learning, applying this improved network to reduce variation among strains in histopathology (Table 8.14).

Table 8.14 Segmentation Using cycle GAN based Models.

Reference	Region of Interest	Modality	Dataset	Performance
Israel et al. (2017)	Retinal anomaly	OCT	K's dataset	DSC = 0.8239
Kessler et al. (2020)	Breast lesions	Breast ultrasound	Private	DSC = 0.92
Schlegl et al. (2019)	Bladder	CT	Private	DSC = 0.93
	Prostate			DSC = 0.88
	Rectum	MRI		DSC = 0.88
	left femoral heads			DSC = 0.94
	right femoral heads			DSC = 0.94
Wei et al. (2020)	Colon tissue	Cell (2D)	Private	DSC = 0.66
	kidney tissue			DSC = 0.85

Table 8.15 Segmentation Using other GAN based Models.

Reference	Region of Interest	Modality	Dataset	Performance
Man et al. (2019)	Left atrium (LA)	CMRI	Private	DSC = 0.946
	atrial scars			DSC = 0.821
Shen et al. (2019)	Femur	X-ray	Private	DSC = 0.9762
	femoral head			DSC = 0.9786
Song et al. (2017)	Head	CT MRI	PDDCA	(brainstem, optical chiasm, mandible, optical nerves) DSC = 0.916, 0.589, 0.816, 0.703
	Neck			(larynx, pharynx, parotid glands) DSC = 0.799, 0.706, 0.845
Sultana et al. (2020)	Abdomen (liver, right kidney, left kidney, spleen)	MRI	CHAOS2019	(Liver, right kidney, left kidney, spleen) DSC = 0.8820, 0.8396, 0.8348, 0.8047
	Brain			DSC = 0.4471
Tong et al. (2019)	Craniomaxillofacial bony structures	MRI, CT	CQ500	Craniomaxillofacial bony structures DSC = 0.8100
	cardiac substructures		ADNI	Cardiac substructures DSC = 0.751

8.4.3.4 Segmentation Using other GAN Models

Authors in Schlegl et al. (2019) introduced the fast AnoGAN method, effectively identifying abnormal images and executing image segmentation. Authors in Chen et al. (2022) introduced an inter-cascade GAN, performing end-to-end segmentation of the left atrium and atrial scars. Authors in Wei et al. (2020) introduced an enhanced DCGAN for femoral region segmentation, facilitating the evaluation of the femoral neck-shaft angle based on the segmentation outcomes. Authors in Zhang et al. (2018a) introduced TD-GAN (Task Driven GAN), pioneering unsupervised segmentation of multiple organs on X-ray images. In Tong et al. (2019), authors enhanced GAN by incorporating shape constraints and utilized a deep supervised fully convolutional DenseNet as a segmentation network for multiple organ segmentation in the head and neck region. Authors in Yuan et al. (2020) overcame the constraints of 2D segmentation, achieving 3D segmentation of abdominal organs and brain tumors. Authors in Chen et al. (2021) introduced a diverse data augmentation GAN, facilitating the training of a segmentation model for an unannotated target image domain by leveraging information from an annotated source image domain (Table 8.15).

8.5 Conclusion

A review of the GAN-based image segmentation techniques is presented in this paper. We briefly present the principles of GAN and several extensions. Regarding the generative model G, its parameter updates differ from optimizing data likelihood; instead, they involve back propagating gradients from the discriminative model D. Additionally, GAN stands apart from traditional probabilistic generation models by circumventing the Markov chain learning mechanism. Moreover, GANs directly perform sampling and inference, enhancing their efficiency in application and broadening their practical use cases.

We also provide a summary of GAN's application, specifically in medical image segmentation. As a versatile design framework, GAN-based DL models have significantly contributed to enhancing the precision of medical image segmentation. The summary in this section highlights the primary improvements made in these models along two main avenues. First, there is a focus on augmenting or refining the loss function. Given GAN's adaptability, a variety of loss functions can be integrated into the GAN model. Consequently, by tailoring diverse loss functions for specific tasks, the model's performance can be notably enhanced. Second, there is an emphasis on integrating GAN with other neural networks (Yan et al. (2019); Yang et al. (2017); Yang et al. (2020); Yang et al. (2021)). GAN's generation and discriminative models can be parameterized through any differentiable function. This unique learning approach enables GAN to more effectively extract semantic segmentation features, thus elevating the segmentation network's performance.

While GAN's advancements offer new prospects for medical image segmentation, practical implementation faces several limitations. First, research in GAN for medical image segmentation leans heavily toward technological aspects, employing evaluation metrics typical in computer science. Most studies assessed the model's feasibility rather than its effectiveness in practical clinical settings, lacking evaluation against medical standards. Second, GAN, as a generative model, encounters issues like non-convergence, training complexity, mode collapse, and mode jump. When applying GAN's trained outcomes to new applications, the model often requires transfer learning to sustain performance, diminishing the repeatability in clinical contexts. Furthermore, GAN's interpretability is notably poor – it operates as a black-box mapping function, taking random variables as input and generating the desired data distribution as output. This lack of interpretability poses a significant hurdle to its practical adoption in the medical field. Hence, researchers must focus on overcoming GAN's challenges related to instability, low repeatability, and lack of interpretability for its successful integration into medical applications.

Furthermore, gaining acceptance from clinicians and patients regarding the data quality produced by GAN poses a challenge. As highlighted by Mazurowski et al. in Zhao et al. (2020), the clinical adoption of artificial intelligence in radiology remains a topic of debate. When implementing GAN in clinical settings, the primary concern revolves around the potential generation of erroneous information. During data generation, GAN might inadvertently create nonexistent disease information or overlook existing disease features as irrelevant. Consequently, cautious consideration is imperative for employing GAN in clinical practice. Similar to other applications, GAN-based implementations necessitate rigorous validation Zhou et al. (2016). In the short term, segmentation outcomes derived from GAN-based methods should undergo review by seasoned clinicians. Moreover, outcomes relying solely on GAN auto-segmentation ought to be limited to controlled experimental ranges. Furthermore, akin to other DL techniques, ethical and legal considerations come into play when employing GAN in clinical scenarios Zhu and Xie (2016). Despite GAN's limitations, judicious and meticulous use holds the potential to introduce numerous novel possibilities for medical image segmentation.

In summary, GAN holds vast potential in the realm of medical image processing. The diverse array of GAN-based methods and their iterations have garnered significant interest, notably advancing the application and evolution of DL algorithms in this field. Nevertheless, gaining acceptance for these methods among clinicians and patients remains a considerable hurdle. Additionally, GAN exhibits limitations, including instability, low repeatability, and interpretability challenges.

Addressing these issues stands to pave the way for novel pathways and approaches in the development of GAN.

References

Ait Skourt, B., El Hassani, A., and Majda, A. (2018). Lung CT image segmentation using deep neural networks. *Procedia Computer Science* 127: 109–113. Available at: https://doi.org/10.1016/J.PROCS.2018.01.104.

Alex, V., Mohammed Safwan K. P., Chennamsetty, S.S., Krishnamurthi, G. (2017) 'Generative adversarial networks for brain lesion detection', *Medical Imaging* https://doi.org/10.1117/12.2254487, 10133, pp. 113–121.

Alsinan, A.Z., Patel, V.M., and Hacihaliloglu, I. (2020). Bone shadow segmentation from ultrasound data for orthopedic surgery using GAN. *International Journal of Computer Assisted Radiology and Surgery* 15 (9): 1477–1485. Available at: https://doi.org/10.1007/S11548-020-02221-Z/METRICS.

Altun Güven, S. and Talu, M.F. (2023). Brain MRI high resolution image creation and segmentation with the new GAN method. *Biomedical Signal Processing and Control* 80: 104246. Available at: https://doi.org/10.1016/J.BSPC.2022.104246.

Arjovsky, M., Chintala, S., and Bottou, L. (2017). Wasserstein GAN. *Arxiv(Cornell University)* Available at:http://arxiv.org/abs/1701.07875.

Barra, V. and Boire, J.Y. (2002). Segmentation of fat and muscle from MR images of the thigh by a possibilistic clustering algorithm. *Computer Methods and Programs in Biomedicine* 68 (3): 185–193. Available at: https://doi.org/10.1016/S0169-2607(01)00172-9.

Borne, L., Rivière, D., Mangin, J. F. (n.d.) Combining 3D U-Net and bottom-up geometric constraints for automatic cortical sulci recognition | OpenReview (no date). Available at: https://openreview.net/forum?id=ryl0VTZCtV (Accessed: 27 December 2023).

Brion, E., Léger, J., Barragán-Montero, A.M. et al. (2021). Domain adversarial networks and intensity-based data augmentation for male pelvic organ segmentation in cone beam CT. *Computers in Biology and Medicine* 131: 104269. Available at: https://doi.org/10.1016/J.COMPBIOMED.2021.104269.

Chartsias, A., Joyce, T., Papanastasiou, G., Semple, S., Williams, M., Newby, D., Dharmakumar, R. and Tsaftaris, S.A., (2018) 'Factorised spatial representation learning: Application in semi-supervised myocardial segmentation', *Lecture Notes in Computer Science (including subseries Lecture Notes in Artificial Intelligence and Lecture Notes in Bioinformatics)*, 11071 LNCS, pp. 490–498. Available at: https://doi.org/10.1007/978-3-030-00934-2_55/TABLES/1.

Chen, C., Dou, Q., Chen, H. and Heng, P.A., (2018a) 'Semantic-aware generative adversarial nets for unsupervised domain adaptation in chest X-ray segmentation',

Lecture Notes in Computer Science (including subseries Lecture Notes in Artificial Intelligence and Lecture Notes in Bioinformatics), 11046 LNCS, pp. 143–151. Available at: https://doi.org/10.1007/978-3-030-00919-9_17/COVER.

Chen, H. et al. (2018b). VoxResNet: Deep voxelwise residual networks for brain segmentation from 3D MR images. *NeuroImage* 170: 446–455. Available at: https://doi.org/10.1016/J.NEUROIMAGE.2017.04.041.

Chen, J., Yang, G., Khan, H. et al. (2022). JAS-GAN: Generative Adversarial Network Based Joint Atrium and Scar Segmentations on Unbalanced Atrial Targets. *IEEE Journal of Biomedical and Health Informatics* 26 (1): 103–114. Available at: https://doi.org/10.1109/JBHI.2021.3077469.

Chen, X., Niemeijer, M., Zhang, L. et al. (2012). 3D Segmentation of Fluid-Associated Abnormalities in Retinal OCT: Probability Constrained Graph-Search–Graph-Cut. *IEEE transactions on medical imaging* 31 (8): 1521. Available at: https://doi.org/10.1109/TMI.2012.2191302.

Chen, X., Duan, Y., Houthooft, R. et al. (2016). InfoGAN: Interpretable Representation Learning. *Arxiv(Cornell University)* Available at: https://arxiv.org/abs/1606.03657.

Chen, X., Lian, C., Wang, L. et al. (2020). One-shot generative adversarial learning for MRI segmentation of craniomaxillofacial bony structures. *IEEE Transactions on Medical Imaging* 39 (3): 787–796. Available at: https://doi.org/10.1109/TMI.2019.2935409.

Chen, X. et al. (2021). Diverse data augmentation for learning image segmentation with cross-modality annotations. *Medical Image Analysis* 71: 102060. Available at: https://doi.org/10.1016/J.MEDIA.2021.102060.

Cheng, G., Ji, H., and He, L. (2021). Correcting and reweighting false label masks in brain tumor segmentation. *Medical Physics* 48 (1): 169–177. Available at: https://doi.org/10.1002/MP.14480.

Christ, P.F., Ji, H., and He, L. (2017). Automatic Liver and Tumor Segmentation of CT and MRI Volumes using Cascaded Fully Convolutional Neural Networks. *Arxiv (Cornell University)* Available at: https://arxiv.org/abs/1702.05970v2(Accessed: 27 December 2023).

Conte, G.M., Weston, A.D., Vogelsang, D.C. et al. (2021). Generative adversarial networks to synthesize missing T1 and FLAIR MRI sequences for use in a multisequence brain tumor segmentation model. *Radiology* 299 (2): 313–323. Available at: https://doi.org/10.1148/RADIOL.2021203786/ASSET/IMAGES/LARGE/RADIOL.2021203786.FIG 6.JPEG.

Conze, P.H., Noblet, V., Rousseau, F. et al. (2017). Scale-adaptive supervoxel-based random forests for liver tumor segmentation in dynamic contrast-enhanced CT scans. *International Journal of Computer Assisted Radiology and Surgery* 12 (2): 223–233. Available at: https://doi.org/10.1007/S11548-016-1493-1/METRICS.

Conze, P.H., Kavur, A.E., Cornec-Le Gall, E. et al. (2021). Abdominal multi-organ segmentation with cascaded convolutional and adversarial deep networks. *Artificial Intelligence in Medicine* 117: 102109. Available at: https://doi.org/10.1016/J.ARTMED.2021.102109.

Cui, H., Yuwen, C., Jiang, L. et al. (2021). Bidirectional cross-modality unsupervised domain adaptation using generative adversarial networks for cardiac image segmentation. *Computers in Biology and Medicine* 136: 104726. Available at: https://doi.org/10.1016/J.COMPBIOMED.2021.104726.

Dai, W., Dong, N., Wang, Z., et al. (2018) 'Scan: Structure correcting adversarial network for organ segmentation in chest x-rays', *Lecture Notes in Computer Science (including subseries Lecture Notes in Artificial Intelligence and Lecture Notes in Bioinformatics)*, 11045 LNCS, pp. 263–273. Available at: https://doi.org/10.1007/978-3-030-00889-5_30/TABLES/4.

de Bel, T., Bokhorst, J.M., van der Laak, J., and Litjens, G. (2021). Residual cyclegan for robust domain transformation of histopathological tissue slides. *Medical Image Analysis* 70: 102004. Available at:https://doi.org/10.1016/J.MEDIA.2021.102004.

Decourt, C. and Duong, L. (2020). Semi-supervised generative adversarial networks for the segmentation of the left ventricle in pediatric MRI. *Computers in Biology and Medicine* 123: 103884. Available at: https://doi.org/10.1016/J.COMPBIOMED.2020.103884.

Delannoy, Q., Pham, C.H., Cazorla, C. et al. (2020). SegSRGAN: Super-resolution and segmentation using generative adversarial networks — Application to neonatal brain MRI. *Computers in Biology and Medicine* 120: 103755. Available at: https://doi.org/10.1016/J.COMPBIOMED.2020.103755.

Delisle, P.L., Anctil-Robitaille, B., Desrosiers, C. et al. (2021). Realistic image normalization for multi-Domain segmentation. *Medical Image Analysis* 74: 102191. Available at: https://doi.org/10.1016/J.MEDIA.2021.102191.

Dong, S., Luo, G., Wang, K., et al. (2018) 'VoxelAtlasGAN: 3D Left Ventricle Segmentation on Echocardiography with Atlas Guided Generation and Voxel-to-Voxel Discrimination', *Lecture Notes in Computer Science (including subseries Lecture Notes in Artificial Intelligence and Lecture Notes in Bioinformatics)*, 11073 LNCS, pp. 622–629. Available at: https://doi.org/10.1007/978-3-030-00937-3_71/TABLES/1.

Dong, X. et al. (2019). Automatic multiorgan segmentation in thorax CT images using U-net-GAN. *Medical Physics* 46 (5): 2157–2168. Available at: https://doi.org/10.1002/MP.13458.

Fei-Fei, L., Deng, J., and Li, K. (2010). ImageNet: Constructing a large-scale image database. *Journal of Vision* 9 (8): 1037–1037. Available at: https://doi.org/10.1167/9.8.1037.

Finck, T. et al. (2020). Deep-Learning Generated Synthetic Double Inversion Recovery Images Improve Multiple Sclerosis Lesion Detection. *Investigative Radiology* 55 (5): 318–323. Available at: https://doi.org/10.1097/RLI.0000000000000640.

Gadermayr, M. et al. (2019). Domain-specific data augmentation for segmenting MR images of fatty infiltrated human thighs with neural networks. *Journal of Magnetic Resonance Imaging* 49 (6): 1676–1683. Available at: https://doi.org/10.1002/JMRI.26544.

Gaj, S., Yang, M., Nakamura, K., and Li, X. (2020). Automated cartilage and meniscus segmentation of knee MRI with conditional generative adversarial networks. *Magnetic Resonance in Medicine* 84 (1): 437–449. Available at: https://doi.org/10.1002/MRM.28111.

Gilbert, A., Marciniak, M., Rodero, C. et al. (2021). Generating Synthetic Labeled Data from Existing Anatomical Models: An Example with Echocardiography Segmentation. *IEEE Transactions on Medical Imaging* 40 (10): 2783–2794. Available at: https://doi.org/10.1109/TMI.2021.3051806.

Gong, H., Liu, J., Li, S., and Chen, B. (2021). Axial-SpineGAN: simultaneous segmentation and diagnosis of multiple spinal structures on axial magnetic resonance imaging images. *Physics in Medicine & Biology* 66 (11): 115014. Available at: https://doi.org/10.1088/1361-6560/ABFAD9.

Goodfellow, I., Pouget-Abadie, J., Mirza, M. et al. (2020). Generative adversarial networks. *Communications of the ACM* 63 (11): 139–144. Available at: https://doi.org/10.1145/3422622.

Guo, S., Wang, K., Kang, H. et al. (2019). BTS-DSN: Deeply supervised neural network with short connections for retinal vessel segmentation. *International Journal of Medical Informatics* 126: 105–113. Available at: https://doi.org/10.1016/J.IJMEDINF.2019.03.015.

Guo, Y., Zhao, W., Li, S. et al. (2020). Automatic segmentation of the pectoral muscle based on boundary identification and shape prediction. *Physics in Medicine & Biology* 65 (4): 045016. Available at: https://doi.org/10.1088/1361-6560/AB652B.

Han, L., Huang, Y., Dou, H. et al. (2020). Semi-supervised segmentation of lesion from breast ultrasound images with attentional generative adversarial network. *Computer Methods and Programs in Biomedicine* 189: 105275. Available at: https://doi.org/10.1016/J.CMPB.2019.105275.

Han, Z., Wei, B., Mercado, A. et al. (2018). Spine-GAN: Semantic segmentation of multiple spinal structures. *Medical Image Analysis* 50: 23–35. Available at: https://doi.org/10.1016/J.MEDIA.2018.08.005.

Heimann, T. and Meinzer, H.P. (2009). Statistical shape models for 3D medical image segmentation: A review. *Medical Image Analysis* 13 (4): 543–563. Available at: https://doi.org/10.1016/J.MEDIA.2009.05.004.

Huang, L., Li, M., Gou, S., Zhang, X. and Jiang, K., (2021) 'Automated Segmentation Method for Low Field 3D Stomach MRI Using Transferred Learning Image

Enhancement Network', *Bio Med Research International*, 2021. Available at: https://doi.org/10.1155/2021/6679603.

Huo, Y., Xu, Z., Bao, S., Assad, A., et al. (2018a) 'Adversarial synthesis learning enables segmentation without target modality ground truth', *Proceedings - International Symposium on Biomedical Imaging*, 2018-April, pp. 1217–1220. Available at: https://doi.org/10.1109/ISBI.2018.8363790.

Huo, Y., Xu, Z., Bao, S., Bermudez, C., et al. (2018b) 'Splenomegaly segmentation using global convolutional kernels and conditional generative adversarial networks', https://doi.org/10.1117/12.2293406, 10574, pp. 45–51. Available at: https://doi.org/10.1117/12.2293406.

Iqbal, T. and Ali, H. (2018). Generative Adversarial Network for Medical Images (MI-GAN). *Journal of Medical Systems* 42 (11): 1–11. Available at: https://doi.org/10.1007/S10916-018-1072-9/METRICS.

Israel, S.A., Goldstein, J.H., Klein, J.S., et al. (2017) 'Generative adversarial networks for classification', *Proceedings - Applied Imagery Pattern Recognition Workshop*, 2017-Octob, pp. 1–4. Available at: https://doi.org/10.1109/AIPR.2017.8457952.

Jain, S., Indora, S., and Atal, D.K. (2021). Lung nodule segmentation using Salp Shuffled Shepherd Optimization Algorithm-based Generative Adversarial Network. *Computers in Biology and Medicine* 137: 104811. Available at: https://doi.org/10.1016/J.COMPBIOMED.2021.104811.

Javanmardi, M. and Tasdizen, T. (2018) 'Domain adaptation for biomedical image segmentation using adversarial training', *Proceedings - International Symposium on Biomedical Imaging*, 2018-April, pp. 554–558. Available at: https://doi.org/10.1109/ISBI.2018.8363637.

Jia, H. et al. (2020). 3D APA-Net: 3D Adversarial Pyramid Anisotropic Convolutional Network for Prostate Segmentation in MR Images. *IEEE Transactions on Medical Imaging* 39 (2): 447–457. Available at: https://doi.org/10.1109/TMI.2019.2928056.

Jiang, H. et al (2018) 'cGAN-Based Lacquer Cracks Segmentation in ICGA Image', *Lecture Notes in Computer Science (including subseries Lecture Notes in Artificial Intelligence and Lecture Notes in Bioinformatics)*, 11039 LNCS, pp. 228–235. Available at: https://doi.org/10.1007/978-3-030-00949-6_27/TABLES/1.

Jiang, H. et al. (2019). Improved cGAN based linear lesion segmentation in high myopia ICGA images. *Biomedical Optics Express* 10 (5): 2355–2366. Available at: https://doi.org/10.1364/BOE.10.002355.

Jin, D. et al. (2018) 'CT-realistic lung nodule simulation from 3D conditional generative adversarial networks for robust lung segmentation', *Lecture Notes in Computer Science (including subseries Lecture Notes in Artificial Intelligence and Lecture Notes in Bioinformatics)*, 11071 LNCS, pp. 732–740. Available at: https://doi.org/10.1007/978-3-030-00934-2_81/FIGURES/5.

Joyce, T., Chartsias, A. and Tsaftaris, S. (2018) 'Deep Multi-Class Segmentation Without Ground-Truth Labels'. Available at: https://www.research.ed.ac.uk/en/

publications/deep-multi-class-segmentation-without-ground-truth-labels(Accessed: 27 December 2023).

Kadambi, S., Wang, Z., and Xing, E. (2020). WGAN domain adaptation for the joint optic disc-and-cup segmentation in fundus images. *International Journal of Computer Assisted Radiology and Surgery* 15 (7): 1205–1213. Available at: https://doi.org/10.1007/S11548-020-02144-9/METRICS.

Kamnitsas, K. et al. (2017) 'Unsupervised domain adaptation in brain lesion segmentation with adversarial networks', *Lecture Notes in Computer Science (including subseries Lecture Notes in Artificial Intelligence and Lecture Notes in Bioinformatics)*, 10265 LNCS, pp. 597–609. Available at: https://doi.org/10.1007/978-3-319-59050-9_47/COVER.

Kan, C.N.E., Gilat-Schmidt, T., and Ye, D.H. (2021). Enhancing reproductive organ segmentation in pediatric CT via adversarial learning. *Medical Imaging 2021: Image Processing* 11596: 282–287. Available at: https://doi.org/10.1117/12.2582127.

Kazeminia, S. et al. (2020). GANs for medical image analysis. *Artificial Intelligence in Medicine* 109: 1–41. Available at: https://doi.org/10.1016/j.artmed.2020.101938.

Kessler, D.A. et al. (2020). The optimisation of deep neural networks for segmenting multiple knee joint tissues from MRIs. *Computerized Medical Imaging and Graphics* 86: 101793. Available at: https://doi.org/10.1016/J.COMPMEDIMAG.2020.101793.

Khaled, A., Han, J.J., and Ghaleb, T.A. (2022). 'Multi-Model Medical Image Segmentation Using Multi-Stage Generative Adversarial Networks'. *IEEE Access* 10: 28590–28599. Available at: https://doi.org/10.1109/ACCESS.2022.3158342.

Kim, B., & Ye, J. C. (2018).Cycle-consistent adversarial network with polyphase U-Nets for liver lesion segmentation|OpenReview (no date). Available at: https://openreview.net/forum?id=SyQtAooiz (Accessed: 28 December 2023).

Kim, S. et al. (2017). Automatic segmentation of supraspinatus from MRI by internal shape fitting and autocorrection. *Computer Methods and Programs in Biomedicine* 140: 165–174. Available at: https://doi.org/10.1016/J.CMPB.2016.12.008.

Knyaz, V.A., Kniaz, V. V. and Remondino, F. (2019) 'Image-to-voxel model translation with conditional adversarial networks', *Lecture Notes in Computer Science (including subseries Lecture Notes in Artificial Intelligence and Lecture Notes in Bioinformatics)*, 11129 LNCS, pp. 601–618. Available at: https://doi.org/10.1007/978-3-030-11009-3_37.

Kohl, S. et al. (2017) 'Adversarial Networks for the Detection of Aggressive Prostate Cancer'. *Arxiv (Cornell University)*. Available at: https://arxiv.org/abs/1702.08014v1(Accessed: 28 December 2023).

Kuang, H., Menon, B.K., and Qiu, W. (2020). Automated stroke lesion segmentation in non-contrast CT scans using dense multi-path contextual generative adversarial network. *Physics in Medicine & Biology* 65 (21): 215013. Available at: https://doi.org/10.1088/1361-6560/ABA166.

Kurutach, T. et al. (2018). Learning plannable representations with causal infogan. *Advances in Neural Information Processing Systems* 31: 8733–8744.

La Rosa, F., Yu, T., Barquero, G. et al. (2021). MPRAGE to MP2RAGE UNI translation via generative adversarial network improves the automatic tissue and lesion segmentation in multiple sclerosis patients. *Computers in Biology and Medicine* 132: 104297. Available at: https://doi.org/10.1016/J.COMPBIOMED.2021.104297.

Lahiri, A.,Ayush, K., Kumar Biswas, P., et al. (2017) 'Generative Adversarial Learning for Reducing Manual Annotation in Semantic Segmentation on Large Scale Miscroscopy Images: Automated Vessel Segmentation in Retinal Fundus Image as Test Case', pp. 42–48. Available at: https://github.com/carpedm20/DCGAN- ().

Ledig, C. et al. (2017) 'Photo-Realistic Single Image Super-Resolution Using a Generative Adversarial Network', *Cvpr*, 2(3), p. 4. Available at: http://openaccess.thecvf.com/content_cvpr_2017/papers/Ledig_Photo-Realistic_Single_Image_CVPR_2017_paper.pdf https://ieeexplore.ieee.org/abstract/document/8099502.

Lei, Y. et al. (2021). Male pelvic CT multi-organ segmentation using synthetic MRI-aided dual pyramid networks. *Physics in Medicine & Biology* 66 (8): 085007. Available at: https://doi.org/10.1088/1361-6560/ABF2F9.

Li, B., You, X., Wang, J. et al. (2021a). IAS-NET: Joint intraclassly adaptive GAN and segmentation network for unsupervised cross-domain in neonatal brain MRI segmentation. *Medical Physics* 48 (11): 6962–6975. Available at: https://doi.org/10.1002/MP.15212.

Li, M., Lian, F., Wang, C., and Guo, S. (2021b). Dual adversarial convolutional networks with multilevel cues for pancreatic segmentation. *Physics in Medicine & Biology* 66 (17): 175025. Available at: https://doi.org/10.1088/1361-6560/AC155F.

Li, Y., Chen, Y. and Shi, Y. (2020) 'Brain Tumor Segmentation Using 3D Generative Adversarial Networks', *International Journal of Pattern Recognition and Artificial Intelligence*, 35(4). Available at: https://doi.org/10.1142/S0218001421570020.

Li, Y., Zhao, G., Zhang, Q. et al. (2021c). SAP-cGAN: Adversarial learning for breast mass segmentation in digital mammogram based on superpixel average pooling. *Medical Physics* 48 (3): 1157–1167. Available at: https://doi.org/10.1002/MP.14671.

Li, Z., Wang, Y. and Yu, J. (2018) 'Brain tumor segmentation using an adversarial network', *Lecture Notes in Computer Science (including subseries Lecture Notes in Artificial Intelligence and Lecture Notes in Bioinformatics)*, 10670 LNCS, pp. 123–132. Available at: https://doi.org/10.1007/978-3-319-75238-9_11/COVER.

Lin, D.Y. et al. (2017) 'Synthesizing remote sensing images by conditional adversarial networks', *International Geoscience and Remote Sensing Symposium (IGARSS)*, 2017-July, pp. 48–50. Available at: https://doi.org/10.1109/IGARSS.2017.8126890.

Liskowski, P. and Krawiec, K. (2016). Segmenting Retinal Blood Vessels with Deep Neural Networks. *IEEE Transactions on Medical Imaging* 35 (11): 2369–2380. Available at: https://doi.org/10.1109/TMI.2016.2546227.

Liu, F. (2019). SUSAN: segment unannotated image structure using adversarial network. *Magnetic Resonance in Medicine* 81 (5): 3330–3345. Available at: https://doi.org/10.1002/MRM.27627.

Liu, J. et al. (2019a). Multi-sequence myocardium segmentation with cross-constrained shape and neural network-based initialization. *Computerized Medical Imaging and Graphics* 71: 49–57. Available at: https://doi.org/10.1016/J.COMPMEDIMAG.2018.11.001.

Liu, J. et al. (2021). Active Cell Appearance Model Induced Generative Adversarial Networks for Annotation-Efficient Cell Segmentation and Identification on Adaptive Optics Retinal Images. *IEEE Transactions on Medical Imaging* 40 (10): 2820–2831. Available at: https://doi.org/10.1109/TMI.2021.3055483.

Liu, X., Cao, J. et al. (2019c). 'Semi-Supervised Automatic Segmentation of Layer and Fluid Region in Retinal Optical Coherence Tomography Images Using Adversarial Learning'. *IEEE Access* 7: 3046–3061. Available at: https://doi.org/10.1109/ACCESS.2018.2889321.

Liu, X., Guo, S. et al. (2019b). Accurate colorectal tumor segmentation for CT scans based on the label assignment generative adversarial network. *Medical Physics* 46 (8): 3532–3542. Available at: https://doi.org/10.1002/MP.13584.

Luo, L. et al. (2021). Joint optic disc and optic cup segmentation based on boundary prior and adversarial learning. *International Journal of Computer Assisted Radiology and Surgery* 16 (6): 905–914. Available at: https://doi.org/10.1007/S11548-021-02373-6/METRICS.

Ma, X. et al. (2020). Automated fibroglandular tissue segmentation in breast MRI using generative adversarial networks. *Physics in Medicine & Biology* 65 (10): 105006. Available at: https://doi.org/10.1088/1361-6560/AB7E7F.

Mahapatra, D. et al. (2017) 'Image super resolution using generative adversarial networks and local saliency maps for retinal image analysis', *Lecture Notes in Computer Science (including subseries Lecture Notes in Artificial Intelligence and Lecture Notes in Bioinformatics)*, 10435 LNCS, pp. 382–390. Available at: https://doi.org/10.1007/978-3-319-66179-7_44/FIGURES/4.

Man, Y. et al. (2019). Deep Q Learning Driven CT Pancreas Segmentation with Geometry-Aware U-Net. *IEEE Transactions on Medical Imaging* 38 (8): 1971–1980. Available at: https://doi.org/10.1109/TMI.2019.2911588.

Mirza, M. and Osindero, S. (2014). Conditional Generative Adversarial Nets. *Arxiv (Cornell University)* 1–7. Available at: http://arxiv.org/abs/1411.1784.

Moeskops, P. et al. (2017) 'Adversarial training and dilated convolutions for brain MRI segmentation', *Lecture Notes in Computer Science (including subseries Lecture Notes in Artificial Intelligence and Lecture Notes in Bioinformatics)*, 10553 LNCS, pp. 56–64. Available at: https://doi.org/10.1007/978-3-319-67558-9_7/COVER.

Mondal, A.K., Dolz, J. and Desrosiers, C. (2018) 'Few-shot 3D Multi-modal Medical Image Segmentation using Generative Adversarial Learning'. *Arxiv (Cornell*

University). Available at: https://arxiv.org/abs/1810.12241v1 (Accessed: 27 December 2023).

Nema, S. et al. (2020). RescueNet: An unpaired GAN for brain tumor segmentation. *Biomedical Signal Processing and Control* 55: 101641. Available at: https://doi.org/10.1016/J.BSPC.2019.101641.

Nishiyama, D. et al. (2021). Deep generative models for automated muscle segmentation in computed tomography scanning. *PLOS ONE* 16 (9): e0257371. Available at: https://doi.org/10.1371/JOURNAL.PONE.0257371.

Odena, A., Olah, C. and Shlens, J. (2017) 'Conditional image synthesis with auxiliary classifier gans', *34th International Conference on Machine Learning, ICML 2017*, 6, pp. 4043–4055.

Oh, K.T. et al. (2020). Semantic Segmentation of White Matter in FDG-PET Using Generative Adversarial Network. *Journal of Digital Imaging* 33 (4): 816–825. Available at: https://doi.org/10.1007/S10278-020-00321-5/METRICS.

Ouyang, J. et al. (2019). Accurate tissue interface segmentation via adversarial pre-segmentation of anterior segment OCT images. *Biomedical Optics Express* 10 (10): 5291–5324. Available at: https://doi.org/10.1364/BOE.10.005291.

Poomeshwaran, J.M. et al. (2019) 'Polyp Segmentation using Generative Adversarial Network', *Proceedings of the Annual International Conference of the IEEE Engineering in Medicine and Biology Society, EMBS*, pp. 7201–7204. Available at: https://doi.org/10.1109/EMBC.2019.8857958.

Purushwalkam, S. et al. (2013) 'Automatic segmentation of adipose tissue from thigh magnetic resonance images', *Lecture Notes in Computer Science (including subseries Lecture Notes in Artificial Intelligence and Lecture Notes in Bioinformatics)*, 7950 LNCS, pp. 451–458. Available at: https://doi.org/10.1007/978-3-642-39094-4_51/COVER.

Radford, A., Metz, L. and Chintala, S. (2016) 'Unsupervised representation learning with deep convolutional generative adversarial networks', *4th International Conference on Learning Representations, ICLR 2016 - Conference Track Proceedings*, pp. 1–16.

Rezaei, M., Yang, H., and Meinel, C. (2018b). Whole heart and great vessel segmentation with context-aware of generative adversarial networks. *Informatik aktuell* 0: 353–358. Available at: https://doi.org/10.1007/978-3-662-56537-7_89/COVER.

Rezaei, M. et al. (2018a) 'A conditional adversarial network for semantic segmentation of brain tumor', *Lecture Notes in Computer Science (including subseries Lecture Notes in Artificial Intelligence and Lecture Notes in Bioinformatics)*, 10670 LNCS, pp. 241–252. Available at: https://doi.org/10.1007/978-3-319-75238-9_21/COVER.

Ronneberger, O., Fischer, P. and Brox, T. (2015) 'U-net: Convolutional networks for biomedical image segmentation', *Lecture Notes in Computer Science (including subseries Lecture Notes in Artificial Intelligence and Lecture Notes in Bioinformatics)*, 9351, pp. 234–241. Available at: https://doi.org/10.1007/978-3-319-24574-4_28/COVER.

Ruan, Y. et al. (2020). MB-FSGAN: Joint segmentation and quantification of kidney tumor on CT by the multi-branch feature sharing generative adversarial network. *Medical Image Analysis* 64: 101721. Available at: https://doi.org/10.1016/J.MEDIA.2020.101721.

Santarossa, M., Kilic, A., von der Burchard, C., et al. (2022) 'MedRegNet: unsupervised multimodal retinal-image registration with GANs and ranking loss', *Medical Imaging 2022: Image Processing*, 12032, pp. 321–333. Available at: https://doi.org/10.1117/12.2607653.

Schlegl, T. et al. (2017) 'Unsupervised anomaly detection with generative adversarial networks to guide marker discovery', *Lecture Notes in Computer Science (including subseries Lecture Notes in Artificial Intelligence and Lecture Notes in Bioinformatics)*, 10265 LNCS, pp. 146–147. Available at: https://doi.org/10.1007/978-3-319-59050-9_12/COVER.

Schlegl, T. et al. (2019). f-AnoGAN: Fast unsupervised anomaly detection with generative adversarial networks. *Medical Image Analysis* 54: 30–44. Available at: https://doi.org/10.1016/J.MEDIA.2019.01.010.

Sekuboyina, A. et al. (2018) 'Btrfly Net: Vertebrae Labelling with Energy-Based Adversarial Learning of Local Spine Prior', *Lecture Notes in Computer Science (including subseries Lecture Notes in Artificial Intelligence and Lecture Notes in Bioinformatics)*, 11073 LNCS, pp. 649–657. Available at: https://doi.org/10.1007/978-3-030-00937-3_74/TABLES/2.

Senthilkumaran, N. and Vaithegi, S. (2016). Image segmentation by using thresholding techniques for medical images. *Computer Science & Engineering: An International Journal (CSEIJ)* 6 (1): Available at: https://doi.org/10.5121/cseij.2016.6101.

Shah, A.V. (n.d.) 'Boundary Detection Algorithm Implementation for Medical Images'. Available at: www.ijert.org ().

Shamshad, F. et al. (2023). Transformers in medical imaging: A survey. *Medical Image Analysis* 88: 102802. Available at: https://doi.org/10.1016/j.media.2023.102802.

Shankaranarayana, S.M. et al. (2017) 'Joint optic disc and cup segmentation using fully convolutional and adversarial networks', *Lecture Notes in Computer Science (including subseries Lecture Notes in Artificial Intelligence and Lecture Notes in Bioinformatics)*, 10554 LNCS, pp. 168–176. Available at: https://doi.org/10.1007/978-3-319-67561-9_19/COVER.

Shen, T. et al. (2019). Learning from adversarial medical images for X-ray breast mass segmentation. *Computer Methods and Programs in Biomedicine* 180: 105012. Available at: https://doi.org/10.1016/J.CMPB.2019.105012.

Shi, X., Du, T., Chen, S., et al. (2020) 'UENet: A Novel Generative Adversarial Network for Angiography Image Segmentation', *Proceedings of the Annual International Conference of the IEEE Engineering in Medicine and Biology Society, EMBS*, 2020-July, pp. 1612–1615. Available at: 10.1109/EMBC44109.2020.9175334.

Shi, Y., Cheng, K., and Liu, Z. (2019). Hippocampal subfields segmentation in brain MR images using generative adversarial networks. *BioMedical Engineering Online* 18 (1): 1–12. Available at: https://doi.org/10.1186/S12938-019-0623-8/TABLES/1.

Son, J., Park, S.J., and Jung, K.H. (2019). Towards Accurate Segmentation of Retinal Vessels and the Optic Disc in Fundoscopic Images with Generative Adversarial Networks. *Journal of Digital Imaging* 32 (3): 499–512. Available at: https://doi.org/10.1007/S10278-018-0126-3/TABLES/6.

Song, R., Zhang, Z., and Liu, H. (2017). Edge connection based Canny edge detection algorithm. *Pattern Recognition and Image Analysis* 27 (4): 740–747. Available at: https://doi.org/10.1134/S1054661817040162/METRICS.

Spurr, A., Aksan, E. and Hilliges, O. (2017) 'Guiding InfoGAN with Semi-supervision', *Lecture Notes in Computer Science (including subseries Lecture Notes in Artificial Intelligence and Lecture Notes in Bioinformatics)*, 10534 LNAI, pp. 119–134. Available at: https://doi.org/10.1007/978-3-319-71249-9_8.

Stiehl, B. et al. (2021). Scalable quorum-based deep neural networks with adversarial learning for automated lung lobe segmentation in fast helical free-breathing CTs. *International Journal of Computer Assisted Radiology and Surgery* 16 (10): 1775–1784. Available at: https://doi.org/10.1007/S11548-021-02454-6/METRICS.

Sultana, S., Robinson, A., Song, D.Y., and Lee, J. (2020). CNN-based hierarchical coarse-to-fine segmentation of pelvic CT images for prostate cancer radiotherapy. *Medical Imaging 2020: Image-Guided Procedures, Robotic Interventions, and Modeling* 11315: 394–401. Available at: https://doi.org/10.1117/12.2549979.

Tan, J., Jing, L., Huo, Y. et al. (2021). LGAN: Lung segmentation in CT scans using generative adversarial network. *Computerized Medical Imaging and Graphics* 87: 101817. Available at: https://doi.org/10.1016/J.COMPMEDIMAG.2020.101817.

Tan, S., Li, L., Choi, W. et al. (2017). Adaptive region-growing with maximum curvature strategy for tumor segmentation in 18F-FDG PET. *Physics in Medicine & Biology* 62 (13): 5383. Available at: https://doi.org/10.1088/1361-6560/AA6E20.

Tennakoon, R. Gostar, A.K., Hoseinnezhad, R. and Bab-Hadiashar, A., (2018) 'Retinal fluid segmentation in OCT images using adversarial loss based convolutional neural networks', *Proceedings - International Symposium on Biomedical Imaging*, 2018-April, pp. 1436–1440. Available at: https://doi.org/10.1109/ISBI.2018.8363842.

Tong, N. et al. (2019). Shape constrained fully convolutional DenseNet with adversarial training for multiorgan segmentation on head and neck CT and low-field MR images. *Medical Physics* 46 (6): 2669–2682. Available at: https://doi .org/10.1002/MP.13553.

Trullo, R., Petitjean, C., Dubray, B., and Ruan, S. (2019). Multiorgan segmentation using distance-aware adversarial networks. *Journal of Medical Imaging* 6 (1): 014001. Available at: https://doi.org/10.1117/1.JMI.6.1.014001.

Upendra, R.R., Dangi, S. and Linte, C.A. (2019) 'An Adversarial Network Architecture Using 2D U-Net Models for Segmentation of Left Ventricle from Cine Cardiac MRI', *Lecture Notes in Computer Science (including subseries Lecture Notes in Artificial Intelligence and Lecture Notes in Bioinformatics)*, 11504 LNCS, pp. 415–424. Available at: https://doi.org/10.1007/978-3-030-21949-9_45/COVER.

Van Leemput, K. et al. (1999). Automated model-based tissue classification of MR images of the brain. *IEEE Transactions on Medical Imaging* 18 (10): 897–908. Available at: https://doi.org/10.1109/42.811270.

Wang, C. et al. (2020). Adversarial convolutional network for esophageal tissue segmentation on OCT images. *Biomedical Optics Express* 11 (6): 3095–3110. Available at: https://doi.org/10.1364/BOE.394715.

Wang, J., Li, W., Chen, Y. et al. (2021a). Weakly supervised anomaly segmentation in retinal OCT images using an adversarial learning approach. *Biomedical Optics Express* 12 (8): 4713–4729. Available at: https://doi.org/10.1364/BOE.426803.

Wang, S. et al. (2019). Patch-Based Output Space Adversarial Learning for Joint Optic Disc and Cup Segmentation. *IEEE Transactions on Medical Imaging* 38 (11): 2485–2495. Available at: https://doi.org/10.1109/TMI.2019.2899910.

Wang, W. et al. (2021b). Automatic segmentation of prostate magnetic resonance imaging using generative adversarial networks. *Clinical Imaging* 70: 1–9. Available at: https://doi.org/10.1016/J.CLINIMAG.2020.10.014.

Wei, Q., Han, J., Jia, Y., et al. (2020) 'An approach for fully automatic femoral neck-shaft angle evaluation on radiographs', *Review of Scientific Instruments*, 91(1). Available at: https://doi.org/10.1063/1.5089738/1021302.

Wittke, C., Mayer, J., and Schweiggert, F. (2007). On the classification of prostate carcinoma with methods from spatial statistics. *IEEE Transactions on Information Technology in Biomedicine* 11 (4): 406–414. Available at: https://doi.org/10.1109/TITB.2006.888703.

Wu, H., Lu, X., Lei, B., and Wen, Z. (2021). Automated left ventricular segmentation from cardiac magnetic resonance images via adversarial learning with multi-stage pose estimation network and co-discriminator. *Medical Image Analysis* 68: 101891. Available at: https://doi.org/10.1016/J.MEDIA.2020.101891.

Xia, Q., Yao, Y., Hu, Z. and Hao, A., (2019) 'Automatic 3D Atrial Segmentation from GE-MRIs Using Volumetric Fully Convolutional Networks', *Lecture Notes in Computer Science (including subseries Lecture Notes in Artificial Intelligence and Lecture Notes in Bioinformatics)*, 11395 LNCS, pp. 211–220. Available at: https://doi.org/10.1007/978-3-030-12029-0_23/COVER.

Xing, J., Li, Z., Wang, B. et al. (2021). Lesion Segmentation in Ultrasound Using Semi-Pixel-Wise Cycle Generative Adversarial Nets. *IEEE/ACM Transactions on*

Computational Biology and Bioinformatics 18 (6): 2555–2565. Available at: https://doi.org/10.1109/TCBB.2020.2978470.

Xu, C., Howey, J., Ohorodnyk, P. et al. (2020). Segmentation and quantification of infarction without contrast agents via spatiotemporal generative adversarial learning. *Medical Image Analysis* 59: 101568. Available at: https://doi.org/10.1016/J.MEDIA.2019.101568.

Xu, Z., Wu, Z. and Feng, J. (2018) 'CFUN: Combining Faster R-CNN and U-net Network for Efficient Whole Heart Segmentation'. *Arxiv (Cornell University).* Available at: https://arxiv.org/abs/1812.04914v1 (Accessed: 27 December 2023).

Xue, Y., Xu, T., Zhang, H. et al. (2018). SegAN: Adversarial Network with Multi-scale L 1 Loss for Medical Image Segmentation. *Neuroinformatics* 16 (3–4): 383–392. Available at: https://doi.org/10.1007/S12021-018-9377-X/METRICS.

Yahyatabar, M., Jouvet, P. and Cheriet, F. (2020) 'Dense-Unet: A light model for lung fields segmentation in Chest X-Ray images', *Proceedings of the Annual International Conference of the IEEE Engineering in Medicine and Biology Society, EMBS*, 2020-July, pp. 1242–1245. Available at: https://doi.org/10.1109/EMBC44109.2020.9176033.

Yan, Z., Yang, X., and Cheng, K.T. (2019). A Three-Stage Deep Learning Model for Accurate Retinal Vessel Segmentation. *IEEE Journal of Biomedical and Health Informatics* 23 (4): 1427–1436. Available at: https://doi.org/10.1109/JBHI.2018.2872813.

Yang, D., Xu, D., Zhou, S.K. et al. (2017) 'Automatic liver segmentation using an adversarial image-to-image network', Lecture Notes in Computer Science (including subseries Lecture Notes in Artificial Intelligence and Lecture Notes in Bioinformatics), 10435 LNCS, pp. 507–515. Available at: https://doi.org/10.1007/978-3-319-66179-7_58/FIGURES/4.

Yang, T., Wu, T., Li, L., and Zhu, C. (2020). SUD-GAN: Deep Convolution Generative Adversarial Network Combined with Short Connection and Dense Block for Retinal Vessel Segmentation. *Journal of Digital Imaging* 33 (4): 946–957. Available at: https://doi.org/10.1007/S10278-020-00339-9/METRICS.

Yang, X., Zhang, Y., Lo, B. et al. (2021). DBAN: Adversarial Network with Multi-Scale Features for Cardiac MRI Segmentation. *IEEE Journal of Biomedical and Health Informatics* 25 (6): 2018–2028. Available at: https://doi.org/10.1109/JBHI.2020.3028463.

Yıldız, E., Arslan, A.T., Taş, A.Y. et al. (2021). 'Generative Adversarial Network Based Automatic Segmentation of Corneal Subbasal Nerves on In Vivo Confocal Microscopy Images', *Translational Vision. Science & Technology* 10 (6): 33–33. Available at: https://doi.org/10.1167/TVST.10.6.33.

Yuan, W., Wei, J., Wang, J., et al. (2019) 'Unified Attentional Generative Adversarial Network for Brain Tumor Segmentation from Multimodal Unpaired Images', *Lecture Notes in Computer Science (including subseries Lecture Notes in Artificial*

Intelligence and Lecture Notes in Bioinformatics), 11766 LNCS, pp. 229–237. Available at: https://doi.org/10.1007/978-3-030-32248-9_26/COVER.

Yuan, W., Wei, J., Wang, J. et al. (2020). Unified generative adversarial networks for multimodal segmentation from unpaired 3D medical images. *Medical Image Analysis* 64: 101731. Available at: https://doi.org/10.1016/J.MEDIA.2020.101731.

Zhang, H., Xu, T., Li, H. et al. (2019). StackGAN++: Realistic Image Synthesis with Stacked Generative Adversarial Networks. *IEEE Transactions on Pattern Analysis and Machine Intelligence* 41 (8): 1947–1962. Available at: https://doi.org/10.1109/TPAMI.2018.2856256.

Zhang, Y., Miao, S., Mansi, T. and Liao, R. (2018a) 'Task driven generative modeling for unsupervised domain adaptation: Application to X-ray image segmentation', *Lecture Notes in Computer Science (including subseries Lecture Notes in Artificial Intelligence and Lecture Notes in Bioinformatics)*, 11071 LNCS, pp. 599–607. Available at: https://doi.org/10.1007/978-3-030-00934-2_67/TABLES/1.

Zhang, Z., Yang, L. and Zheng, Y. (2018b) 'Translating and Segmenting Multimodal Medical Volumes With Cycle- and Shape-Consistency Generative Adversarial Network', pp. 9242–9251.

Zhang, Z., Zhao, T., Gay, H. et al. (2021). ARPM-net: A novel CNN-based adversarial method with Markov random field enhancement for prostate and organs at risk segmentation in pelvic CT images. *Medical Physics* 48 (1): 227–237. Available at: https://doi.org/10.1002/MP.14580.

Zhao, W., Jiang, D., Queralta, J.P., and Westerlund, T. (2020). MSS U-Net: 3D segmentation of kidneys and tumors from CT images with a multi-scale supervised U-Net. *Informatics in Medicine Unlocked* 19: 100357. Available at: https://doi.org/10.1016/J.IMU.2020.100357.

Zhou, S., Wang, J., Zhang, S. et al. (2016). Active contour model based on local and global intensity information for medical image segmentation. *Neurocomputing* 186: 107–118. Available at: https://doi.org/10.1016/J.NEUCOM.2015.12.073.

Zhu, W. and Xie, X. (2016) 'Adversarial Deep Structural Networks for Mammographic Mass Segmentation', *bioRxiv*, p. 095786. Available at: https://doi.org/10.1101/095786.

9

A Collaborative Cell Image Segmentation Model Based on the Multilevel Improvement of Data

Ishfaq Sheikh, Manzoor Chachoo, and Aijaz Mir

Department of computer science, University of Kashmir, Srinagar, Jammu and Kashmir, India

9.1 Introduction

Computational advancements in cell biology have transformed the medical field by providing unprecedented insights into morphological cell patterns. Cell image segmentation is pivotal for extracting meaningful patterns from biomedical images, facilitating a deeper comprehension of cellular processes. Precise segmentation of biological cells is crucial for personalized medication, enabling treatments tailored to individual cell characteristics and aiding in the early diagnosis of diseases by identifying abnormal cell patterns. Recently, numerous computational solutions have emerged for automatically segmenting cell images, categorized into three classes: image thresholding techniques, clustering approaches, and deep learning methods. The thresholding technique segments medical images by generating a filter to distinguish between foreground and background pixel categories, calculated based on the pixel intensities of various components within the image. Finding the optimal value for this filter is highly challenging due to inherent preset conditions in the method, which may potentially alter the morphological properties (such as perimeter, intensity, eccentricity, and major arc) of cells (Sheikh and Chachoo 2022a). Consequently, this approach risks damaging the morphological features of the cells. Clustering methods assign identities to data points based on their proximity to the nearest cluster, determined through Euclidean and Manhattan distance measurements. These methods typically employ k-means and fuzzy c-means for medical image segmentation. However, it has been observed that these approaches can suffer from both over-sampling and under-sampling of data points (Sheikh and Chachoo 2022b). Nevertheless, these approaches may suffer from over- or under-sampling of data points. Deep learning models are extensively utilized in cell tracking and

Deep Learning Applications in Medical Image Segmentation: Overview, Approaches, and Challenges, First Edition. Edited by Sajid Yousuf Bhat, Aasia Rehman, and Muhammad Abulaish.

segmentation tasks due to their efficient data representation. Despite addressing major deficiencies in existing techniques, deep learning encounters challenges related to data quantity and quality. The quality of biological data notably impedes the generalization of appropriate data representations (Xu et al. 2022; Long 2020).

Strategies have been developed to improve the quality of biological data in response to existing challenges. These strategies are broadly categorized into representative and nonrepresentative learning approaches. In the nonrepresentative approach, a common method involves employing a multiscale transformation (MST) strategy, where data observations transform into high and low frequency data patches (Candès et al. 2006; Bhutada et al. 2011; Do and Vetterli 2005). These decomposed patches are then integrated using inverse transformation techniques, employing spatial fusion strategies. Despite its effectiveness in enhancing data quality, this transformation process often encounters misclassification issues due to inherent conditions within the MST approach. In contrast, the representative learning technique aims to minimize the misregistration of data points by linearly decomposing input observations into local and global geometric features. Fusion of these decomposed observations follows spatial fusion rules, resulting in the generation of improved medical images capable of discerning substructural data patterns (Li et al. 2020; Jia et al. 2021; Makem and Tiedeu 2020).

The refined medical observations are fed into the deep learning model for semantic segmentation of cell images. We opted for the U-net model for the subsequent fusion process due to its effectiveness in preserving both local and global geometric characteristics. This fully convolutional neural network is widely

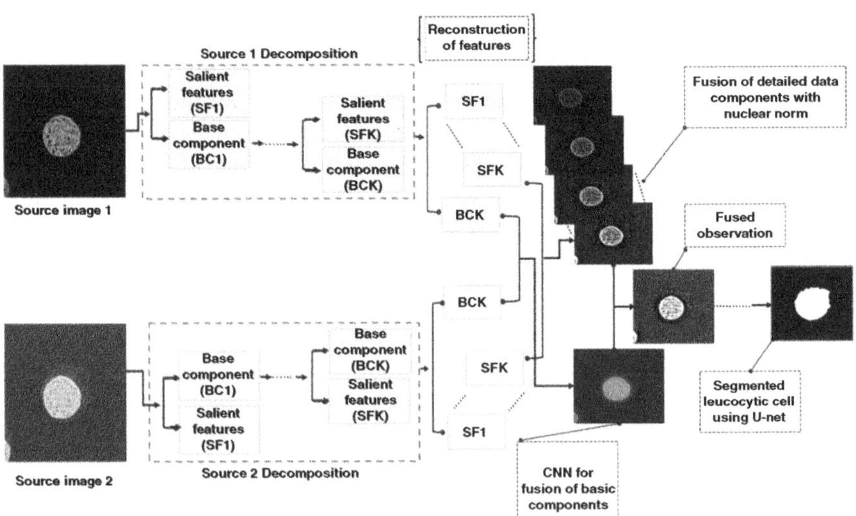

Figure 9.1 Framework of a proposed medical image fusion model.

employed for semantic segmentation tasks in medical imaging and has achieved success in competitions such as the cell tracking and segmentation challenge (ISBI challenge) (Xu et al. 2022). The model architecture consists of various layers, including an input layer, encoding path, bottleneck, and decoding path. The input layer handles data of varying sample sizes, accommodating either RGB images with three channels or grayscale images with a single channel. Following this, the encoder stage employs repeated convolution and max-pooling operations to extract contextual features. Subsequently, deconvolution and upsampling operations are applied to the resulting feature map to preserve local features. Our research has introduced several enhancements for cell fusion and segmentation tasks, such as isolating substructural data patterns, reducing data distortion, improving coefficient representation, and accurately extracting leukocytes. The framework of our proposed approach is illustrated in Figure 9.1.

9.2 Methodology

The framework of the proposed approach comprises three distinct stages: pre-processing, data enhancement, and post-processing. During the pre-processing phase, resampling and data generation procedures are carried out. As a result, the image enhancement operation boosts the identification rate of subcomponents, while post-processing conducts segmentation of the enhanced cell images. Pre-processing operations were conducted on three biomedical databases: Acute Lymphoblastic Leukemia International Database (ALL-IDB) (ALL-IDB 2024), JTSC (Zheng et al. 2018), and CellaVision (Zheng et al. 2018). The image samples from these datasets encompass leucocytes of five different types (lymphocytes, monocytes, neutrophils, basophils, and eosinophils), featuring varying dimensions that were standardized through resampling to a common size. Subsequently, once the resampling process is complete, two distinct appearances (Magenta and Saturation) of biological images are generated. These color channels contain high luminance information crucial for discriminating cells from background textures (Makem and Tiedeu 2020).

The outcomes of pre-processing are directed toward the multilevel decomposition and fusion phase, where a significant enhancement in the quality of biological data occurs. We have constrained the data improvement process to four distinct levels due to the risk of image quality deterioration with further enhancements. This operation involves data decomposition and integration strategies. The medical observation decomposition is executed using latent low-rank due to its resilience to noise and its ability to minimize insufficiently sampled features (Liu and Yan 2011). This process, illustrated in Figure 9.2, generates two different components (basic and detailed) at each level, with one addressing local features (structural properties) and the other encompassing

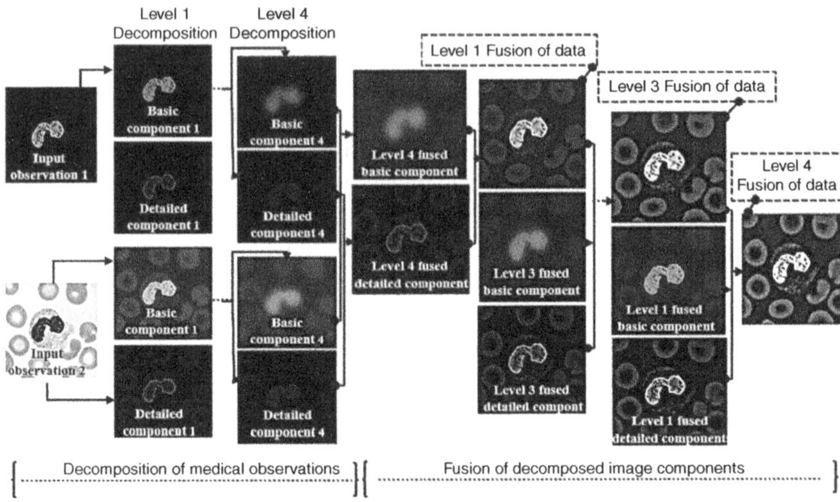

Figure 9.2 An example of a cell image that depicts four-level decomposition and integration of image components.

global features (luminance features). Subsequently, fusion of local features is conducted using the nuclear norm approach, while the global components are fused utilizing the CNN approach. This fusion process, depicted in Figure 9.3, has demonstrated the most effective performance in overall data representation (Sheikh and Chachoo 2023).

The enhanced medical images are fed into a deep learning model for semantic segmentation. Various models are available for analyzing medical images, one of which is the U-net model, a fully convolutional neural network. Its architecture is segmented into encoder and decoder paths. The encoder path captures contextual information (the content of the image), while the decoder portion preserves spatial features (the location of information within the image). The encoder component consists of a sequence of convolutional and max-pooling layers. A convolutional layer serves as a fundamental unit for processing image data and detecting patterns and spatial features in the input data. The convolutional operation involves sliding a small filter (kernel) over the input data, resulting in a dot product between the filter's weights and the values in the receptive field of the input domain. The inputs provided to the convolutional operation include a cell imaging sample of size (n x n x channels) and a set of filters, each with a size of (i x i x channels). The output of the convolution yields an image or feature map with a size of (n-out x n-out x k).

Following the convolution operation, a max-pooling layer is applied to perform downsampling on the feature map. The size of the feature map is regulated by two hyperparameters: filter and strides. The pooling operation process is illustrated in

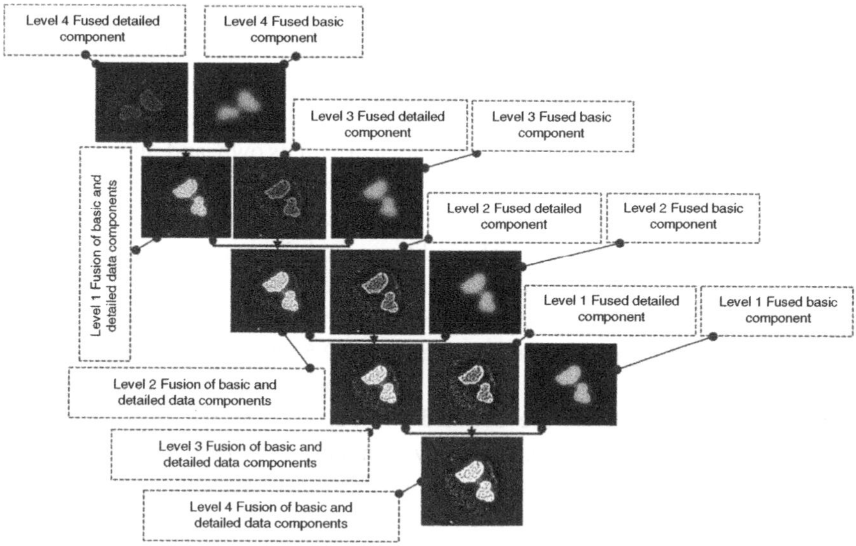

Figure 9.3 Four-level data integration operation on cell imaging sample.

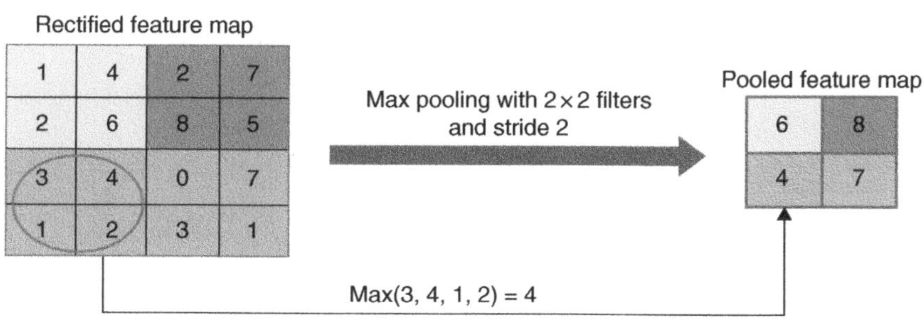

Figure 9.4 Max-pooling operation.

Figure 9.4, where input features (4*4) are downsampled to a (2*2) feature map dimension. This is achieved by selecting the maximum value from each 2*2 block. The convolution operation is iterated multiple times within the network; as we progress deeper into the neural network, the size of the data matrix decreases. This reduction enables the filters of deeper layers to perceive a larger context of the data. While the height and width of the input data gradually diminish in convolution, the number of data filters increases, facilitating the extraction of complex patterns from the data.

The process of downsampling focuses on contextual features of the data and does not address spatial features. However, for medical cell segmentation, both contextual and spatial features are necessary. This requirement is met by the upsampling operation, which preserves spatial information by converting a low-resolution image to a higher resolution one. Various upsampling techniques are available, such as bilinear interpolation, cubic interpolation, nearest neighbor interpolation, and transposed convolution. Most of these methods are based on interpolation, meaning the network does not learn on its own, and manual feature engineering is required. To achieve optimal upsampling, transposed convolution has been identified as the preferred method. Unlike other techniques, transposed convolution does not rely on preset conditions, and the network contains learnable parameters. Transposed convolution has been widely utilized in semantic segmentation to reconstruct the original sample size.

The U-net architecture is illustrated in Figure 9.5 and does not include dense layers, allowing it to accept data samples of any dimension. In our classical U-net design, various parameters are denoted by specific symbols, each carrying a distinct meaning. For instance, "2@Conv" denotes a pair of consecutive convolutional layers, while the output tensors of these convolutions are represented by "c1, c2,..., cn." The output tensors of the upsampling layers are prefixed with "u" (e.g. "u6, u7, u8, and u9"), and those of the downsampling layers are indicated by "p1, p2, p3, and p4." The output of the encoder corresponds to an image size of 8*8*256, while that of the decoder segment is 128*128*1. This signifies that the contraction path reduces the image dimensions and increases

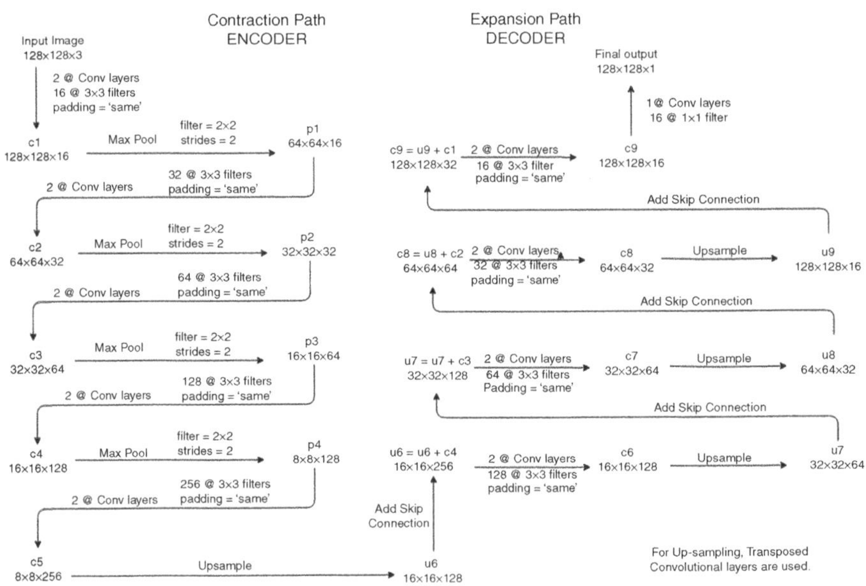

Figure 9.5 Detailed U-net architecture.

the filter depth in deeper layers of the network, whereas the decoder segment reconstructs the original image size by incorporating skip connections with the upconvolutional layers. For example, the output of the upsampling layer u6 is obtained by concatenating the convolutional (c4) and deconvolution tensors (u6), denoted as u6 = u6 + c4. This process generates an image containing both local and global geometric features. We employed an Adam optimizer for model compilation, while the loss of the model is governed by binary cross-entropy due to the presence of only two classes: leucocytic cells and background. Learning rate decay is implemented for three consecutive epochs, and an early stopping condition is triggered if there is no improvement for five consecutive epochs. The operation of the U-net at various enhanced levels is depicted in Figure 9.6.

The U-net architecture is illustrated in Figure 9.5 and does not include dense layers, allowing it to accept data samples of any dimension. In our classical U-net design, various parameters are denoted by specific symbols, each carrying a distinct meaning. For instance, "2@Conv" denotes a pair of consecutive convolutional layers, while the output tensors of these convolutions are represented by "c1, c2,…, cn." The output tensors of the upsampling layers are prefixed with "u" (e.g. "u6, u7, u8, and u9"), and those of the downsampling layers are indicated by "p1, p2, p3, and p4." The output of the encoder corresponds to an image size of 8*8*256, while that of the decoder segment is 128*128*1. This signifies that the contraction path reduces the image dimensions and increases the filter depth in deeper layers of the network, whereas the decoder segment reconstructs the original image size by incorporating skip connections with the upconvolutional layers. For example, the output of the upsampling layer u6 is obtained by concatenating the convolutional (c4) and deconvolution tensors (u6), denoted as u6 = u6 + c4. This process generates an image containing both local and global geometric features. We

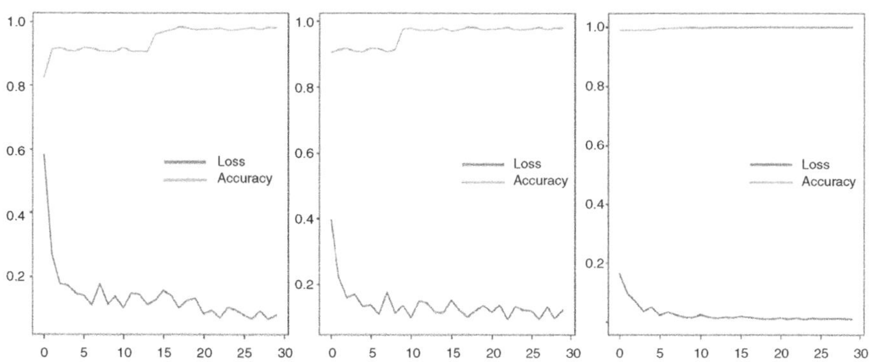

Figure 9.6 Performance of U-net on the different data enhancement levels.

employed an Adam optimizer for model compilation, while the loss of the model is governed by binary cross-entropy due to the presence of only two classes: leucocytic cells and background. Learning rate decay is implemented for three consecutive epochs, and an early stopping condition is triggered if there is no improvement for five consecutive epochs. The operation of the U-net at various enhanced levels is depicted in Figure 9.6.

9.3 Result and Discussion

Medical images often suffer from various types of outliers, leading to inappropriate discrimination of cell imaging subcomponents. Additionally, many relevant studies have recognized the challenges associated with processing biomedical imaging datasets (Jia et al. 2021; Makem and Tiedeu 2020). Some automated approaches, such as pattern-based segmentation and boundary cell segmentation, result in under-segmentation and over-segmentation of data points due to noisy data clusters. To address this issue, we have devised an improvement in our research that focuses on segmenting enhanced biological images. The objective of this approach is to mitigate misregistration of data points to enable smooth extraction of leucocytic cells.

The proposed approach is evaluated using three different biological databases: the ALL-IDB dataset, CellaVision dataset, and the JTSC database. The ALL-IDB contains lymphocytes from acute leukemia patients, with segmented and non-segmented subsets available. For evaluation purposes, we utilized the non-segmented samples from this subset. The medical samples in this subset vary in dimension, necessitating resampling to a common size. The CellaVision and JTSC datasets comprise leucocytes of five different types: basophils, eosinophils, monocytes, lymphocytes, and neutrophils. These datasets are publicly accessible, and manual annotation files are provided for all of them. We adopted a specific ratio (80 : 20) for training and testing the model.

Evaluation metrics: The performance of the model is assessed using various metrics (Dice 1945; Muthu and Murali 2021), including the Jaccard Index (J), F1 measure, accuracy, precision, recall, and specificity. The Jaccard Index (J) gauges the degree of overlap between the model's results and the annotation file masks, ranging from 0 (indicating imperfect segmentation) to 1 (denoting perfect segmentation). The F1 measure strikes a balance between precision and recall, with values ranging from 0 (signifying an imbalanced harmonic mean) to 1 (representing a balanced harmonic mean).

Accuracy is a metric that computes the overall correctness of the model, where perfect accuracy is indicated by a value of 1 and imperfect accuracy by 0. Precision, also known as the true positive rate, evaluates the accuracy of true positive (TP) predictions relative to the total positive predictions (TP + FP [false positive]), with values between 0 and 1. Higher precision values correspond to lower false positive rates. Specificity, also referred to as the true negative rate, measures the accuracy of true negatives (TN) relative to the total negative predictions (TN + FN [false negative]). A higher specificity value suggests a lower false positive rate. Recall, or sensitivity, evaluates the correctness of all relevant instances and ranges from 0 to 1, with higher values indicating fewer false negatives. It is computed by dividing true positives (TP) by the sum of false negatives (FN) and true positives (TP).

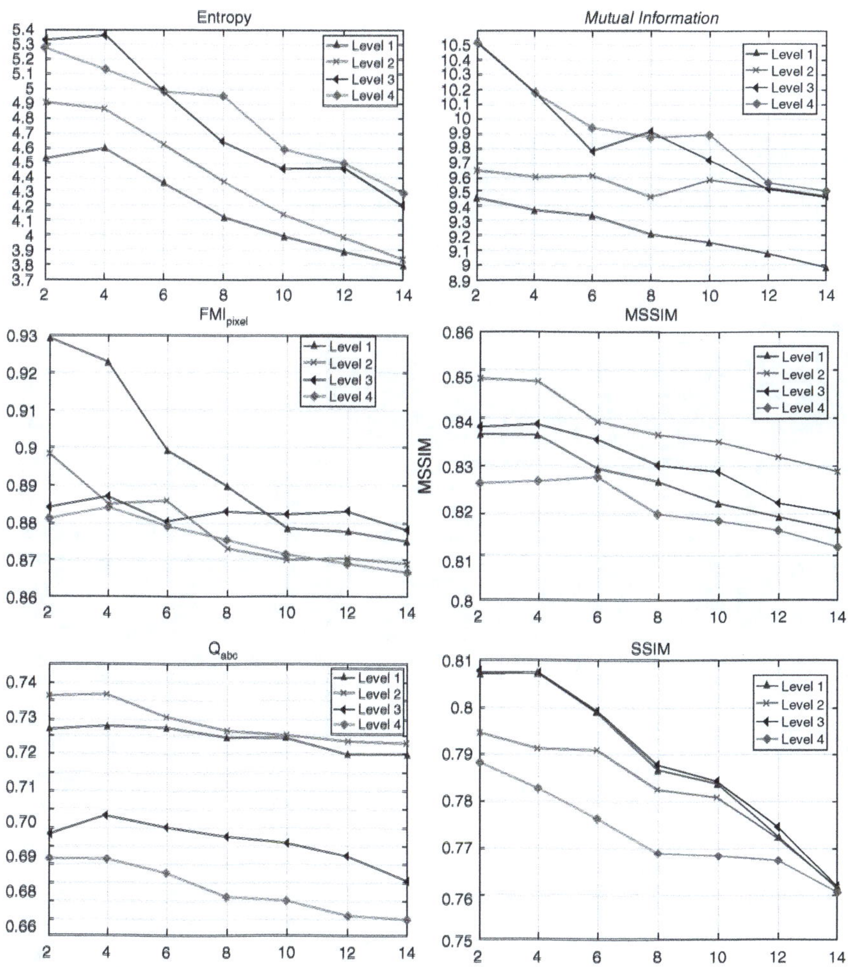

Figure 9.7 Performance of data integration operation for different metrics, which include SSIM (structural similarity), MSSIM (maximum structural similarity), FMI (fast mutual information), and Qabc (quality metrics).

Quantitative comparison: We have conducted both qualitative and quantitative evaluations of the model. The qualitative assessments reveal visual enhancements in the appearance of various cellular substructures (RBC, WBC, platelets, and background). Four levels of improvement were generated for each biological database, aiming to enhance the identification of leucocytes for smoother extraction, while retaining fine-grained and detailed information on morphological subpatterns. Visual representations of the proposed approach are depicted in three separate figures (Figures 9.7–9.9), where Figures 9.7 and 9.8 showcase the outcomes of the data integration operation, and Figure 9.9 presents the segmentation results. Through qualitative analysis, it is evident that our generated results exhibit enhanced brightness and clarity compared

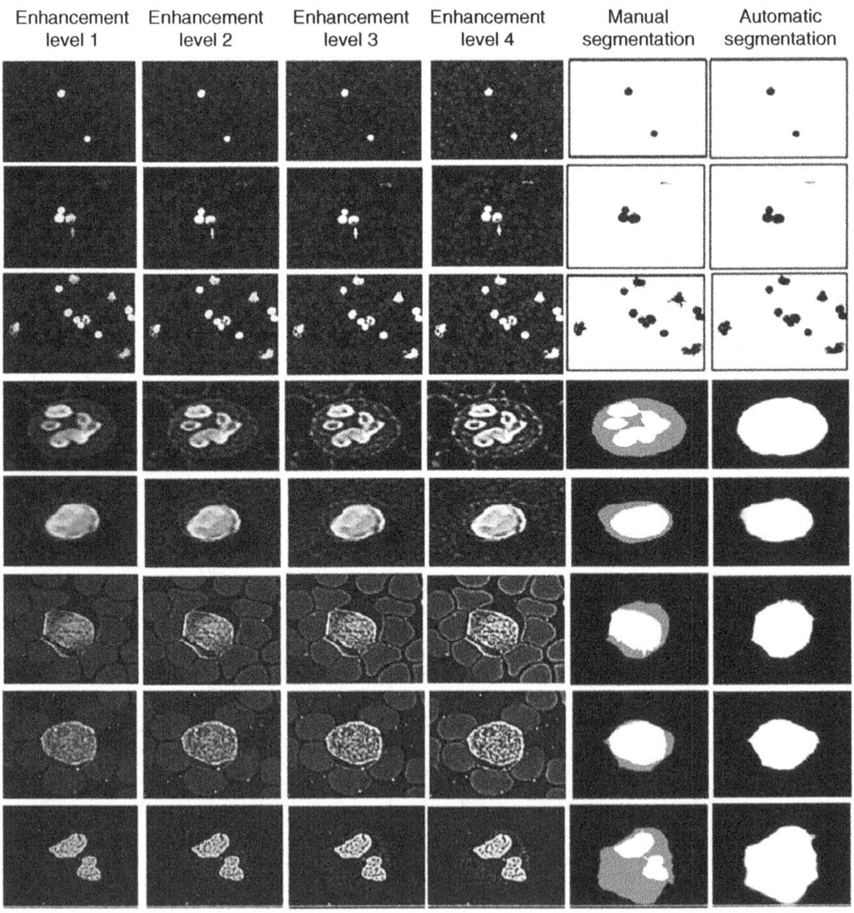

Figure 9.8 An example of medical images selected for collaborative fusion strategy.

to related techniques. Quantitative results of the proposed approach are presented in two tables (Tables 9.1 and 9.2), and their comparative analysis is conducted against state-of-the-art methods. Our adopted approach demonstrates superior performance metrics, as evidenced by the highest and second-highest values achieved across various performance metrics, surpassing those of related techniques.

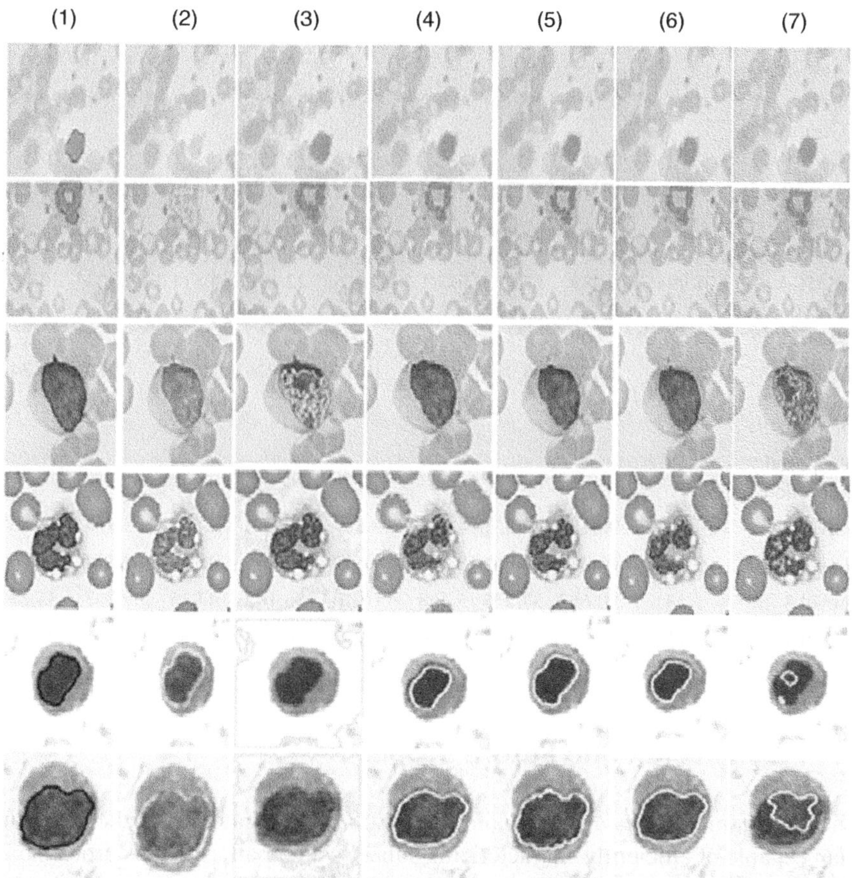

Figure 9.9 Qualitative comparison of different cell image segmentation methods on some cell images collected from different datasets, which include CellaVision, JTSC and BloodSeg. Column (1)represents the expert segmentation, column (2) represents the results of the proposed method, column (3) is the segmentation of Source: Abdeldaim et al. 2018, column (4) is the segmentation by Source: Vincent et al. 2015, column (5) by Source: Makem and Tiedeu 2020, column (6) is segmented by Source: Vogado et al. 2016, and column (7) by Source: Abdul Nasir et al. 2011.

Table 9.1 Quantitative comparison of data integration operation (image fusion phase).

	CellaVision			ALL-IDB			JTSC		
Dataset Model	**Entropy**	**MI**	**SD**	**Entropy**	**MI**	**SD**	**Entropy**	**MI**	**SD**
LRR-NSST (Li et al. 2018)	4.545	9.071	29.516	4.725	9.187	30.389	4.405	8.869	28.756
LRR-Wavelet (Li et al. 2018)	4.554	9.071	29.659	4.791	9.253	30.758	4.419	8.749	28.958
NSST (Guorong et al. 2013)	4.544	9.109	29.653	4.542	8.931	29.531	4.394	8.708	28.353
LP-CNN (Liu et al. 2017)	5.098	10.196	21.412	5.463	**10.927**	21.9876	**5.555**	**9.431**	38.254
CSMCA (Zhu et al. 2019)	4.994	9.989	17.796	5.081	10.162	22.1006	4.811	9.3224	18.984
NSST-PC-LLE (Liu et al. 2019)	**5.873**	**10.547**	28.982	5.198	10.396	22.9263	2.494	4.9891	**38.346**
Proposed approach									
Level 1	4.907	9.818	32.931	4.932	9.367	33.536	4.608	8.918	31.838
Level 2	5.168	10.336	37.061	5.013	9.633	33.751	4.718	9.334	32.561
Level 3	5.331	10.663	37.258	5.468	10.403	36.162	4.915	9.763	35.257
Level 4	5.115	10.551	37.385	5.136	9.732	36.347	4.865	9.201	38.438

9.4 Conclusion and Future Scope

The amalgamation of diverse biological features generates a robust decision map capable of efficiently characterizing subclass data patterns. This process has demonstrated enhancements in the identification of cellular components. As data fusion was conducted across four different levels, it was observed that higher enhancement levels resulted in improved segmentation performance. By employing a collaborative strategy on cell imaging samples, fine-grained characteristics of various components were observed. This work exhibits broad applicability for application on multimodal medical images such as CT scans, X-ray images, POSET images, knee images, and X-ray images. Computational analysis of these

Table 9.2 Quantitative comparison of post-fusion operation.

Dataset	Approach	Recall	Specificity	Precision	Accuracy	f-measure	J
ALL-IDB	OTSU (Safuan et al. 2017)	0.8234	–	0.8902	–	0.8554	0.747
	FC (Alférez et al. 2019)	0.6137	–	0.6008	–	0.6071	0.435
	Shahzad et al. (2020)	–	–	–	0.9334	0.3309	0.198
	Sudha and Geetha (2020)	**0.9805**	–	**0.9932**	–	**0.9867**	**0.973**
	Garcia et al. (2021)	0.7671	**0.9997**	0.9857	**0.9924**	0.8628	0.758
	Proposed Approach	**0.9951**	**0.9865**	**0.9901**	**0.9989**	**0.9715**	**0.944**
CellaVision	SVR	0.8592	–	0.9655	–	0.9242	0.867
	OTSU (Safuan et al. 2017)	0.861	–	0.9781	–	0.9161	0.845
	FC Alférez et al. 2019)	0.848	–	0.9025	–	0.8746	0.777
	Makem and Tiedeu (2020)	**0.970**	–	0.9737	**0.9937**	0.9475	**0.900**
	Sudha and Geetha (2020)	0.8791	–	**0.9963**	–	**0.9341**	0.876
	Proposed Approach	**0.9825**	**0.9794**	**0.9875**	**0.9968**	**0.9597**	**0.922**
JTSC	Vincent et al. (2015)	0.753	0.4772	0.5115	0.7921	0.4833	0.318
	Vogado et al. (2016)	0.971	**0.8318**	**0.9355**	**0.9899**	0.8768	0.780
	Kumar and Kumar (2017)	0.9677	0.8186	0.9343	**0.9897**	0.8653	0.762
	Abdeldaim et al. (2018)	0.6598	0.4544	0.1679	0.6849	0.1913	0.106
	Makem and Tiedeu (2020)	**0.972**	–	0.9101	0.9312	**0.9079**	**0.830**
	Proposed approach	**0.9845**	**0.9721**	**0.9742**	0.9651	**0.9389**	**0.884**

databases holds potential for diagnosing various biological diseases including Alzheimer's disease, brain tumors, and COVID-19. The multilevel fusion rules of the adopted approach can also be leveraged for integrating multiomics data such as RNA-seq, DNA methylation, whole slide imaging (WSI), and copy number variation data. This integration not only minimizes insufficient sampling features but also yields new insights into disease prediction.

Acknowledgments

All authors have contributed equally.

References

Abdeldaim, A.M., Sahlol, A.T., Elhoseny, M., and Hassanien, A.E. (2018). Computer-aided acute lymphoblastic leukemia diagnosis system based on image analysis. In: *Advances in Soft Computing and Machine Learning in Image Processing*, 131–147. Cham: Springer International Publishing.

A.S. Abdul Nasir, M.Y. Mashor, and H. Rosline (2011). Unsupervised colour segmentation of white blood cell for acute leukaemia images', in *IEEE International Conference on Imaging Systems and Techniques*, Batu Ferringhi, Malaysia.

Alférez, S., Merino, A., Acevedo, A. et al. (2019). Color clustering segmentation framework for image analysis of malignant lymphoid cells in peripheral blood. *Med. Biol. Eng. Comput.* 57 (6): 1265–1283.

ALL-IDB. (2024) Acute Lymphoblastic Leukemia Image Database for Image Processing [Online]. Available: https://homes.di.unimi.it/scotti/all/. [Accessed: 25 Mar 2024].

Bhutada, G.G., Anand, R.S., and Saxena, S.C. (2011). Edge preserved image enhancement using adaptive fusion of images denoised by wavelet and curvelet transform. *Digital Signal Processing* 21 (1): 118–130.

Candès, E., Demanet, L., Donoho, D., and Ying, L. (2006). Fast Discrete Curvelet Transforms. *Multiscale Modeling and Simulation* 5 (3): 861–899.

Dice, L.R. (1945). Measures of the amount of ecologic association between species. *Ecology* 26 (3): 297–302.

Do, M.N. and Vetterli, M. (2005). The contourlet transform: an efficient directional multiresolution image representation. *IEEE Transactions on Image Processing* 14 (12): 2091–2106.

Garcia, F.L., Alvarado, M., and Cervantes, J. (2021). Systematic segmentation method based on PCA of image hue features for white blood cell counting. *PLoS One* 16 (12): e0261857.

Guorong, G., Luping, X., and Dongzhu, F. (2013). Multi-focus image fusion based on non-subsampled shearlet transform. *IET Image Processing* 7 (6): 633–639.

D. Jia, S. Gao, Q. Chen, X. Luo, and X. Zhuang. (2021). A low-rank representation for unsupervised registration of medical images, *Arxiv (Cornell University) arXiv [cs.CV]*.

Kumar, P.S. and Kumar, S. (2017). Automated diagnosis of acute lymphocytic leukemia and acute myeloid leukemia using multi-SV. *Journal of Biomedical Imaging and Bioengineering* 1 (1): 20–24.

H. Li, X.-J. Wu, and T. Durrani. (2018). 'Multi-focus noisy image fusion using low-rank representation', *Arxiv (Cornell University) arXiv [cs.CV]*.

Li, Z., Dong, A., and Zhou, J. (2020). Research of low-rank representation and discriminant correlation analysis for Alzheimer's disease diagnosis. *Computational and Mathematical Methods in Medicine* 2020: 1–8.

G. Liu and S. Yan. (2011). Latent Low-Rank Representation for subspace segmentation and feature extraction', in *2011 International Conference on Computer Vision*, Barcelona, Spain.

Liu, Y., Chen, X., Peng, H., and Wang, Z. (2017). Multi-focus image fusion with a deep convolutional neural network. *Information Fusion* 36: 191–207.

Liu, Y., Chen, X., Ward, R.K., and Wang, Z.J. (2019). Medical image fusion via convolutional sparsity-based morphological component analysis. *IEEE Signal Processing Letters* 26 (3): 485–489.

F. Long. (2020). Microscopy cell nuclei segmentation with enhanced U-Net, *BMC Bioinformatics*, vol. 21, no. 1 Dec. 2020.

M. Makem and A. Tiedeu. (2020). An efficient algorithm for detection of white blood cell nuclei using adaptive three stage PCA-based fusion, *Informatics in Medicine Unlocked*, vol. 20, no. 100416, p. 100416, 2020.

Muthu, J.S. and Murali, P. (2021). Review of chaos detection techniques performed on chaotic maps and systems in image encryption. *SN Computer Science* 2 (5): 1–24.

S.N.M. Safuan, R. Tomari, W.N.W. Zakaria, and N. Othman. (2017). White blood cell counting analysis of blood smear images using various segmentation strategies, *Presented at the advances in electrical and electronic engineering: from theory to applications: Proceedings of the International Conference on Electrical and Electronic Engineering (IC3E 2017).*

Shahzad, M., Umar, A.I., Khan, M.A. et al. (2020). Robust method for semantic segmentation of whole-slide blood cell microscopic images. *Computational and mathematical methods in medicine* 2020 (1): 4015323.

Sheikh, I. M., and Chachoo, M. A. (2022a). Leukocytic Cell Nucleus Identification Using Boundary Cell Detection Algorithm with Dilation and Erosion Based

Morphometry. In *Springer e-books* (pp. 79–102) Cham: Springer International Publishing. http://dx. doi.org/10.1007/ 978-3-030-96569-3_4.

Sheikh, I.M., and Chachoo, M.A.(2022b). An enforced block diagonal low-rank representation method for the classification of medical image patterns. *International Journal of Information Technology*, 14(3), 1221–1228. /https://doi.org/ 10.1007/s41870-021-00841-5.

Sheikh, I.M. and Chachoo, M.A. (2023). A novel cell image fusion approach based on the collaboration of multilevel latent Low-Rank representation and the convolutional neural network. *Biomedical Signal Processing and Control* 83 (104654): 104654.

Sudha, K. and Geetha, P. (2020). A novel approach for segmentation and counting of overlapped leukocytes in microscopic blood images. *Biocybernetics and Biomedical Engineering* 40 (2): 639–648.

I. Vincent, K.-R. Kwon, S.-H. Lee, and K.-S. Moon. (2015). Acute lymphoid leukemia classification using two-step neural network classifier, in *21st Korea-Japan Joint Workshop on Frontiers of Computer Vision (FCV)*, Mokpo, South Korea.

Vogado, L.H., ds MS Veras, R., Andrade, A.R., e Silva, R.R., De Araujo, F.H. and De Medeiros, F.N., (2016). Unsupervised leukemia cells segmentation based on multi-space color channels, *in IEEE International Symposium on Multimedia (ISM)*, San Jose, CA, USA.

Xu, J., Zhou, D., Deng, D. et al. (2022). Deep learning in cell image analysis. *Intelligent Computing*.

Zheng, X., Wang, Y., Wang, G., and Liu, J. (2018). Fast and robust segmentation of white blood cell images by self-supervised learning. *Micron* 107: 55–71.

Zhu, Z., Zheng, M., Qi, G. et al. (2019). A phase congruency and local Laplacian energy based multi-modality medical image fusion method in NSCT domain. *IEEE Access* 7: 1–1.

10

Challenges and Future Directions for Segmentation of Medical Images Using Deep Learning Models

Roshan Birjais

Department of Electrical, Computer and Software Engineering, Faculty of Engineering, The University of Auckland, Auckland, New Zealand

10.1 Introduction

Healthcare professionals, including clinicians and radiologists, predominantly handle the interpretation of medical images. However, the constrained availability of human specialists, combined with the exhaustion and inexact methods they use for estimation, limits the efficiency of image interpretation among proficient healthcare practitioners. Challenges arise from variations among experts and the complexities inherent in medical images, making precise disease diagnosis a significant obstacle for these professionals.

Automated computer techniques have simplified the challenging process of image analysis, enabling both semi- and fully automatic procedures. These methods aid experts in achieving objective, rapid, and precise diagnoses. As a result, the ongoing exploration and advancement of deep learning-based approaches for analyzing medical images continue to be a compelling and dynamic area of research.

Integrating deep learning (DL) techniques into medical image analysis is captivating, yet progress faces various challenges. A key limitation hindering DL in medical images is the inherent variation within the data, encompassing factors, such as contrast, resolution, and signal-to-noise ratio, often arising from clinical practice procedures. Nonstandardized acquisition of medical data further complicates the analysis, and the demand for detailed medical image labeling constrains the utilization of DL in this domain.

A significant challenge arises from the scarcity of data, particularly in contrast to other datasets, and the intricate nature of sharing medical datasets. Handling the privacy of medical data is both a technological and sociological concern that requires examination from both perspectives. Constructing Deep Learning

Deep Learning Applications in Medical Image Segmentation: Overview, Approaches, and Challenges, First Edition. Edited by Sajid Yousuf Bhat, Aasia Rehman, and Muhammad Abulaish.

Algorithms (DLAs) necessitate a substantial amount of annotated data, and the annotation process is time consuming due to the requisite domain knowledge of radiologists.

To tackle the challenge of limited labeled data, the implementation of semi-supervised learning can leverage existing labeled data alongside extensive unlabeled data. Additionally, developing few-shot learning methods with a significantly reduced dataset presents a potential remedy for the challenge of limited data availability.

In spite of the accomplishments of the DLA, numerous restrictions and hurdles persist in the medical field. DL offers the possibility to decrease medical expenses, enhance efficiency in healthcare, and boost patient satisfaction in healthcare remains uncertain. Nevertheless, conducting clinical trials that show the effectiveness of DL algorithms and establishing guidelines for their application in the analysis of medical images is imperative.

10.2 Types of Medical Datasets

In the domain of medical imaging and healthcare research, the accessibility of diverse and meticulously curated datasets assumes a pivotal role in propelling the advancements of DLA. These datasets serve as the fundamental basis for researchers to develop and evaluate novel methods for analyzing the medical images, aiding in the generation of diagnoses, prognoses, and treatment strategies. The expanse of medical datasets is extensive, encapsulating a multitude of imaging modalities and analyzing anatomical structures and pathological conditions. Figure 10.1 illustrates the various modalities employed in assessing the medical images. The information was gathered using Kaggle and paperwithcode .com. Each dataset represents a reservoir of information, presenting distinctive challenges and prospects for the development of algorithms. Within this section, we intricately examine the multifaceted nature of medical datasets, scrutinizing their categorizations, intrinsic attributes, and the invaluable contributions they bestow upon the forefront of medical inquiry and computational healthcare.

10.2.1 X-Ray

X-rays are electromagnetic radiations distinguished by wavelengths that are shorter than ultraviolet (UV) rays but longer than gamma rays. Possessing the capacity to penetrate matter to varying extents, X-rays have extensive applications in medical imaging for diagnostic purposes. They serve as a valuable tool for detecting and visualizing internal structures within the human body. Figure 10.2 demonstrates the difference between Normal lung anatomy and

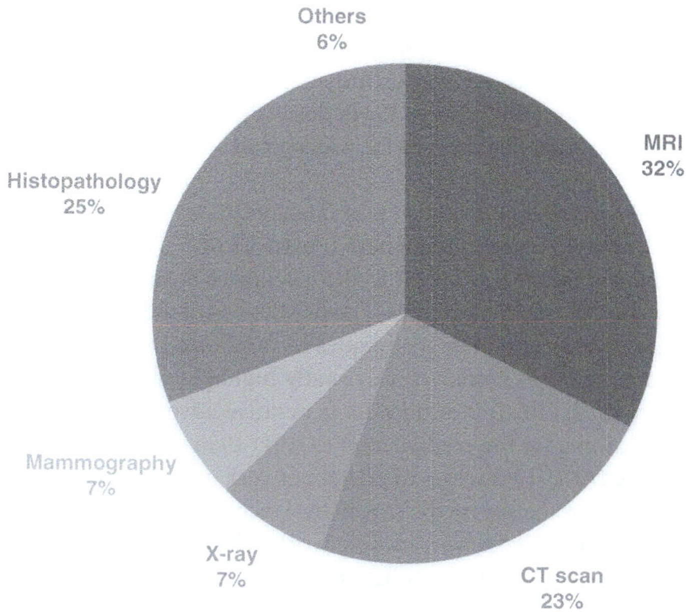

Figure 10.1 The distribution of modalities utilized in medical imaging expressed as percentages.

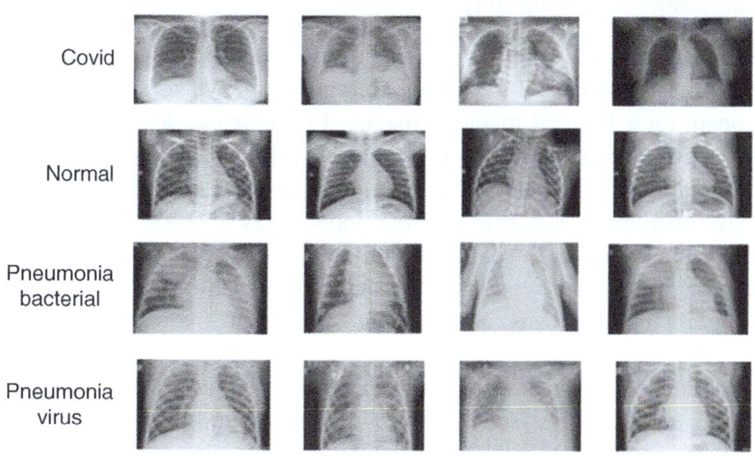

Figure 10.2 Chest X-ray samples. Source: Loey et al. (2020)/MDPI/CC BY 4.0.

other pathological conditions. Chest radiography is crucial in diagnosing lung diseases and heart pathologies, including tuberculosis, pleural effusion atelectasis, consolidation, pneumothorax, and hypercardiac inflation. These images are widely available, cost-effective, and involve lower doses than alternative imaging methods, making them an effective method for widespread screening (Candemir et al. 2018).

The initial tuberculosis screening system was introduced, leveraging transfer learning techniques and deep convolutional neural network (CNN) (Hwang et al. 2016). Rajaraman and Antani (2020a) introduced a specialized ensemble learning approach to identify chest X-ray irregularities. The predictions of these models are consolidated through diverse ensemble techniques to minimize prediction variance. Class-selective mapping is employed to visually highlight affected regions in these images. Loey et al. (2020) introduced a generative adversarial network (GAN) with transfer training for the prediction of COVID-19 in chest X-rays. Due to the limited data on COVID-19 disease, the GAN network generates additional chest X-ray images. The introduction to the CovidGAN technique is dependent on the Auxiliary Classifier Generative Adversarial Network, which produces artificial chest X-ray images for the COVID-19 classification (Waheed et al. 2020). Rajaraman and Antani (2020b) implemented a labeled data augmentation technique to elaborate the dataset for training purposes, thereby improving the prediction of COVID-19 in chest X-ray images.

10.2.2 Computerized Tomography

Computed tomography (CT) images are diagnostic medical images generated through a technology called CT scanning, commonly known as CT scanning. CT scans constitute a form of medical imaging that employs X-rays to create comprehensive cross-sectional body images. This technique facilitates the creation of a three-dimensional perspective of internal structures, enabling a more comprehensive assessment compared to traditional X-ray imaging. The various features of CT images are high spatial resolution, contrast enhancement, multiplanar imaging, and dense and soft tissue differentiation. These images are highly used for diagnosis and staging, treatment planning, vascular imaging, etc.

In 2016, researchers pioneered the introduction of a deep CNN designed to detect three nodule types: solid, semisolid, and ground-glass opacity (Li et al. 2016). Balagourouchetty et al. (2019) proposed a liver lesion classification ensemble FCNet classifier based on GoogLeNet. The fundamental GoogLeNet architecture underwent three modifications to enhance feature extraction. Masood et al. (2020) introduced the multidimensional region-based fully convolutional network for detecting and classifying lung nodules, achieving an impressive accuracy of 97.91%. Their emphasis was particularly on the detection of micronodules (less than 3 mm) in lung nodule identification without compromising performance metrics. In 2019, Zhao and Zeng introduced a Deep Learning Architecture (DLA) based on supervised MSS U-Net and 3DU-Net for the automatic segmentation of kidneys and associated tumors (Zhao and Zeng 2019). Fan et al. (2020) and Li et al. (2019) applied DL methods to identify COVID-19 from CT images during COVID-19.

10.2.3 Mammography (MG)

MG, a specialized medical imaging technique, plays an important role in screening and diagnosing breast conditions, with a primary focus on breast cancer detection. This procedure utilizes X-rays to generate detailed images of the breast tissue. Mammograms are indispensable in the early prognosis of breast cancer and are recommended as part of routine screening protocols for women, usually commencing at a specific age or based on individual risk factors. The automated classification and early-stage detection of masses in mammography continue to be the areas of active research. Over the last decade, DLAs have made significant strides in overcoming challenges associated with breast cancer detection and classification.

Fonseca et al. (2015) introduced a method for detecting breast composition using a CNN to extract features following the ACR standard. Some researchers suggested a CNN model with 12 layers for detecting breast arterial calcifications and assessing coronary artery disease (Wang et al. 2017). In another research, a computer-aided design (CAD) system employing faster R-CNN, which autonomously classifies lesions into benign and malignant in mammogram images, illustrated in Figure 10.3 (Ribli et al. 2018).

A deep CNN trained on more than 1,000,000 mammogram data for the classification of breast cancer (Wu et al. 2019). Another deep CNN-based system has been developed for detecting AQ lesions, including calcified and soft tissue abnormalities, in digital breast tomosynthesis images (Conant et al. 2019). The proposed architecture of fuzzy completely connected layer architecture integrates fused fuzzy rules along with conventional CNN for semantic BI-RADS scoring (Kang et al. 2020). This framework demonstrated superior performance in BI-RADS scoring for both triple and multi-class classifications.

10.2.4 Histopathology

Histopathological images are high-resolution microscopic images capturing tissue specimens that undergo processing and staining for examination under a microscope. This imagery is integral to pathology, a medical specialty focused

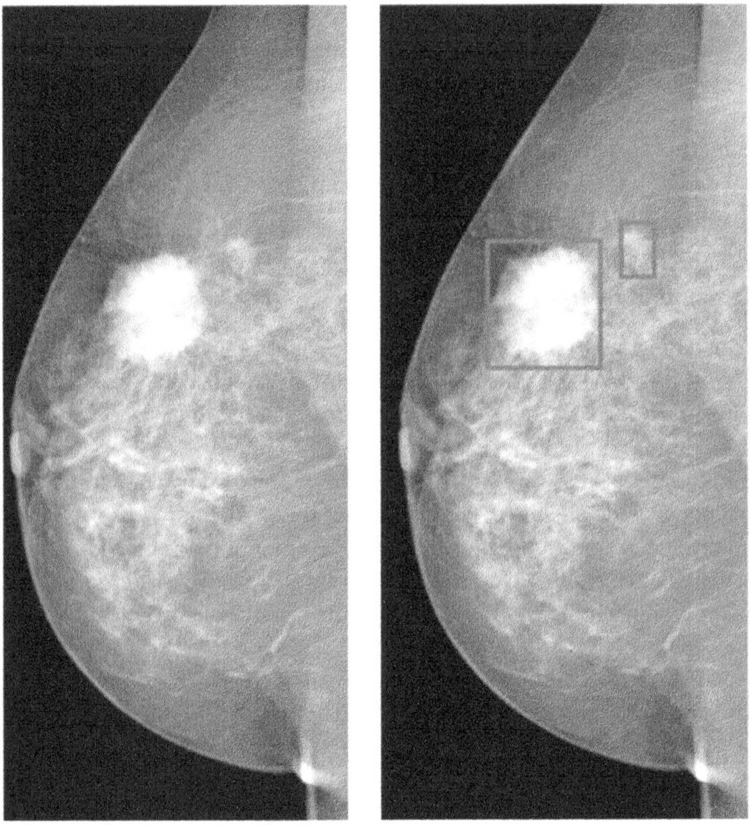

Figure 10.3 Detection of lesions using mammogram images. Source: Ribli et al. (2018)/Springer Nature/CC BY 4.0.

on studying and diagnosing diseases by examining tissues, organs, and cells. Figure 10.4 shows four different magnification factors of the histopathological images from the BreakHis database (Spanhol et al. 2016).

DL is gaining prominence as a powerful method for analyzing histopathology images and tackling tasks such as nucleus detection, image classification, and cell and tissue segmentation (Xing et al. 2018). The domain of digital pathology analysis of images shows significant advancement of whole slide imaging (WSI), enabling the digitization of glass slides containing stained tissue sections at high resolution. In another research, Dimitriou et al. (2019) offered an overview of challenges associated with analyzing WSI images of multi-gigabytes to construct DL models.

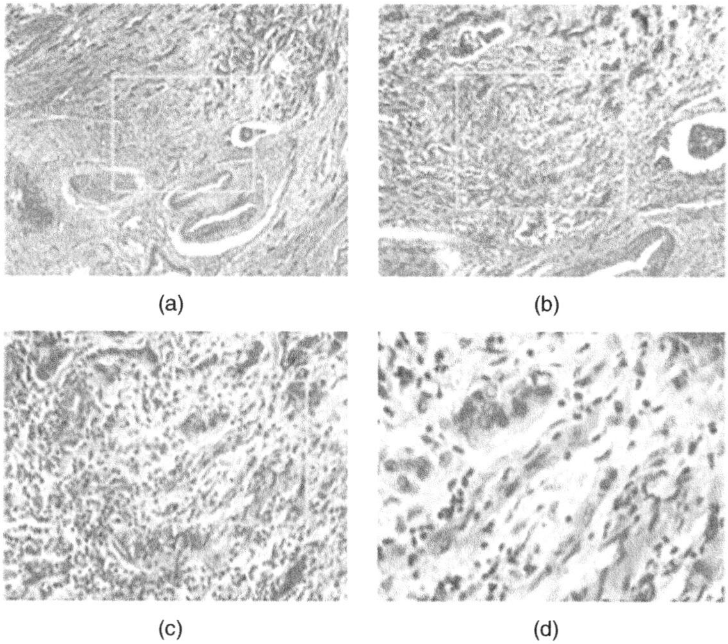

Figure 10.4 Microscopic image of breast tumor tissue with four different magnification factors. (a) 40X, (b) 100X, (c) 200X, and (d) 400X. Source: Spanhol et al. (2016)/with permission of IEEE.

10.2.5 Magnetic Resonance Imaging (MRI)

Utilizing magnetic resonance, it captures electromagnetic signals emitted by human organs and subsequently reconstructs information about the structure of these organs. MRIs with high resolution provide improved structural details, significantly contributing to the precise localization of lesions and accurate diagnosis of diseases. Segmenting MRI images presents various challenges in medical image processing. The intricacies of brain tissue, coupled with artifacts like motion artifacts, ring artifacts, and noise, contribute to the difficulty of achieving accurate segmentation (Prakasha et al. 2023). Furthermore, challenges such as partial volume effects, asymmetrical grayscale, and additional noise further complicate the segmentation process (Veeramalla et al. 2023). In the context of rectum MRI segmentation, the irregular shape of the organ and the proximity of nearby nodes and organs pose challenges in isolating the rectum area accurately (Srivaramangai 2023). Additionally, the intrinsic heterogeneity stemming from different MRI scanners, vendors, acquisition sequences, and diverse stages of neurodevelopment increase the complexity of segmenting infant brain MRI across various ages, modalities, and sites (Zhang et al. 2023).

Overall, MRI segmentation faces challenges related to artifacts, tissue complexity, irregular shapes, and heterogeneity in data acquisition.

10.2.6 Other Images

Endoscopy entails inserting a long, nonsurgical tube into the body to visually examine internal organs or tissues in detail. This technique is valuable for studying various systems within the human body, including the respiratory, gastrointestinal, urinary, and female reproductive tract (Jani and Srivastava 2019; Münzer et al. 2018).

Wireless capsule endoscopy is an innovative device designed for painless and noninvasive examination to detect and diagnose diseases such as ulcers and bleeding in the gastrointestinal tract. Soffer et al. systematically analyzed the literature on DL in WCE (Soffer et al. 2020). He et al. (2018) introduced the first deep learning based framework for hookworm detection in WCE images, incorporating two CNN networks for edge extraction and hookworm classification. Some researchers created a CNN model for early gastric cancer identification and prediction of invasion depth, which is crucial for determining the appropriate treatment method (Yoon et al. 2019). Nakagawa et al. (2019) applied DL techniques based on CNN to enhance the diagnosis of an esophageal wall using endoscopy, while Choi et al. (2020) discussed the features and aspects of DL in endoscopy.

Positron emission tomography (PET) is a tool for nuclear imaging that visualizes molecular-level activities within tissues by injecting specific radioactive tracers. Wang et al. (2020) examined the use of machine learning in PET attenuation correction and low-count PET reconstruction, emphasizing the benefits of DL compared to conventional machine learning in PET image tasks. Another research provides an overview of PET image reconstruction, highlighting its direct use in DL or incorporated within conventional reconstruction techniques (Reader et al. 2020).

10.3 Challenges Related to the Dataset

The segmentation of medical images contributes to understanding an image, feature extraction, recognition, and the assessment of abnormalities or lesions. It offers crucial information for analyzing pathologies and, in turn, aids in diagnosing and planning a treatment. The main objective of segmentation is to divide an image into distinct regions that exhibit sturdy correlations. This process entails separating an image I into a finite set of regions $R_1, R_2, \ldots, R_s$, as expressed in Eq. (10.1).

$$I = \cup_{i=1}^{s} R_i, R_i \cap R_j = \emptyset \quad \text{and} \quad i \neq j \tag{10.1}$$

The efficient operation of machine learning techniques hinges on extracting descriptive features. Identifying these features is often challenging, particularly in applications related to image understanding, an area still under active research. A strategic approach to address this challenge is the development of intelligent machines capable of autonomously learning and extracting the requisite features for image understanding. The CNN model stands out as an intelligent and successful model in this regard, and advancements in various architectures such as U-Net, SegNet, and W-Net have enabled the automatic learning and extraction of essential features for medical image understanding (Badrinarayanan et al. 2017; Ronneberger et al. 2015; Xia and Kulis 2017). Researchers have effectively utilized CNNs in various medical image understanding applications, including tumor detection and classification into benign and malignant categories (Ovalle et al. 2016). Skin lesion detection and identification of anomalies in optical coherence tomography images can also be detected using CNN (Kermany et al. 2018; Nasr-Esfahani et al. 2016). Many researchers have also shown colon cancer detection, blood cancer detection, and heart abnormalities (Kiranyaz et al. 2016; Sirinukunwattana et al. 2016). Kallenberg et al. (2016) have shown how breast abnormalities are detected using CNN. Notably, CNN-based models like CheXNet, employed for classifying 14 different chest-related ailments, have demonstrated superior performance compared to the average expertise of human practitioners (Philips et al. 2020; Rajpurkar et al. 2017).

CNNs have emerged as a predominant force in the realm of COVID-19 detection through the analysis of chest X-rays and CT scans. COVID-19, a global pandemic, is rapidly spreading across the world. The commonly utilized test for detecting COVID-19 infection is reverse transcription polymerase chain reaction (RT-PCR). While RT-PCR is considered the gold standard for COVID-19 testing, it is a complex, time-consuming, and labor-intensive process with limited availability and accuracy. In places facing a shortage of RT-PCR kits, chest X-rays could serve as an initial screening tool for COVID-19, offering a more accurate diagnosis. DL techniques have been employed by many researchers to classify chest infections and distinguish between COVID-19 and other ailments. An early model suggested for COVID-19 detection involved utilizing a basic pre-trained AlexNet model, which was fine-tuned using chest X-ray images. To improve the performance of the models, more training samples and better segmenting techniques are required (Hasan et al. 2022). Various factors like insufficient details about the study participants, the randomization process, and the absence of external validation have led individuals to reconsider the use of these diagnostic techniques for this disease (Montazeri et al. 2021).

In the quest to advance methodologies for medical image segmentation, the significance of high-quality datasets cannot be emphasized enough. The challenges

Table 10.1 Challenges concerning datasets and their solutions.

Issues	Solutions
Limited annotated data	• Augmentation • Use transfer learning
Sparse annotations	• Weighted loss function
Class imbalance	• Oversampling • Modifying evaluation metric • Data augmentation • Combining minority classes
Intensity inhomogeneities	• Prefiltering operations • Better scanning devices
Image texture complexities	• Use image enhancement techniques

associated with datasets play a crucial role in shaping the effectiveness and applicability of segmentation algorithms. Table 10.1 shows various issues and their solutions pertaining to datasets during the segmentation. Issues ranging from data variability and annotation complexities to concerns about dataset size and diversity are pivotal factors that researchers must navigate. Tackling these challenges is vital to ensuring the robustness and reliability of segmentation models. This section delves into the multifaceted landscape of challenges related to datasets, exploring the intricacies that researchers contend with to unleash the full potential of medical image segmentation technologies. Addressing these challenges is not only imperative for algorithmic development but also establishes the foundation for translating cutting-edge research into practical and impactful clinical applications. The different challenges related to the dataset are shown in Figure 10.5 and described below.

10.3.1 Limited Annotated Dataset

DL network models necessitate a substantial volume of data, and the prerequisite for well-annotated training data underscores the dataset's importance in various deep learning-based medical procedures (Srinivasu et al. 2021). Nevertheless, the endeavor to amass a large repository of annotated medical images for medical image processing encounters challenges (ÇiÇek et al. 2016). Annotating new medical images is labor-intensive and costly and requires a high level of expertise. While several large-scale datasets are publicly available, the need persists for more challenging datasets to further enhance the training of DL models, especially in scenarios involving complex objects. Existing 3D datasets, in particular, are frequently insufficient in size, with some being synthetic, emphasizing the ongoing requirement for more challenging datasets (Levin et al. 1988).

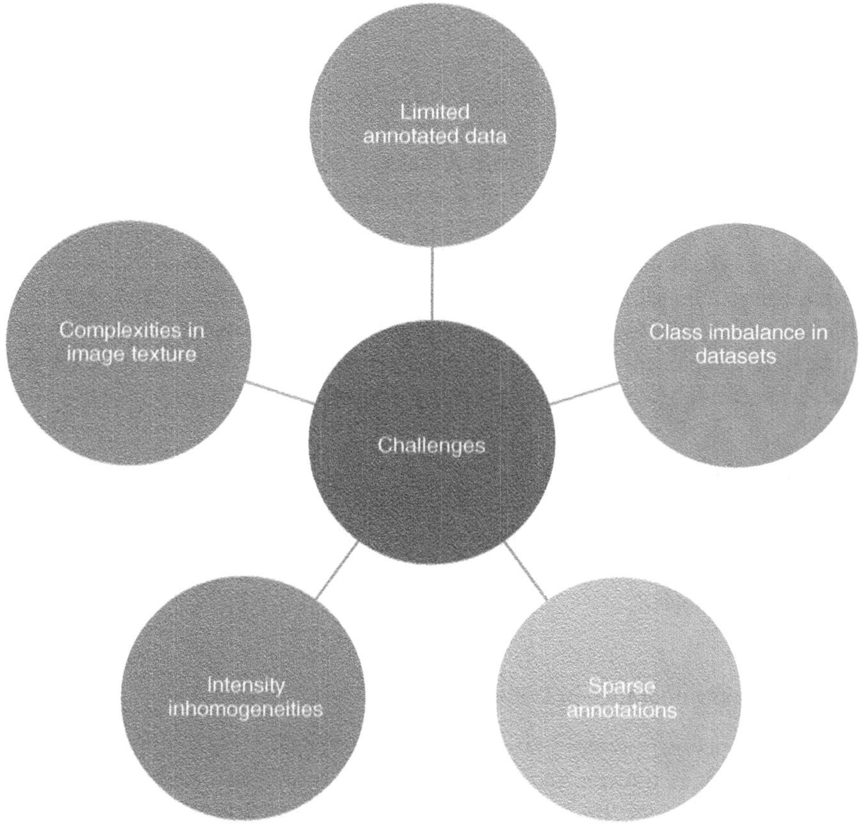

Figure 10.5 The various challenges related to the datasets.

10.3.1.1 Solution

Expanding the size of existing medical image datasets can be accomplished through various strategies:

(I) Employing image augmentation transformations, such as rotating images at different angles, flipping images vertically or horizontally, cropping, and shearing images. These augmentation techniques contribute to the enhanced performance of the system.
(II) Leveraging transfer learning from efficient models can provide a viable solution to the limited data problem (Bhattacharya et al. 2021).
(III) Synthesizing data collected from various sources offers an additional avenue for augmenting dataset size (Bhattacharya et al. 2021).

10.3.2 Sparse Annotations

Sparse annotation in medical image segmentation refers to situations where only a limited subset of the available data has been annotated or labeled. Fully annotating information, especially for 3D images, is a time-intensive task and is not consistently feasible. Consequently, partial labeling of information slices within 3D images is common. Training DL models using these sparsely annotated 3D images presents considerable challenges (ÇiÇek et al. 2016). This means limited training data, increased annotation burden, and bias in the model results. It can also lead to challenges in handling rare cases. In medical imaging, certain pathological conditions or anatomical variations may be relatively rare. Sparse annotation might inadequately represent these less common cases, making it challenging for the model to accurately segment such instances when encountered in clinical practice.

10.3.2.1 Solution

In cases of sparsely annotated datasets, applying a weighted loss function is a viable solution. In this method, the weights for the unlabeled data in the dataset are all set to zero, enabling the model to focus exclusively on learning from the pixels that are labeled.

10.3.3 Class Imbalance in Datasets

Class imbalance in a dataset occurs when the distribution of instances across different classes is uneven, meaning that some classes have significantly more instances than others. In the context of medical image segmentation, where each class may correspond to a specific anatomical structure or pathological condition, class imbalance can have several implications: model biases, reduced sensitivity to minority class, misleading evaluation metrics, and reduced model performance.

Imbalances in class distribution are inherent in various publicly available medical image datasets, posing a significant challenge in training DL models and potentially leading to misleading model accuracy. For example, in the patient data, where a disease is relatively rare, occurring in only 10% of screened patients, the overall model accuracy can be inflated, reaching local minima, as most patients do not have the disease (Bhattacharya et al. 2020; Merkow et al. 2016).

10.3.3.1 Solution

To address the issue of class imbalance, several strategies can be employed:

(I) Oversampling the data and adjusting the extent of oversampling based on the degree of imbalance in the dataset.

(II) Modifying the evaluation or performance metric to alleviate the impact of dataset imbalance.
(III) Applying data augmentation techniques to create new data samples.
(IV) Handling the dataset class imbalance problem by combining minority classes.

10.3.4 Intensity Inhomogeneities

Intensity inhomogeneities, also known as shading or nonuniformity, refer to variations in pixel intensity across an image that are not related to the underlying anatomical structures. These variations can be caused by factors such as variations in tissue thickness, patient positioning, or imperfections in imaging equipment. The impact of intensity inhomogeneities on medical image segmentation can be significant, leading to various challenges such as inaccurate segmentation boundaries, misleading texture information, difficulty in differentiating tissues, increased false positives and negatives, and compromised qualitative analysis. In images related to pathology, variations in color and intensity are commonly observed (Roy et al. 2011). Intensity inhomogeneities contribute to shading effects on the image, particularly in the segmentation of MR images. Additionally, TEM images may display brightness variations due to the presence of nonuniform support films, posing challenges in the segmentation process.

10.3.4.1 Solution

To mitigate intensity inhomogeneities, various algorithms are employed, and numerous nonparametric techniques are proposed in the literature (Roy et al. 2011). The use of prefiltering operations before segmentation is one approach to eliminate inhomogeneities. Moreover, advancements in scanning devices contribute to addressing and enhancing intensity inhomogeneities.

10.3.5 Complexities in Image Texture

The complexities in image texture refer to the intricate and detailed patterns and variations present in the visual appearance of an image. Understanding and handling these complexities is essential for image segmentation. In the realm of medical images, diverse artifacts may arise during image manipulation, primarily attributed to the use of different sensors and electronic components for image capture (Guo and Ashour 2019; Hesamian et al. 2019). The captured images often exhibit closely situated grey levels, resulting in indistinct image boundaries. Overlapping tissues and irregularities such as skin lines and hair in dermoscopic images add complexity to the identification of the region of interest in medical images.

10.3.5.1 Solution

Diverse image enhancement techniques (such as histogram equalization, Sobel filter, and Canny edge detector) are applied before segmentation to mitigate the impact of various artifacts and noise in the images. These techniques are designed to suppress image noise while preserving the information on the image edges.

10.4 Challenges Concerning the DL Models

The incorporation of deep neural networks (DNNs) has transformed medical image segmentation by providing unmatched capabilities for learning intricate patterns and representations from complex imaging data. However, this transformative shift presents its own set of challenges that demand careful examination. Challenges associated with DNNs in medical image segmentation include issues, such as model interpretability, the requirement for large and diverse datasets, computationally intensive training processes, and the risk of overfitting, as listed in Table 10.2. As researchers endeavor to leverage the potential of DNNs for precise segmentation tasks, it becomes crucial to comprehend and address these challenges. This section explores the nuanced complexities related to the application of DNNs in medical image segmentation, shedding light on both the hurdles and opportunities for refinement in this rapidly evolving field.

The key and difficult challenges concerning the training of DNNs for robust segmentation of medical images include:

10.4.1 Overfitting

Overfitting is a common challenge in DL tasks, including medical image segmentation. Overfitting makes the model learn the intricacies and patterns in the

Table 10.2 Challenges concerning deep learning models and their solutions.

Issues	Solutions
Overfitting the model	• Expand the dataset size through augmentation techniques • Use dropout technique
Space complexity	• Use batch normalization • Incorporating pooling (if using CNN)
Vanishing gradient	• Use deconvolution and softmax • Thoughtfully initialization of weights
Computational complexity	• Filter visualization • Regularization • Layer-wise relevance propagation (LRP)

training dataset too well, potentially surpassing its performance on unprocessed data instances. This problem is especially noticeable when training the model with a small-sized dataset (Shen et al. 2017).

10.4.1.1 Solution

To tackle overfitting, two essential strategies can be utilized:

(I) Expanding the dataset size through augmentation techniques (Merkow et al. 2016).
(II) Applying dropout techniques, which entail discarding the output of a random set of network neurons during each iteration, helps to alleviate overfitting (Cui et al. 2016).

10.4.2 Space Complexity of Models

Medical image segmentation models necessitate a substantial amount of memory (Srivastava et al. 2014). To ensure compatibility with specific devices, like mobile phones, simplification is imperative.

10.4.2.1 Solution

Simplifying models and employing techniques involving model compression techniques can effectively diminish the memory requirements of a DL model.

In terms of training time, DNN architectures demand a significant investment of time. Rapid convergence during training is particularly crucial in image segmentation.

10.4.2.2 Solution

(I) Implementing batch normalization, a technique that centers pixel values around 0 by subtracting them from the mean value. This approach is efficacious in facilitating fast convergence (Srivastava et al. 2014).
(II) Incorporating pooling layers to reduce parameter dimensions can also contribute to expediting convergence.

10.4.3 Vanishing and Exploding Gradient

The deep neural network faces the issue of the vanishing gradient, which refers to the difficulty of the final gradient loss in propagating backward to earlier layers, with this challenge being more noticeable in 3D models (Ioffe and Szegedy 2015).

10.4.3.1 Solution

Various solutions tackle the vanishing gradient problem:

(I) Scaling up the output of intermediate hidden layers using softmax and deconvolution involves combining auxiliary losses and the original loss of hidden layers. This strengthens the gradient value.
(II) Thoughtfully initializing weights for the network represents another strategy to address and alleviate the vanishing gradient problem (Kamnitsas et al. 2017).

10.4.4 Computational Complexity

An efficient DLA focused on feature analysis requires high-performance computing devices and GPUs for optimal operation (Goceri 2019). Some advanced algorithms may even rely on high-performance computers for model training, which might not always be readily available.

10.4.4.1 Solution

In addressing these challenges, researchers should meticulously analyze the number of parameters to achieve the required level of accuracy. Various techniques like filter visualization, regularization, and layer-wise relevance propagation are used to assess the parameters required to train a model.

10.5 Conclusion

DL techniques have shown significant success in medical image segmentation, providing state-of-the-art results in various applications. In the present work, we have explained the distribution of modalities utilized in medical imaging, which are necessary for clinical decisions. From the nuanced textures captured by MRI to the detailed anatomical structures revealed through CT scans, the richness of medical datasets provides a foundation for advancements in computational healthcare. Our exploration of these modalities has underscored the critical role they play in driving innovation and enhancing our understanding of complex medical conditions.

However, medical image segmentation faces many challenges when it comes to the integration of DL algorithms into medical imaging analysis. The scarcity of annotated data, compounded by the inherent variability in anatomical structures and pathologies, presents a formidable hurdle in training robust and generalizable DL models. This chapter separates these challenges based on their association with the dataset and model. The intricate textures and patterns inherent in medical images demand sophisticated approaches, yet the risk of overfitting looms large, threatening the models' ability to extend their learnings to diverse clinical scenarios. The quest for comprehensive datasets representative of the vast spectrum of medical conditions is integral to the success of future endeavors.

As we grapple with challenges, both inherent in the data and embedded in the algorithms, the potential for transformative breakthroughs remains tantalizingly within reach. The integration of modalities, the harnessing of diverse datasets, and the continual refinement of DL models constitute the compass guiding us toward a future where medical image segmentation not only aids diagnosis and treatment planning but fundamentally transforms the paradigm of personalized healthcare.

References

Badrinarayanan, V., Kendall, A., and Cipolla, R. (2017). Segnet: a deep convolutional encoder-decoder architecture for image segmentation. *IEEE Transactions on Pattern Analysis and Machine Intelligence* 39 (12): 2481–2495.

Balagourouchetty, L., Pragatheeswaran, J.K., Pottakkat, B., and Ramkumar, G. (2019). GoogLeNet based ensemble FCNet classifier for focal liver lesion diagnosis. *IEEE Journal of Biomedical and Health Informatics* 2194: 1–1. https://doi.org/10.1109/jbhi.2019.2942774.

Bhattacharya, S., Maddikunta, P.K.R., and Hakaketa, S. (2020). Antlion resampling based deep neural network model for classification of imbalanced multimodal stroke dataset. *Multimedia Tools and Applications* 79: 1–25.

Bhattacharya, S., Maddikunta, P.K.R., and Phametal, Q.V. (2021). Deep learning and medical image processing for coronavirus (COVID-19) pandemic: a survey. *Sustainable Cities and Society* 65: 102589.

Candemir, S., Rajaraman, S., Thoma, G., and Antani, S. (2018). Deep learning for grading cardiomegaly severity in chest X-rays: an investigation. In: *2018 IEEE Life Sciences Conference (LSC)*, pp. 109–113. https://doi.org/10.1109/LSC.2018.8572113

Choi, J., Shin, K., Jung, J. et al. (2020). Convolutional neural network technology in endoscopic imaging: artificial intelligence for endoscopy. *Clinical Endoscopy* 53 (2): 117–126. https://doi.org/10.5946/ce.2020.054.

ÇiÇek, O., Abdulkadir, A., Lienkamp, S.S. et al. (2016). 3D U-Net: learning dense volumetric segmentation from sparse annotation. In: *Proceedings of the International Conference on Medical Image Computing and Computer-Assisted Intervention*, pp. 424–432, Springer, Athens, Greece.

Conant, E.F., Toledano, A.Y., Periaswamy, S. et al. (2019). Improving accuracy and efficiency with concurrent use of artificial intelligence for digital breast tomosynthesis. *Radiology: Artifical Intelligence* 1 (4): e180096. https://doi.org/10.1148/ryai. 2019180096.

Cui, H., Zhang, H., Ganger, G.R. et al. (2016). Geeps: scalable deep learning on distributed gpus with a gpu- specialized parameter server. In: *Proceedings of the Eleventh European Conference on Computer Systems*, pp. 1–16, Lisbon, Portugal (July 2016).

Dimitriou, N., Arandjelović, O., and Caie, P.D. (2019). Deep learning for whole slide image analysis: an overview. *Frontiers in Medicine* 6 (November): 1–7. https://doi.org/10.3389/fmed.2019.00264.

Fan, D.-P., Zhou, T., Ji, G.-P., et al. (2020). Inf-Net: automatic COVID-19 lung infection segmentation from CT scans, pp. 1–10 [Online]. http://arxiv.org/abs/2004.14133

Fonseca, P., Mendoza, J., Wainer, J. et al. (2015) Automatic breast density classification using a convolutional neural network architecture search procedure. In: *Proceedings Volume 9414, Medical Imaging 2015: Computer-Aided Diagnosis*, p. 941428. https://doi.org/10.1117/12.2081576

Goceri, E. (2019). Challenges and recent solutions, for image segmentation in the era of deep learning. In: *Proceedings of the 2019 Ninth International Conference on Image Processing Theory, Tools and Applications (IPTA)* (November 2019), pp. 1–6. Istanbul, Turkey: IEEE.

Guo, Y. and Ashour, A.S. (2019). Neutrosophic sets in dermoscopic medical image segmentation. In: *Neutrosophic Set in Medical Image Analysis*, 229–243. Academic Press.

Hasan, M.K., Alam, M.A., Dahal, L. et al. (2022). Challenges of deep learning methods for COVID-19 detection using public datasets. *Informatics in Medicine Unlocked* 30: 100945. https://doi.org/10.1016/j.imu.2022.100945.

He, J.Y., Wu, X., Jiang, Y.G. et al. (2018). Hookworm detection in wireless capsule endoscopy images with deep learning. *IEEE Transactions on Image Processing* 27 (5): 2379–2392. https://doi.org/10.1109/TIP. 2018.2801119.

Hesamian, M.H., Jia, W., He, X., and Kennedy, P. (2019). Deep learning techniques for medical image segmentation: achievements and challenges. *Journal of Digital Imaging* 32 (4): 582–596.

Hwang, S., Kim, H.-E., Jeong, J., and Kim, H.-J. (2016). A novel approach for tuberculosis screening based on deep convolutional neural networks. In: *Proceedings Volume 9785, Medical Imaging 2016: Computer-Aided Diagnosis; 97852W*. https://doi.org/10.1117/12.2216198

Ioffe, S. and Szegedy, C. (2015). Batch normalization: accelerating deep network training by reducing internal covariate shift. https://arxiv.org/abs/1502.03167.

Jani, K.K. and Srivastava, R. (2019). A survey on medical image analysis in capsule endoscopy. *Current Medical Imaging* 15 (7): 622–636. https://doi.org/10.2174/1573405614666181102152434.

Kallenberg, M., Petersen, K., and Nielsen, M. (2016). Unsupervised deep learning applied to breast density segmentation and mammographic risk scoring. *IEEE Transactions on Medical Imaging* 35 (5): 1322–1331.

Kamnitsas, K., Ledig, C., Newcombe, V.F. et al. (2017). Efficient multi-scale 3D CNN with fully connected CRF for accurate brain lesion segmentation. *Medical Image Analysis* 36: 61–78.

Kang, C., Yu, X., Wang, S.H. et al. (2020). A heuristic neural network structure relying on fuzzy logic for images scoring. *IEEE Transactions on Fuzzy Systems* 29: 34–35. https://doi.org/10.1109/tfuzz.2020.2966163.

Kermany, D.S., Goldbaum, M., Cai, W. et al. (2018). Identifying medical diagnoses and treatable diseases by image-based deep learning. *Cell* 172 (5): 1122–1131.

Kiranyaz, S., Ince, T., and Gabbouj, M. (2016). Real-time patient-specific ECG classification by 1-D convolutional neural networks. *IEEE Transactions on Biomedical Engineering* 63 (3): 664–675.

Levin, D.N., Pelizzari, C.A., Chen, G.T. et al. (1988). Retrospective geometric correlation of MR, CT, and PET images. *Radiology* 169 (3): 817–823.

Li, L., Qin, L., Yin, Y. et al. (2019). Artificial intelligence distinguishes COVID-19 from community acquired pneumonia on chest CT. *Radiology* 2020: 1–5. https://doi.org/10.1007/s10489-020-01714-3.

Li, W., Cao, P., Zhao, D., and Wang, J. (2016). Pulmonary nodule classification with deep convolutional neural networks on computed tomography images. *Computational and Mathematical Methods in Medicine* 2016: https://doi.org/10.1155/2016/6215085.

Loey, M., Smarandache, F., and Khalifa, N.E.M. (2020). Within the lack of chest COVID-19 X-ray dataset: a novel detection model based on GAN and deep transfer learning. *Symmetry (Basel)* 12 (4): https://doi.org/10.3390/SYM12040651.

Masood, A., Sheng, B., Yang, P. et al. (2020). Automated decision support system for lung Cancer detection and classification via enhanced RFCN with multilayer fusion RPN. *IEEE Transactions on Industrial Informatics* 16 (12): 7791–7801. https://doi.org/10.1109/tii.2020.29729187801.

Merkow, J., Marsden, A., Kriegman, D., and Tu, Z. (2016). Dense volume-to-volume vascular boundary detection. In: *Proceedings of the International Conference on Medical Image Computing and Computer-Assisted Intervention* (October 2016), pp. 371–379. Athens, Greece: Springer.

Montazeri, M., ZahediNasab, R., Farahani, A. et al. (2021). Machine learning models for image-based diagnosis and prognosis of COVID-19: systematic review. *JMIR Medical Informatics* 9 (4): e25181. https://doi.org/10.2196/25181.

Münzer, B., Schoeffmann, K., and Böszörmenyi, L. (2018). Content-based processing and analysis of endoscopic images and videos: a survey. *Multimedia Tools and Applications* 77 (1): 1323–1362. https://doi.org/10.1007/s11042-016-4219-z.

Nakagawa, K., Ishihara, R., Aoyama, K., and Ohmori, M. (2019). Classification for invasion depth of esophageal squamous cell carcinoma using a deep neural network compared with experienced endoscopists. *Gastrointestinal Endoscopy* 90 (3): 407–414. https://doi.org/10.1016/j.gie.2019.04.245.

Nasr-Esfahani, E., Samavi, S., and Karimi, N. (2016). Melanoma detection by analysis of clinical images using convolutional neural network. In: *Proceedings of the 38th IEEE Annual International Conference on Engineering in Medicine and Biology Society, EMBC*, pp. 1373–1376.

Ovalle, J.E.A., González, F.A., Ramos-Pollán, R. et al. (2016). Representation learning for mammography mass lesion classification with convolutional neural networks. *Computer Methods and Programs in Biomedicine* 127: 248–257.

Phillips, N.A., Rajpurkar, P., Sabini, M. et al. (2020) Chexphoto: 10,000+ smartphone photos and synthetic photographic transformations of chest X-rays for benchmarking deep learning robustness. https://doi.org/10.48550/arXiv.2007.06199.

Prakasha, S., Bhyri, C., Tawade, C.M., and Kalpana, V. (2023). Segmentation of brain tumor and challenges facing during registration of brain tumor in magnetic resonance images. In: *2023 International Conference on Distributed Computing and Electrical Circuits and Electronics (ICDCECE)*, pp. 1–5. IEEE.

Rajaraman, S. and Antani, S.K. (2020a). Modality-specific deep learning model ensembles toward improving TB detection in chest radiographs. *IEEE Access* 8: 27318–27326. https://doi.org/10.1109/ACCESS.2020.2971257.

Rajaraman, S. and Antani, S. (2020b). Weakly labeled data augmentation for deep learning: a study on COVID-19 detection in chest X-rays. *Diagnostics* 10 (6): 1–17. https://doi.org/10.3390/diagnostics10060358.

Rajpurkar, P., Irvin, J., Zhu, K. et al. (2017). Chexnet: radiologist-level pneumonia detection on chest X-rays with deep learning. CoRR arXiv:1711.05225.

Reader, A.J., Corda, G., Mehranian, A. et al. (2020). Deep learning for PET image reconstruction. *IEEE Transactions on Radiation and Plasma Medical Sciences* 7311 (1): 1–1. https://doi.org/10.1109/trpms. 2020.3014786 25.

Ribli, D., Horváth, A., Unger, Z. et al. (2018). Detecting and classifying lesions in mammograms with deep learning. *Scientific Reports* 8 (1): 1–7. https://doi.org/10.1038/s41598-018-22437-z.

Ronneberger, O., Fischer, P., and Brox, T. (2015). U-net: convolutional networks for biomedical image segmentation. In: *Medical Image Computing and Computer-Assisted Intervention–MICCAI 2015: 18th International Conference, Munich, Germany, October 5–9, 2015, Proceedings, Part III 18*, pp. 234–241. Springer International Publishing.

Roy, S., Carass, A., Bazin, P.L., and Prince, J.L. (2011). Intensity inhomogeneity correction of magnetic resonance images using patches. *Proceedings of SPIE The International Society for Optical Engineering* 7962: 79621F.

Shen, D., Wu, G., and Suk, H.I. (2017). Deep learning in medical image analysis. *Annual Review of Biomedical Engineering* 19: 221–248.

Sirinukunwattana, K., Raza, S.E.A., Tsang, Y. et al. (2016). Locality sensitive deep learning for detection and classification of nuclei in routine colon cancer histology images. *IEEE Transactions on Medical Imaging* 35 (5): 1196–1206.

Soffer, S., Klang, E., Shimon, O. et al. (2020). Deep learning for wireless capsule endoscopy: a systematic review and meta-analysis. *Gastrointestinal Endoscopy* 92 (4): 831–839.e8. https://doi.org/10.1016/j.gie.2020.04.039.

Spanhol, F., Oliveira, L.S., Petitjean, C., and Heutte, L. (2016). A dataset for breast cancer histopathological image classification. *IEEE Transactions on Biomedical Engineering (TBME)* 63 (7): 1455–1462.

Srinivasu, P.N., Bhoi, A.K., Jhaveri, R.H. et al. (2021). Probabilistic deep Q network for real-time path planning in censorious robotic procedures using force sensors. *Journal of Real-Time Image Processing* 18 (5): 1773–1785.

Srivaramangai, R. (2023). Rectal cancer magnetic resonance image segmentation. In: *Computational Intelligence in Image and Video Processing* (ed. M.D. Patil, G.K. Birajdar, and S.S. Chaudhari), 155–173. Chapman and Hall/CRC.

Srivastava, N., Hinton, G., Krizhevsky, A. et al. (2014). Dropout: a simple way to prevent neural networks from overfitting. *Journal of Machine Learning Research* 15 (1): 1929–1958.

Veeramalla, S.K., Hindumathi, V., Reddy, T.V. et al. (2023). Segmentation of MRI images using a combination of active contour modeling and morphological processing. *Journal of Mechanics in Medicine and Biology* 23: 2340002.

Waheed, A., Goyal, M., Gupta, D. et al. (2020). CovidGAN: data augmentation using auxiliary classifier GAN for improved Covid-19 detection. *IEEE Access* 8: 91916–91923. https://doi.org/10.1109/ACCESS.2020.2994762.

Wang, J., Ding, H., Bidgoli, F.A. et al. (2017). Detecting cardiovascular disease from mammograms with deep learning. *IEEE Transactions on Medical Imaging* 36 (5): 1172–1181. https://doi.org/10.1109/TMI.2017.2655486.

Wang, T., Lei, Y., Fu, Y. et al. (2020). Machine learning in quantitative PET: a review of attenuation correction and low-count image reconstruction methods. *Physica Medica* 76 (March): 294–306. https://doi.org/10.1016/j.ejmp. 2020.07.028.

Wu, N., Phang, J., Park, J. et al. (2019). Deep neural networks improve radiologists' performance in breast Cancer screening. *IEEE Transactions on Medical Imaging* 39: 1–1. https://doi.org/10.1109/tmi.2019.2945514 1194.

Xia, X. and Kulis, B. (2017). W-net: a deep model for fully unsupervised image segmentation. *arXiv preprint arXiv:1711.08506*.

Xing, F., Xie, Y., Su, H. et al. (2018). Deep learning in microscopy image analysis: a survey. *IEEE Transactions on Neural Networks and Learning Systems* 29 (10): 4550–4568. https://doi.org/10.1109/TNNLS.2017.2766168.

Yoon, H.J., Kim, S., Kim, J.H. et al. (2019). A lesion-based convolutional neural network improves endoscopic detection and depth prediction of early gastric cancer. *Journal of Clinical Medicine* 8 (9): 1310. https://doi.org/10.3390/jcm8091310.

Zhang, X., Wu, Y., Guo, J. et al. (2023). 3D masked autoencoding and pseudo-labeling for domain adaptive segmentation of heterogeneous infant brain MRI. *arXiv preprint arXiv:2303.09373*.

Zhao, W., and Zeng, Z. (2019). Multi scale supervised 3D U-net for kidney and tumor segmentation. https://doi.org/10.24926/548719.007.

11

Advancements in Deep Learning for Medical Image Analysis: A Comprehensive Exploration of Techniques, Applications, and Future Prospects

Vani Malagar, Navin Mani Upadhyay, and Mekhla Sharma

Model Institute of Engineering and Technology, Department of Computer Science and Engineering, Jammu, India

11.1 Introduction

Medical imaging has played a significant role in modern healthcare and provides extremely useful insights into human anatomy and physiology. There are many techniques available, such as X-ray, computed tomography (CT), magnetic resonance imaging (MRI), and positron emission tomography (PET), which generate huge amount of data for further research in the field of health care. These data are in binary, nominal, and image format. So, extracting the relevant information from these data often necessitates image acquisition and segmentation. The segmentation is a process in which the image is partitioned into distinct regions corresponding to anatomical structures or tissues. Traditionally, medical image segmentation relied on manually generated techniques that involved trained professionals. However, the techniques were prone to the following limitations (Nazir and Kaleem 2023):

- *Time-consuming process:* The manual segmentation can be a tedious and time-consuming task that affects workflow efficiency.
- *Subjectivity and inter-observer variability:* The manual approaches are vulnerable to human error and inconsistencies which may affect the analysis accuracy.
- *Limited scalability:* The manual methods become unsuitable for large datasets or real-time applications.

Deep Learning Applications in Medical Image Segmentation: Overview, Approaches, and Challenges, First Edition. Edited by Sajid Yousuf Bhat, Aasia Rehman, and Muhammad Abulaish.

Today from the deep learning technique, convolutional neural networks (CNNs) have transformative approaches in medical image segmentation and possess the exceptional capabilities like:

- *Extracting features:* These help in learning complex patterns and relationships within medical images, hence eliminating the need for manual feature engineering.
- *Achieving high accuracy:* Exhibiting the demonstrated state-of-the-art performance in various segmentation tasks, surpassing traditional methods in demanding scenarios.

11.2 Significance of Medical Image Segmentation

Medical data involves electronic health records and the medical imaging that has evolved complex tomographic (i.e. cross-sectional) images, such as ultrasound, CT, tomosynthesis, PET, and MRI. The images generated are usually three- or four-dimensional in nature. Medical Image segmentation focuses on two categories in consideration, the first is identifying and isolating specific structures or abnormalities within the medical images including their clinical significance, and the second that discusses how precise segmentation contributes to personalized treatment plans and interventions (Luo et al. 2021).

- *Clinical significance:* Medical image segmentation plays a crucial role in identifying and isolating specific structures or abnormalities within medical images, providing useful insights for diagnosis, involving treatment planning, and keeping track of various medical conditions. Outlining the distinct anatomical structures or pathological regions within the images enables healthcare professionals to better recognize and understand the extent and location of abnormalities, facilitating a more precise diagnosis. Hence, medical image segmentation enables (Said et al. 2023):
  - *Early detection and diagnosis of diseases:* For instance, in radiology, segmenting tumors or lesions from surrounding tissues in CT or MRI scans allows for a precise assessment of their size, shape, and characteristics and is also vital for oncologists to determine the stage of cancer and plan appropriate treatment strategies.
  - *Treatment planning*: By providing a detailed map of the patient's anatomy and suggesting surgeons to use segmented images to plan the optimal approach for surgeries. For instance, in neurosurgery, segmenting brain structures helps surgeons navigate critical areas and avoid damage to healthy tissues.
  - *Monitoring disease progression:* For tracking the changes in the affected areas over time, aiding in the evaluation of treatment effectiveness and the adjustment of therapeutic strategies.

- *Precision medicine:* Precision medicine aims at customizing various medical interventions and treatment plans to individual and distinctive characteristics of each patient. Hence, precise segmentation of medical images plays a significant role in advancing the principles of precision medicine. Detailed personalized treatment plans can be created by healthcare professionals by accurately delineating anatomical structures and pathological regions using precision medicine. As can be seen in the treatment of cancer, oncologists using precise segmentation of tumors are able to customize therapeutic strategies based on the specific characteristics of tumors. Moreover, segmentation also facilitates the monitoring of the disease over a period of time (Alsanea and Dutta 2024). Hence, the amalgamation of the machine learning algorithms helps in recognizing subtle patterns and variations and aids in increasing the efficiency and accuracy of the personalized medicine approaches. Overall, precise and accurate segmentation is used as a foundation in the realization of precision medicine, offering the possibility of optimizing patient outcomes and minimizing adverse effects by tailoring treatments to the distinctive attributes of each patient.

11.2.1 Case Studies

Some of the engrossing case studies covering the application of deep learning models in medical image segmentation are covered below that have led to the transformative outcomes and offer significant advancements in the healthcare sector. These success stories showcase the transformative impact of deep learning models in medical image segmentation (Aljabri and AlGhamdi 2022).

i) *Radiology:* CNNs, the network architecture for deep learning, have shown exceptional results in segmenting brain tumors from various MRI scans facilitating surgical planning and treatment monitoring. Case studies have shown that this has resulted in reduced manual workload for radiologists and hence improved the diagnostic accuracy.
ii) *Cardiology:* The use of deep learning has completely transformed the segmentation of cardiac structures in medical imaging. Some of the applications, like the one used for left ventricle segmentation from cardiac MRI scans, have contributed to more precise assessments of cardiac function and have led to enhanced accuracy in the diagnosis of cardiac diseases.
iii) *Chest CT scans:* Deep learning models have been used in detecting and segmenting the pulmonary modules from chest CT scans which help in early detection of lung cancer. Case studies have shown that using these models has led to timely interventions for improving the survival rates.
iv) *Diabetes:* Deep learning models have been used in retinal vessel segmentation for diagnosing and monitoring diabetic retinopathy, which has the ability to

identify the subtle vascular changes leading to early intervention and prevention of vision loss in patients suffering from diabetes.

v) *Multi-parametric MRI:* Multi-parametric MRI data for prostate cancer localization use deep learning models for improving biopsy targeting and treatment planning and has shown enhanced diagnostic accuracy and more informed clinical decision-making (Lateef and Ruichek 2019).
vi) *Melanoma detection:* Deep learning models have been used in skin lesion segmentation for melanoma detection and the success stories have shown that these models have the ability to differentiate between benign and malignant lesions resulting in timely and accurate diagnosis.
vii) *Musculoskeletal imaging:* Deep learning models are applied to musculoskeletal imaging enabling joint segmentation and quantification of structures such as cartilage and bones, and have contributed to improved assessments of arthritis progression and treatment efficacy.
viii) *Automated fetal brain segmentation in ultrasound:* Deep learning models aid in the assessment of fetal neurodevelopment. These models have the ability to provide quick and precise measurements, leading to early identification of developmental abnormalities (Salman and Bahrani 2010).

11.3 Deep Learning Techniques for Medical Image Segmentation

Deep learning has emerged as an important advancement in medical image analysis and segmentation. This section provides a basic understanding of deep learning which is necessary for medical image segmentation challenges and future advancements. The steps are classified in the following stages (Luo et al. 2021).

11.3.1 Building Blocks for Medical Image Segmentation

After pre-processing of the medical images, the segmentation phase starts. All the individual images are divided into different sets of pixels by applying image segmentation algorithm. The image segmentation involves converting an image into a collection of pixels that are represented by a mask or a labeled image. By dividing an image into segments, one can process only the important segments of the image instead of processing the entire image. This chapter discusses various techniques for segmentation, such as Clustering which combines pixels that are related in some way, Region expanding expands regions until they reach a boundary, and thresholding used as an end-to-end solution for image segmentation. This chapter also uses K-means, histogram-based bundling, and active contours. By delving into these fundamental components, this chapter provides the information required to understand the inner workings and enormous potential of deep learning in this critical healthcare application. The important concepts involved in the concept of deep learning are explained below.

11.3.1.1 Activation Functions

Activation functions add nonlinearity to the network, allowing it to learn complicated correlations between input and output data. Common activation functions utilized in CNNs are:

- *Rectified linear unit (ReLU):* This function is computationally efficient and avoids the vanishing gradient problem that can hinder training in deeper networks. The representation of the ReLU function is shown in below equation:

  $$f(x) = \max(0, x)$$

  where $f(x)$ is the computationally efficient set of functions that returns 0 if it receives any negative input otherwise it returns x.
- *Sigmoid:* The sigmoid function guarantees that the output of the neural network will always be 0 and 1. This function is applied to each layer of the neural network. A sigmoid function is a bounded, differentiable real function that defines all the real input values and has a non-negative derivative at each point. The sigmoid function is defined as the below equation:

  $$f(x) = \frac{1}{1 + e^{-x}}$$
- *Hyperbolic tangent (TanH)*: The TanH is a nonlinear activation function having a center at 0 and all the values range between −1 and 1. This activation function helps to de-center the hidden layers of neural networks because the mean of each TanH function is 0 or near 0.

  $$f(x) = \frac{\exp(x) - \exp(-x)}{\exp(x) + \exp(-x)}$$

11.3.1.2 Loss Functions

Loss functions measure how well the predictions of the model deviate from the actual truth labels. Minimizing the loss function during training guides the network toward learning optimal parameters.

Common loss functions used in image segmentation include:

- *Binary cross-entropy:* Suitable for binary classification tasks (e.g. pixel-wise classification between background and foreground).
- *Dice loss:* Penalizes the model for both false positives (classifying background as foreground) and false negatives (classifying foreground as background).

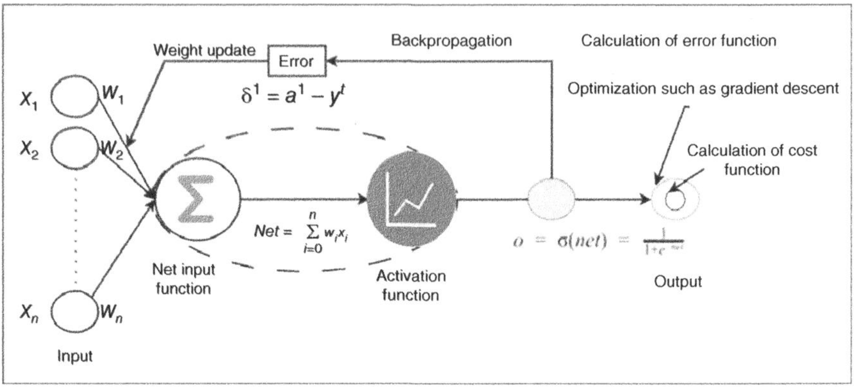

Figure 11.1 Gradient descent with backpropagation.

11.3.1.3 Gradient Descent with Backpropagation

Gradient descent is an optimization approach for training the CNN model. It iteratively modifies the network's weights and biases to reduce the loss function, as shown in Figure 11.1.

- *Forward pass:* The input data is passed through the network layers, resulting in a prediction.
- *Loss calculation:* The loss function compares the predicted output with the ground truth label.
- *Backpropagation:* The mistake (loss) is propagated backward through the network, calculating gradients (slopes) for each weight and bias.
- *Weight update:* The gradients are used to adjust the weights and biases in a way that minimizes loss.

11.3.2 Common Architectures

11.3.2.1 U-Net

U-Net is a fully convolutional network (FCN) developed exclusively for medical image segmentation. It uses an encoder–decoder architecture with skip connections.

11.3.2.2 Components

- *Encoder:* Extracts features from the input image through repeated convolutional and pooling operations.
- *Decoder:* Upsamples the extracted features and combines them with corresponding features from the encoder path (via skip connections) for precise localization.

- *Skip connections:* Connect corresponding encoder and decoder layers directly to preserve spatial information and aid in precise segmentation of small structures.

11.3.2.3 Convolutional Neural Networks (CNNs)

CNNs are a type of deep neural network design that work particularly well with image data. These are skilled in capturing spatial characteristics and relationships within an image. CNNs are a broad category of architectures that use convolutional layers to extract features from images. They can be utilized for a variety of segmentation tasks. A complete image processing is shown in Figure 11.2.

The key components are as follows (Gudhe et al. 2023):

- *Input layer:* Receives the pre-processed image data, typically a 3D tensor representing the image width, height, and color channels (e.g. RGB).
- *Convolutional layer:* Applies filters (kernels) that slide across the input, extracting local features like edges, shapes, and textures.
- *Pooling layer:* Downsampling the feature maps created by the convolutional layer reduces data size and processing expense while keeping critical information. Maximum and average pooling are two common pooling operations.
- *Activation layer:* This introduces non-linearity to the network, allowing it to learn complex patterns. Popular activation functions include ReLU and sigmoid.
- *Fully connected layer:* Flattens the output from the previous layers into a vector and performs traditional neural network operations for classification or regression tasks.

11.3.2.4 Fully Convolutional Network (FCN)

The FCNs are a type of CNN where all layers depend on convolutional function, which enables end-to-end segmentation. The end-to-end segmentation is a cluster of pixel-wise selection of images. The participating components of FCN are as follows:

- *Encoder:* Similar to a general CNN encoder, extracting features.
- *Upsampling layers:* Increase the feature map resolution to match the input image size.
- *Output layer:* Produces a probability map for each pixel belonging to a specific class.

11.3.2.5 SegNet

SegNet is an encoder–decoder architecture similar to U-Net, but utilizes pooling indices for upsampling instead of DE convolutions. Table 11.1 contains a detailed description of CNN layers. The components of SegNet are as follows:

- *Encoder:* Similar to U-Net's encoder, extracting features.

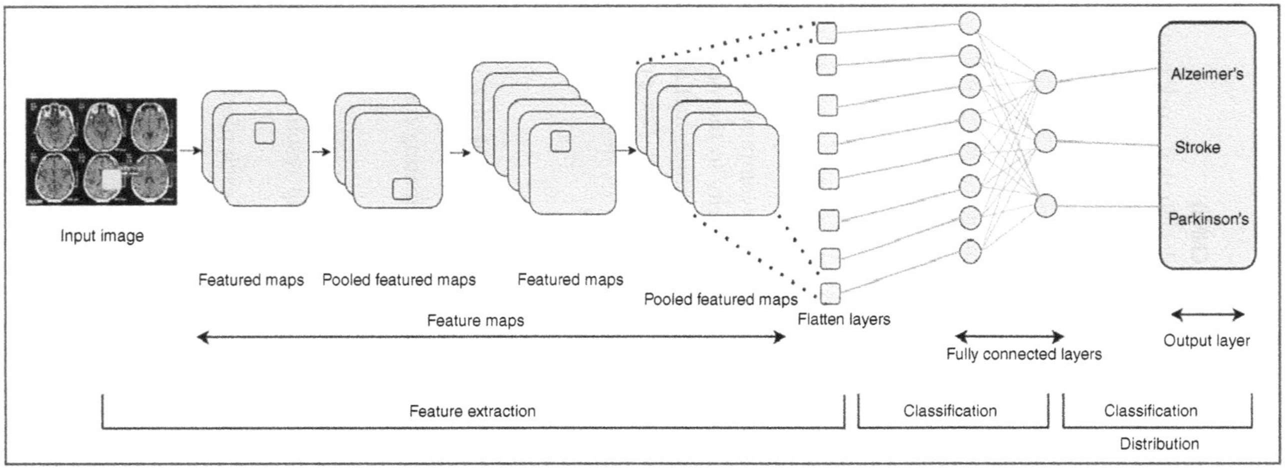

Figure 11.2 Basic CNN architecture.

Table 11.1 Detailed description of CNN layers.

Layer	Description
Input	Receives pre-processed image data.
Convolutional	Extracts local features using filters.
Pooling	Reduces dimensionality of feature maps.
Activation	Introduces nonlinearity.
Fully connected	Performs final classification or regression.

- *Decoder:* Employs pooling indices from the encoder path for upsampling, reducing the number of parameters compared to U-Net.
- *Output layer:* Produces a segmentation map.

11.3.2.6 DeepLabv3+

DeepLabv3+ utilizes atrous convolutions (also known as dilated convolutions) to capture multi-scale information efficiently. The components of DeepLabv3+ are listed below (Luo et al. 2021):

- *Atrous convolution:* Applies the filter with a specific dilation rate, capturing information from a wider range without increasing parameter count significantly.
- *Encoder–decoder:* Similar to U-Net, with atrous convolutions replacing standard convolutions.

11.3.3 Advanced Techniques

This section explores advanced techniques that hold promise for further enhancing the capabilities of medical image segmentation using deep learning, as shown in Figure 11.3.

11.3.3.1 Generative Adversarial Networks (GANs) for Data Augmentation

Data scarcity is a significant challenge in medical image segmentation. GANs offer a potential solution by generating synthetic medical images that can augment existing datasets. The GANs comprise two competing neural networks, as listed below:

- *Generator*: Learns to generate realistic synthetic images that closely reflect the real data distribution.
- *Discriminator*: Attempts to distinguish between real and synthetic images, making the generator improve its creations.

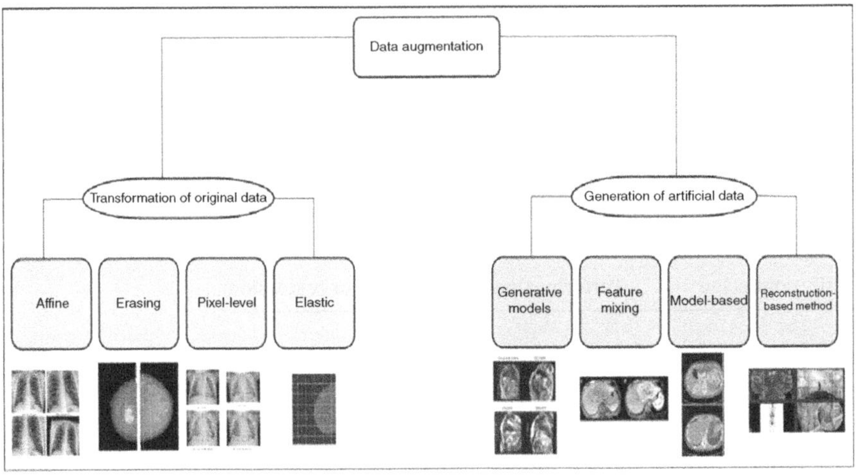

Figure 11.3 Data augmentation in medical images.

Based on the above networks, the advantages of segmentation in medical image are as follows:

- *Augments datasets:* Generates additional training data, addressing data scarcity and improving model generalizability.
- *Reduces bias:* Allows the production of synthetic data with specified features to reduce potential biases in real-world datasets.

11.3.3.2 Transformers for Medical Image Segmentation

Transformers, which have proven successful in natural language processing, are being investigated for potential applications in medical image segmentation. Transformers rely on self-attention processes to detect long-range dependencies in data. The steps are shown in Figure 11.3. This can be useful for applications such as medical image segmentation, which requires understanding the relationships between distant image regions. The advantages of transforming medical images into segmentation are as follows:

- Transformers can capture complex relationships in medical images, resulting in better segmentation accuracy.
- Transformer architectures may perform more efficiently than the classic CNNs for particular segmentation.

11.3.3.3 Ensemble Learning for Improved Performance

Ensemble learning combines numerous deep learning models to provide a more robust and accurate predictor. Different models are trained independently, and

Table 11.2 Summary of advanced techniques.

Description	Technique	Benefits in medical image segmentation
Two competing neural networks: generator creates synthetic images, discriminator evaluates them.	Generative adversarial networks (GANs)	Augments datasets reduces bias
Utilize self-attention mechanisms for long-range dependency modeling.	Transformers	Potentially captures complex relationships in images, and improves accuracy and efficiency.
Combines predictions from multiple models.	Ensemble Learning	Improves accuracy and reduces variance

then their predictions are combined using techniques such as averaging or voting. Table 11.2 shows a detailed summary of used advanced techniques. This method takes advantage of the capabilities of multiple models while minimizing the impact of any single model's shortcomings. The two main benefits of ensemble learning are as follows (Alemi Koohbanani et al. 2020):

- *Improved accuracy:* Combining varied designs can outperform individual models.
- *Reduced variance:* Combining various models reduces variation and leads to more consistent findings.

11.4 Applications of Deep Learning in Medical Image Segmentation

11.4.1 Diagnostic Applications

Deep learning has transformed medical image segmentation, unlocking enormous potential in a variety of diagnostic applications. This section discusses how deep learning supports healthcare professionals in:

11.4.1.1 Improved Tumor Segmentation and Characterization

Early and precise tumor diagnosis is essential for effective therapy for cancer treatment. Deep learning models are very effective at segmenting tumors in medical images, such as mammograms and CT scans. Precise segmentation enables early detection of cancers, leading to more effective treatments.

- *Tumor characterization:* Analyzing size, shape, and texture can help in distinguishing between benign and malignant tumors and guide for more treatment options.
- *Treatment planning:* Segmentation helps plan precise radiation therapy or surgical procedures by properly identifying tumor-specific areas and their extent.

11.4.1.2 Lesion Detection and Analysis

Deep learning algorithms can effectively identify and analyze various lesions in medical images. Examples are included in Table 11.3.

11.4.1.3 Organ Segmentation

Precise organ segmentation is essential for several diagnostic techniques. Preoperative planning for complex procedures is made easier by precise segmentation of organs such as the brain, kidneys, and liver. The surgeons can receive visual guidance during surgery through real-time segmentation, which increases

Table 11.3 Detailed description, applications of lesion detection analysis, and benefits.

Application	Description	Benefit
Skin cancer detection	• Segment suspicious lesions in dermoscopic images. • Aid in early melanoma detection. • Models can analyze features like asymmetry, border irregularity, color variation, and diameter (ABCD rule) to identify potentially malignant lesions.	• Prompt intervention significantly improves treatment success rates.
Diabetic retinopathy analysis	• Automatically detect and characterize diabetic retinopathy (DR) in retinal fundus photographs. • Identify microvascular abnormalities like microaneurysms, hemorrhages, and exudates, which are early signs of DR.	• Timely management of blood sugar levels. • Preventative measures are to be taken, potentially preventing vision loss.
Breast cancer detection	• Models are being investigated for mammogram analysis to identify suspicious masses and microcalcifications. • Analyze mammogram images from multiple views to improve lesion detection accuracy.	• Improved breast cancer detection through deep learning can lead to more targeted biopsies and potentially earlier intervention.
Lung nodule detection	• Analyze chest X-rays and CT scans for lung nodule detection. • Identify subtle changes in lung density that might indicate the presence of nodules, which could be cancerous.	• Early detection of lung nodules allows for prompt investigation and potentially curative treatment for lung cancer.

Table 11.4 Applications of organ segmentation in preoperative planning.

Organ	Preoperative planning
Liver	Planning for liver resection surgery and transplantation
Kidneys	Precise targeting during kidney transplant procedures
Brain	Assists in surgical planning for brain tumor removal and aneurysm clipping
Heart	Enables evaluation of cardiac structures for valve replacement surgery
Lungs	Planning for lung volume reduction surgery, lobectomy
Spine	Facilitates preoperative assessment for spinal fusion surgery

accuracy and minimizes tissue damage. Table 11.4 shows applications of organ segmentation in preoperative planning.

11.4.1.4 Medical Image Analysis for Disease Progression Monitoring

Deep learning models can be used to track the progression of various diseases over time by analyzing serial medical images. This allows for:

- *Monitoring treatment response:* Assessing the effectiveness of treatment by observing changes in the size and characteristics of lesions or abnormalities.
- *Early detection of recurrence:* Identifying signs of disease recurrence through subtle changes in medical images, enabling early intervention.

Overall, deep learning for medical image segmentation provides a number of benefits for diagnostic applications. These methods provide accurate tumor segmentation, lesion detection, organ delineation, and disease monitoring, enabling medical personnel to identify patients more accurately, plan better treatments, and eventually improve patient outcomes.

11.4.2 Therapeutic Applications

- *Image-guided intervention:* Providing real-time segmentation for operations, such as robotic surgery or radiation therapy.
- *Personalized medicine:* Enabling the creation of personalized treatment regimens according to individual patient information and segmentation outcomes.

11.5 Challenges and Future Prospects

11.5.1 Challenges and Limitations

The complexity of medical data, as well as the need for precise and robust results, provide various problems for medical image segmentation. One significant problem is the inherent variety in anatomical structures and diseases, which requires models that perform well across varied populations. The lack of annotated datasets, as well as the significant cost and effort associated with manual segmentation, make it difficult to design and train successful models. Handling multi-modal images, such as merging data from CT and MRI scans, is very challenging. Furthermore, the prevalence of noise, artifacts, and low contrast in medical images require robust segmentation methods. Finally, the interpretability of deep learning models in the medical arena remains an issue. Clinicians demand transparency in the decision-making process for universal acceptance and trust in these technologies. Addressing these problems is essential for the effective implementation of accurate and clinically useful medical image segmentation technologies (Chanu 2020).

A) *Data Variability*

Medical image segmentation presents major issues due to the inherent diversity found in various imaging modalities, resolutions, and acquisition factors. The combination of data from diverse sources, such as CT, MRI, ultrasound, and X-rays, results in unique properties and imaging artifacts. These modalities capture anatomical components differently, resulting in variations in intensity, contrast, and spatial resolution. Furthermore, variances in acquisition factors, such as slice thickness, field of view, and imaging methods, add to the data's complexity are shown in Figure 11.4.

- *Modality-specific characteristics:* Each imaging modality has unique strengths and limits, resulting in a wide range of data properties. For example, CT scans are efficient at depicting bone structures, whereas MRI is better at visualizing soft tissues. Adapting segmentation models to address these modality-specific properties is an intimidating challenge.
- *Resolution disparities:* Variations in spatial resolution between imaging modalities or within the same modality pose challenges. Handling data with changing resolutions requires the use of robust pre-processing techniques, interpolation methods, or resolution-invariant models.
- *Acquisition parameter variability:* Variations in contrast agents, imaging methods, and patient positioning affect the consistency of segmentation models. Developing algorithms that are resistant to these parameter changes is critical for generalizability.

B) *Anatomical Variability*

The complexity of segmenting structures with inherent anatomical variability presents a second layer of challenges in medical image segmentation. Natural variances in organ shape, size, position, and patient-specific factors all contribute to anatomical variability shown in Figure 11.5.

- *Patient-specific anatomy:* Variations in anatomy among individuals, impacted by factors such as age, gender, and underlying health issues,

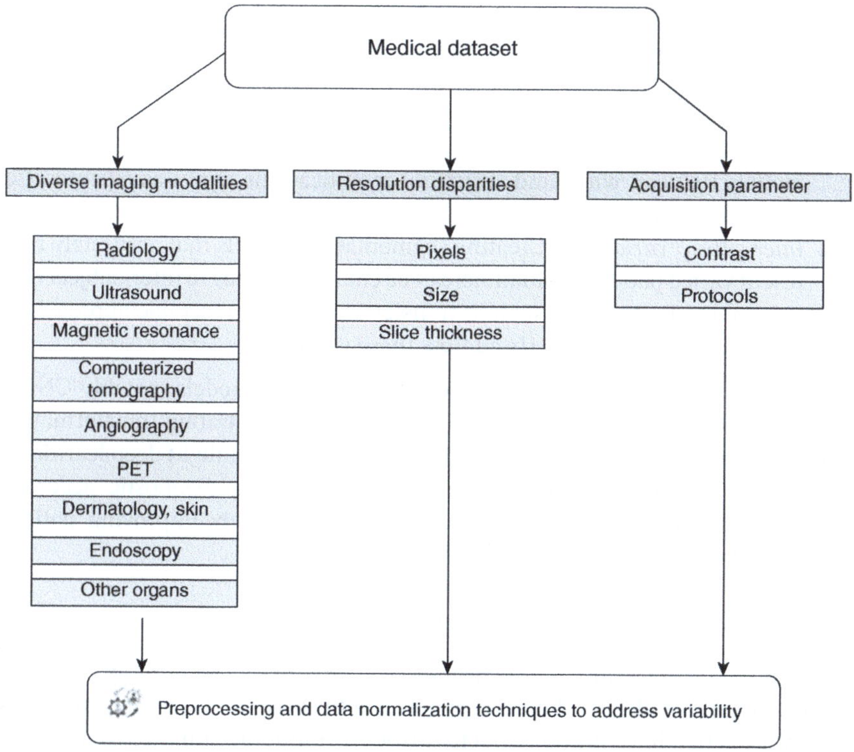

Figure 11.4 Flow diagram for handling data variability.

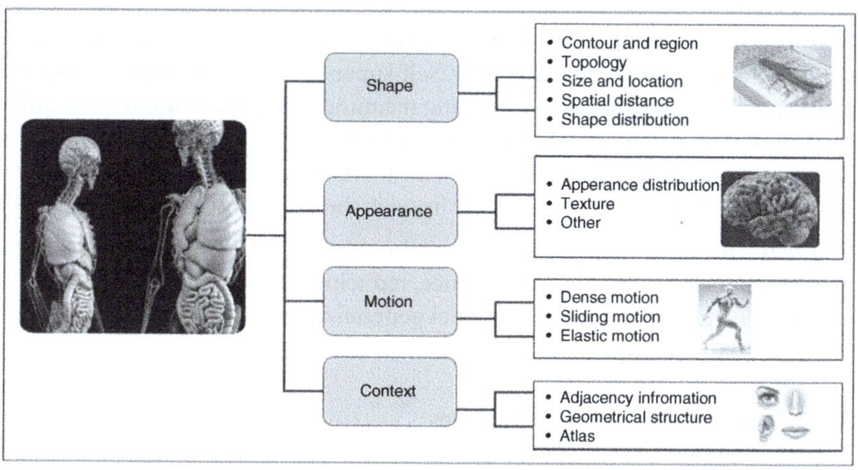

Figure 11.5 Anatomical information.

necessitate segmentation models that can accommodate this intrinsic diversity. Diverse patient anatomy may be difficult to adapt to one-size-fits-all techniques.

- *Structural deformations:* Natural organ deformations, such as those caused by aging, disease, or surgery, complicate segmentation efforts. Developing models that can withstand structural modifications serves as essential for accurate delineation.
- *Inter-subject variability:* Creating segmentation models that accurately represent varied patient populations can be challenging due to inter-subject heterogeneity. Techniques, such as transfer learning or ensemble approaches, may be required to properly address these variables.

With the challenges mentioned above, deep learning models, notably CNNs, have revolutionized medical image segmentation, demonstrating transformative results in a variety of clinical contexts. These difficulties highlight deep learning's potential to transform healthcare practices by boosting diagnostic accuracy and enabling personalized treatment strategies, ultimately improving patient outcomes (Pranathi et al. 2024).

11.5.2 Future Trends and Advancements

The future of deep learning in medical image segmentation is entirely complete with exciting possibilities. This section delves into some of the significant trends and advances that have the potential to further revolutionize this area of work.

11.5.2.1 Self-Supervised Learning

Data scarcity has been a significant challenge in medical image segmentation. Self-supervised learning, which uses unlabeled data for model training, is a promising way to address this difficulty. Self-supervised learning approaches train models on challenges aimed at extracting meaningful representations from unlabeled input. These representations can subsequently be used for downstream tasks such as medical image segmentation, even with insufficient labeled data. The benefits of medical image segmentation are listed in the following (Osmani et al. 2024):

- *Decreases dependency on labeled data:* Allows for the utilization of a large number of unlabeled medical images, hence, reducing data scarcity.
- *Model generalization:* Improves model generalizability by learning representations from unlabeled data.

11.5.2.2 Explainable AI (XAI) Techniques

Deep learning models frequently operate as "black boxes," making it difficult to understand their decision-making processes. Explainable AI (XAI) methods seek to address this by providing insights into how models make their predictions. Table 11.5 presents a detailed description with advantages and disadvantages.

Table 11.5 Explainable AI techniques for deep learning models.

Technique	Description	Advantages	Disadvantages
Local Interpretable Model-Agnostic Explanations (LIME)	Explains individual predictions of any black-box model by learning an interpretable model locally around the prediction.	* Model-agnostic: works with any machine learning model. * Generates explanations for individual predictions.	* Can be computationally expensive for complex models. * Local explanations might not generalize well to other data points.
SHapley Additive exPlanations (SHAP)	Explains how each feature contributes to a specific prediction by distributing the prediction credit among all features.	* Provides insights into feature importance. * Offers different explanation modes (summary, dependence plots).	* Can be computationally expensive for large datasets. * Interpretation of SHAP values might require domain knowledge.
Feature importance techniques (permutation importance, feature ablation)	Ranks the features based on the drop in model performance when a feature is permuted or removed.	* Simple to implement and understand. * Identifies the most important features of the model.	* Does not explain how features interact. * Can be misleading for correlated features.
Partial dependence plots (PDP)	Visualizes the marginal effect of a single feature on the model's prediction, averaging over the other features.	* Easy to interpret visually. * Shows how the model's prediction changes with a single feature.	* Can be cumbersome to generate for many features. * Does not account for feature interactions.
Gradient-based techniques (Grad-CAM, integrated gradients)	Highlights image regions that contribute most to the model's prediction.	* Provides visual explanation for image classification models. * Helps identify which parts of the image the model focuses on.	* Limited to image data. * Interpretation might be subjective.

- *Importance of medical applications:* XAI is critical for increasing confidence and adoption of deep learning models in medical settings. Healthcare practitioners need to understand the reason behind predictions from models in order to make informed decisions.
- *Approaches to explain ability:* Analyzing feature importance to determine which image attributes have the most impact on model predictions. Visualize which image regions receive the most attention from the model during segmentation.

11.5.2.3 Federated Learning

Federated learning provides a mechanism for training deep learning models on distributed private datasets while protecting patient privacy. Model training takes place on individual devices or local servers containing patient data, as shown in Figure 11.6. Instead of exchanging raw data, only model updates are transmitted to achieve global improvement while maintaining patient privacy. Some of the major benefits of segmentation in federated learning are listed in the following (Ye et al. 2022):

- *Promotes collaboration:* Allows for training on data from multiple institutions without the need for centralized data storage, encouraging collaboration while protecting privacy.

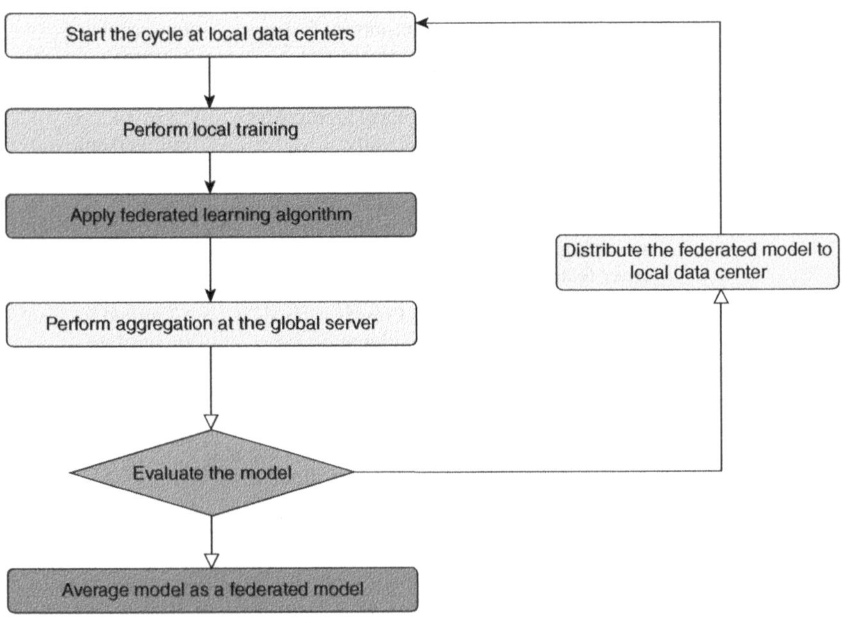

Figure 11.6 Flowchart of federated learning for medical image segmentation.

- *Improves generalizability:* Exploring heterogeneous datasets from diverse healthcare centers enhances model generalizability.

11.5.2.4 Integration with AI for Comprehensive Medical Decision Support Systems

Deep learning for image segmentation has the potential to be used with other AI components to form comprehensive medical decision support systems. By merging deep learning models with other AI features (e.g. disease classification, and risk prediction), healthcare practitioners can gain a more comprehensive perspective for making informed clinical decisions (Drioua et al. 2023).

Potential applications: Integrating segmentation results with patient data enables personalized approaches to treatment. AI systems improve workflow efficiency by automating operations and providing real-time image analysis for healthcare personnel.

The future of deep learning in medical image segmentation seems promising. By solving obstacles, such as data scarcity, interpretability, and privacy, as well as fostering collaboration and integration with other AI technologies, we can unlock the enormous potential of this field to revolutionize healthcare and improve patient outcomes.

11.6 Conclusion

In conclusion, the future of medical image segmentation using deep learning models has enormous potential for revolutionizing healthcare diagnosis and treatment planning. Despite the challenges caused by restricted data availability, class imbalances, variability in patient circumstances, and computing resource limits, the proposed path ahead involves a comprehensive and collaborative effort. By utilizing advanced techniques, such as data augmentation, domain adaptation, and multi-modal fusion, the area aims to tackle data scarcity challenges, increase model generalization, and improve segmentation accuracy across varied patient populations. Integrating self-supervised learning and uncertainty estimation techniques provides to reduce reliance on labeled data while improving model interpretability. Furthermore, optimizing models for real-time, on-device processing ensures that crucial medical applications are delivered on time. Collaboration among machine learning researchers and healthcare practitioners, combined with continuous training on ethical issues plays a very critical role in the responsible development and implementation of deep learning models in medical image segmentation. The objective of these collaborative efforts is to develop robust, transparent, and broadly applicable models that dramatically increase the precision and efficiency of medical image interpretation, ultimately leading to better patient outcomes.

References

Alemi Koohbanani, N., Jahanifar, M., Zamani Tajadin, N., and Rajpoot, N. (2020). NuClick: a deep learning framework for interactive segmentation of microscopic images. *Medical Image Analysis* 65: 101771.

Aljabri, M. and AlGhamdi, M. (2022). A review on the use of deep learning for medical images segmentation. *Neurocomputing* 506: 311–335.

Alsanea, M. and Dutta, A.K. (2024). Detecting cardiovascular diseases from radiographic images using deep learning techniques. *Expert Systems* e13542.

Chanu, M.M. (2020). A review on brain tumor segmentation and classification from magnetic resonance images using deep learning methods. *Journal of Advanced Research in Dynamical and Control Systems* 12 (SP3): 87–94.

Drioua, W.R., Benamrane, N., and Sais, L. (2023). Breast cancer histopathological images segmentation using deep learning. *Sensors* 23 (17): 7318.

Gudhe, N.R., Kosma, V.-M., Behravan, H., and Mannermaa, A. (2023). Nuclei instance segmentation from histopathology images using Bayesian dropout based deep learning. *BMC Medical Imaging* 23 (1).

Lateef, F. and Ruichek, Y. (2019). Survey on semantic segmentation using deep learning techniques. *Neurocomputing* 338: 321–348.

Luo, X., Wang, G., Song, T. et al. (2021). MIDeepSeg: minimally interactive segmentation of unseen objects from medical images using deep learning. *Medical Image Analysis* 72: 102102.

Nazir, S. and Kaleem, M. (2023). Federated learning for medical image analysis with deep neural networks. *Diagnostics* 13 (9): 1532.

Osmani, N., Rezayi, S., Esmaeeli, E., and Karimi, A. (2024). Transfer learning from non-medical images to medical images using deep learning algorithms. *Frontiers in Health Informatics* 13: 177.

Pranathi, V., Vignan, D., Akshay, B. et al. (2024). Semantic segmentation of remote sensing images of urban areas using deep learning methods. *International Journal of Research Publication and Reviews* 5 (3): 3799–3804.

Said, Y., Alsheikhy, A.A., Shawly, T., and Lahza, H. (2023). Medical images segmentation for lung cancer diagnosis based on deep learning architectures. *Diagnostics* 13 (3): 546.

Salman, S.D. and Bahrani, A.A. (2010). Segmentation of tumor tissue in gray medical images using watershed transformation method. *International Journal of Advancements in Computing Technology* 2 (4): 123–127.

Ye, E.Z., Ye, E.H., Bouthillier, M., and Ye, R.Z. (2022). DeepImageTranslator V2: analysis of multimodal medical images using semantic segmentation maps generated through deep learning. *HighTech and Innovation Journal* 3 (3): 319–325.

Index

Deep Learning Applications in Medical Image Segmentation: Overview, Approaches, and Challenges,
First Edition. Edited by Sajid Yousuf Bhat, Aasia Rehman, and Muhammad Abulaish.

Printed and bound by CPI Group (UK) Ltd, Croydon, CR0 4YY
17/09/2026
14964312-0002